Last Minute
MRCP 1
Practi

W Stephe

Consultant P
Scottish Poiso
Royal Infirmai
Edinburgh

The loan period may be shortened if the item is requested.

© 2006 PASTEST LTD
Egerton Court
Parkgate Estate
Knutsford
Cheshire
WA16 8DX

Telephone: 01565 752000

First Published 2006

ISBN: 1 904627 47 1

A catalogue record for this book is available from the British Library.

The information contained within this book was obtained by the author from
reliable sources. However, while every effort has been made to ensure its accuracy,
no responsibility for loss, damage or injury occasioned to any person acting or
refraining from action as a result of information contained herein can be accepted
by the publishers or author.

PasTest Revision Books and Intensive Courses

PasTest has been established in the field of postgraduate medical education
since 1972, providing revision books and intensive study courses for doctors
preparing for their professional examinations.

Books and courses are available for the following specialties:

MRCGP, MRCP Parts 1 and 2, MRCPCH Parts 1 and 2, MRCPsych, MRCS,
MRCOG Parts 1 and 2, DRCOG, DCH, FRCA, PLAB Parts 1 and 2.

For further details contact:

PasTest, Freepost, Knutsford, Cheshire WA16 7BR

Tel: 01565 752000   **Fax: 01565 650264**
www.pastest.co.uk   **enquiries@pastest.co.uk**

Text typeset and designed by Type Study, Scarborough, North Yorkshire

Printed and bound in the UK by Athenaeum Press, Gateshead, Tyne & Wear

CONTENTS

CONTRIBUTORS

Cardiology
Shani Esmail MB BChir BSc MRCP, Specialist Registrar in Cardiology,
York District Hospital, York.

Respiratory Medicine
Elora Mukherjee MBBS MRCP, Senior House Officer, Renal Medicine,
King's College Hospital, London.

Psychiatry
Gayle A. Christie MBChB BSc (Hons), Senior House Officer in Emergency Medicine,
St John's Hospital, Livingstone, Edinburgh.

1005899729

INTRODUCTION

The MRCP(UK) diploma is a recognised entry qualification for higher specialist training in medicine and its related specialties. For many, the MRCP Part 1 examination is the first step towards obtaining the diploma. To be eligible to sit the MRCP Part 1 exam, applicants should normally have been qualified with a primary medical degree for at least 18 months. Candidates sitting the MRCP Part 1 exam are expected to have a broad knowledge and understanding including clinical sciences and features of common and important disorders. The MRCP Part 1 examines factual knowledge around a wide range of topics, and expects the candidate to be able to apply that knowledge to problem solving in the context of clinical scenarios presented in the examination paper.

The style of the MRCP Part 1 examination has evolved over recent years, and there have been a number of important changes. The number of questions has increased, and the 'best of five' format (one answer is chosen from five options) has gradually replaced the more traditional 'multiple choice' format. 'Negative marking' has been phased out and, in the current exam style, a correct answer will score +1, whereas no attempt or an incorrect answer will score 0. The exam is criterion referenced, and a pass mark is set before each diet by experienced clinicians responsible for standard setting. These steps have been taken to create a more reliable assessment of candidates' abilities. Increasing assessment of knowledge as applied to theoretical clinical situations means that the exam has become more relevant to everyday medical practice.

The MRCP Part 1 examination is held three times per year, normally in January, May and September. It consists of two papers, each lasting three hours. Each paper has 100 questions in the 'best of five' question format (one answer is chosen from five options). Questions are chosen to represent each of the main specialty areas, and randomly distributed between both exam papers. The typical numbers of questions appearing in the exam for each specialty are shown below:

Specialties	
Clinical sciences*	25
Clinical pharmacology/therapeutics/toxicology	20
Cardiology	15
Clinical haematology/oncology	15
Respiratory medicine	15
Neurology	15
Nephrology	15
Rheumatology	15
Endocrinology	15
Gastroenterology	15
Infectious diseases, tropical medicine & STDs	15
Psychiatry	8
Dermatology	8
Ophthalmology	4
Total:	*200*

*Clinical science questions are made up of:

Statistics, epidemiology, evidence-based medicine (5)
Clinical biochemistry and metabolism (4)
Clinical physiology (4)
Immunology (4)
Genetics (3)
Clinical anatomy (3)
Cell, molecular and membrane biology (2)

The best way to prepare for the exam will vary according to individual learning styles. It is crucial that candidates are familiar with all the topics outlined above, and that there are no major factual gaps. The knowledge tested in the MRCP Part 1 examination will probably be acquired from a number of different sources during General Professional Training, including ward-round teaching, Grand Rounds, Royal College symposia and local postgraduate educational programmes. Candidates should reinforce these learning opportunities by reading relevant materials in general textbooks and up-to-date scientific journals. In addition, a wide range of textbooks and on-line resources focussed specifically on preparation for the MRCP Part 1 exam are currently available from PasTest. These can be an invaluable resource and allow candidates to become familiar with the style and format of the MRCP exam questions whilst guiding study towards an appropriate depth and breadth of knowledge.

Last Minute MRCP Part 1 Practice Questions gives candidates an opportunity to refresh their knowledge over the very broad range of topics included in the exam syllabus. The book contains 1000 questions written in 'best of five' examination style, and covers topics that are frequently encountered in the MRCP Part 1 exam. The large number of questions and answers provide an exceptional revision tool that is likely to be especially valuable to candidates nearing the exam date. The answers are given as an *aide memoir* rather than an exhaustive summary of individual topics, and this will enable candidates to cover large numbers of questions more quickly.

Useful websites for further information are:

1. http://www.mrcpuk.org/plain/mrcppt1.html
    Further information on the MRCP Part 1 exam regulations and application process.
2. http://www.pastestonline.co.uk/
    Online revision source with practice papers (different questions from those appearing in the book range), including a free demo.

Good luck!

WSW
2006

ABBREVIATIONS

ACE	angiotensin converting enzyme
ACTH	adrenocorticotrophic hormone
ALP	alkaline phosphatase
ALT	alanine transaminase
ANCA	antineutrophil cytoplasmic antibody
APKD	adult polycystic kidney disease
ARDS	adult respiratory distress syndrome
ASCT	autologous stem cell transplantation
AST	aspartate transaminase
5-ASA	5-aminosalicylic acid
ASD	atrial septal defect
AWS	alcohol withdrawal syndrome
BDZ	benzodiazepine
BiPAP	bilevel positive airways pressure
CAPD	continuous ambulatory peritoneal dialysis
CMV	cytomegalovirus
CO	cardiac output
CABG	coronary artery bypass graft
COPD	chronic obstructive pulmonary disease
COX-1	cyclo-oxygenase-1
CPAP	continuous positive airways pressure
CSF	cerebrospinal fluid
CT	computed tomography
CTPA	computed tomography pulmonary angiography
DIC	disseminated intravascular coagulation
ECG	electrocardiography
ECT	electroconvulsive therapy
EEG	electroencephalography
EPS	extrapyramidal symptoms
ESR	erythrocyte sedimentation rate
ESRF	end-stage renal failure
FBN1	fibrillin 1
FEV	forced expiratory volume
FFP	fresh frozen plasma
FNAC	fine needle aspiration cytology
FOC	faecal occult blood
FSH	follicle stimulating hormone
GABA	γ-aminobutyric acid
GFR	glomerular filtration rate
GGT	γ-glutamyl transpeptidase
GI	gastrointestinal
GLP-1	glucagon-like peptide 1
GTN	glyceryl trinitrate
GVHD	graft-versus-host disease
HAV	hepatitis A virus
HCG	human chorionic gonadotrophin
HELLP	haemolysis, elevated liver enzymes, low platelets

HSV	herpes simplex virus
HLA	human leukocyte antigen
HONK	hyperosmotic non-ketotic syndrome
HRT	hormone replacement therapy
HUS	haemolytic uraemic syndrome
IBS	irritable bowel syndrome
ICD	implantable cardiac defibrillator
ICP	intracranial pressure
INR	International Normalised Ratio
JVP	jugular venous pressure
KCO	CO transfer coefficient (= transfer factor divided by alveolar volume)
LDH	lactate dehydrogenase
LH	luteinising hormone
MAOI	monoamine oxidase inhibitor
MCV	mean corpuscular volume
MRI	magnetic resonance imaging
MUGA	multiple gated acquisition
NAC	N-acetylcysteine
NMS	neuroleptic malignant syndrome
NO	nitric oxide
NOS	nitric oxide synthase
NSAIDs	non-steroidal anti-inflammatory drugs
PACS	partial anterior circulation stroke
$PaCO_2$	carbon dioxide pressure
PaO_2	oxygen pressure
pCO_2	partial carbon dioxide pressure
pO_2	partial oxygen pressure
PCR	polymerase chain reaction
PCWP	pulmonary capillary wedge pressure
PDA	patent ductus arteriosus
PET	positron emission tomography
PNH	paroxysmal nocturnal haemoglobinuria
PTH	parathyroid hormone
PTHrP	parathyroid hormone related protein
PTSD	post-traumatic stress disorder
SARS	severe acute respiratory distress syndrome
SBE	subacute bacterial endocarditis
SBGH	sex hormone binding globulin
SIADH	syndrome of inappropriate antidiuretic hormone
SPECT	single photon emission computed tomography
SSRI	selective serotonin reuptake inhibitor
SVT	supraventricular tachycardia
SLE	systemic lupus erythematosus
TACS	total anterior circulation stroke
TB	tuberculosis
TCA	tricyclic antidepressant
TENS	transcutaneous electrical nerve stimulation
THS	thyroid stimulating hormone
TIA	transient ischaemic attack

TNF	tumour necrosis factor
TPO	anti-thyroid peroxidase
TRALI	transfusion-related acute lung injury
TRH	thyroid releasing hormone
TTP	thrombotic thrombocytopenic purpura
VIP	vasoactive intestinal peptide
VMA	vanillyl mandelic acid
VSD	ventricular septal defect
VT	ventricular tachycardia
vWF	von Willebrand factor
VZV	varicella zoster virus

1. CARDIOLOGY

1.1 A 56-year-old man is admitted with palpitations and chest discomfort. His ECG shows a broad complex tachycardia. Which of the following suggest a supraventricular rather than a ventricular origin for the arrhythmia?

- [ ] **A** AV dissociation
- [ ] **B** Capture beats
- [ ] **C** Fusion beats
- [ ] **D** Slowing or termination following carotid sinus massage
- [ ] **E** Ventricular concordance

1.2 A 58-year-old man is admitted with palpitations and dizziness. An ECG shows a broad complex tachycardia. Which is the most appropriate initial treatment?

- [ ] **A** Amiodarone
- [ ] **B** DC cardioversion
- [ ] **C** Digoxin
- [ ] **D** Temporary cardiac pacing
- [ ] **E** Verapamil

1.3 A 44-year-old woman is admitted after a sudden collapse. In the Emergency Department, her ECG shows an appearance consistent with *torsade de pointes*. After initial resuscitation, normal sinus rhythm is restored, and a repeat ECG shows a prolonged QT interval. Which of the following is most likely to be responsible?

- [ ] **A** Amiodarone
- [ ] **B** Atropine
- [ ] **C** Digoxin
- [ ] **D** Epinephrine
- [ ] **E** Furosemide

1.1   Answer: D

SVT may be slowed or terminated by vagal manoeuvres (such as carotid sinus massage) or adenosine. The other answers all suggest ventricular tachycardia.

1.2   Answer: B

Scenario suggests ventricular tachycardia; in view of symptoms, treatment is as for ventricular fibrillation.

1.3   Answer: A

Other drugs commonly associated with prolonged QT interval are sotalol, quinidine and quinine, macrolide antibiotics, disopyramide, phenothiazines, terfenadine and other antihistamines. Non-drug causes include familial Romano–Ward and Jervell–Lange-Nielsen syndromes, ischaemic heart disease and metabolic disturbances.

1.4 A 26-year-old man is referred to Cardiology Outpatients with a history of palpitations and dizziness. His resting ECG shows a slurred up-stroke to the QRS complex, and a 24-h ECG shows episodes of paroxysmal atrial fibrillation. Which of the following conditions is most likely to account for these findings?

☐ A Accessory pathway between the atria and ventricles

☐ B Lown–Ganong–Levine syndrome

☐ C Prolonged QT interval

☐ D Right bundle branch block

☐ E Structural heart disease

1.5 You review a 58-year-old woman in the Cardiology Outpatient Department 1 month after an acute anterior MI. An echocardiogram shows severe left ventricular systolic dysfunction, with an ejection fraction of 30%. Which of the following treatments is most likely to improve long-term survival?

☐ A Digoxin

☐ B Furosemide

☐ C Glyceryl trinitrate

☐ D Lisinopril

☐ E Spironolactone

1.6 Which of the following, when implemented after myocardial infarction, have been shown most convincingly to reduce the risk of further ischaemic cardiac events?

☐ A Beta-carotene

☐ B Cardiac rehabilitation

☐ C Diltiazem

☐ D Hormone replacement therapy

☐ E Warfarin

A

1.4 Answer: A

This is the basis of Wolff–Parkinson–White syndrome, which results in short PR interval and widened QRS complex with a pathognomonic delta wave.

1.5 Answer: D

Spironolactone can also reduce morbidity and mortality in addition to ACE inhibitor treatment. Digoxin has been shown to improve symptoms and reduce hospital admissions in chronic heart failure but is unlikely to improve survival.

1.6 Answer: B

This results in better compliance with medication in addition to ensuring patients are given appropriate lifestyle advice regarding exercise and diet.

1.7   You have been asked to report ECGs requested by GPs to be performed in the ECG Department. One of these has a tall R wave in lateral lead V1. What is the most likely cause?

☐ A Anterior myocardial infarction

☐ B Duchenne muscular dystrophy

☐ C Left bundle branch block

☐ D Left ventricular hypertrophy

☐ E Wolff–Parkinson–White type B

1.8   You are reviewing a 66-year-old man in the Cardiology Outpatient Clinic, who has been taking amiodarone treatment for the past 8 months. Which of the following statements best describes the effects of this drug?

☐ A Increases the plasma concentration of digoxin

☐ B Reduces the anticoagulant effect of warfarin

☐ C Short half-life and a small volume of distribution

☐ D Shortens the refractory period of cardiac tissue

☐ E Superior to implantable cardiac defibrillators in preventing sudden death

1.9   Which of the following features is most likely to be associated with the use of amiodarone?

☐ A Erythema nodosum

☐ B Gingival hyperplasia

☐ C Prolonged PR interval

☐ D Renal failure

☐ E Sodium channel blockade

1.10   You are asked to help at a Paediatric Cardiology Clinic. An 11-month-old boy is referred with a history of failure to thrive and an episode of syncope. His mother mentions he goes blue sometimes. On examination he is cyanosed and has finger clubbing. Which of the following is the most likely underlying diagnosis?

☐ A Atrial septal defect

☐ B Coarctation of the aorta

☐ C Congenital aortic stenosis

☐ D Patent ductus arteriosus

☐ E Tetralogy of Fallot

A

1.7   Answer: B

This is a feature also found in right bundle branch block, right ventricular hypertrophy, posterior MI, dextrocardia, Wolff–Parkinson–White type A, hypertrophic cardiomyopathy.

1.8   Answer: A

Therefore, dose of digoxin must be reduced by around 50% to prevent toxicity. It potentiates the anticoagulant effect of warfarin. Amiodarone has a long half-life (30–110 days) and large volume of distribution, and therefore a loading dose is needed.

1.9   Answer: E

Prolongs refractory period of cardiac tissue hence is considered a class III antiarrhythmic agent and prolongs QT interval. Inhibits potassium, sodium and calcium channel activity, and exhibits α- and β-adrenergic antagonist properties. Adverse effects include skin photosensitivity, slate-grey or blue skin pigmentation, hypothyroidism and hyperthyroidism, ataxia, peripheral neuropathy, hepatitis and liver cirrhosis, pulmonary fibrosis and metallic taste.

1.10   Answer: E

The others all characteristically cause heart disease, but cyanosis would not be an expected feature.

1.11 Which of the following would most strongly support a diagnosis of tetralogy of Fallot?

- ☐ A Left ventricular hypertrophy and left axis deviation on ECG
- ☐ B Pulmonary plethora on CXR
- ☐ C Rib notching on CXR
- ☐ D Systolic thrill and pulmonary ejection systolic murmur
- ☐ E Wide fixed splitting of the second heart sound

1.12 Which of the following features is most typically associated with tetralogy of Fallot?

- ☐ A Absence of cardiac murmur
- ☐ B Arachnodactyly
- ☐ C Cyanosis that resolves during feeding
- ☐ D Fainting episodes
- ☐ E Single palmar crease

1.13 A 32-year-old woman presents to her GP with a history of palpitations. An ECG shows atrial fibrillation, and she is referred for echocardiography. This shows a small ostium secundum atrial septal defect (ASD). Which of the following findings is most typically associated with this condition?

- ☐ A Left axis deviation and right bundle branch block on ECG
- ☐ B Left ventricular hypertrophy
- ☐ C Mitral valve prolapse
- ☐ D Oligaemic lung fields on CXR
- ☐ E Wide fixed splitting of the first heart sound

1.14 You are examining a patient in the Coronary Care Unit and find that he has an added third heart sound. Which of the following is most characteristic of this physical sign?

- ☐ A A feature of severe mitral regurgitation
- ☐ B Atrial fibrillation is not a recognised association
- ☐ C Due to ventricular wall disease
- ☐ D Indicates an underlying pathological cause
- ☐ E Occurs in early systole

1.11   Answer: D

Tetralogy of Fallot is the most common cause of cyanotic congenital heart disease and accounts for 10% of these patients. It usually presents after 6 months. Cardinal features are ventricular septal defect, right ventricular outflow tract obstruction, right ventricular hypertrophy and overriding aorta.

1.12   Answer: D

Patients typically experience cyanosis that worsens during vasodilatation, which results in increased left to right shunt (eg during feeding, crying, fever, hot weather or bathing). Severe cyanosis can cause syncope, convulsions, strokes and occasionally death. Squatting increases peripheral systemic vascular resistance, thereby reducing left to right shunting.

1.13   Answer: C

Also associated with wide fixed splitting of the second heart sound. There may also be a pulmonary ejection systolic murmur and a mid-diastolic (tricuspid) murmur. Chest X-ray may show plethoric lung fields and prominent proximal pulmonary arteries. Right axis deviation and right bundle branch block may be seen in young patients.

1.14   Answer: A

Third heart sound occurs in early diastole and results from rapid ventricular filling. It may be physiological (young adults) or a pathological finding associated with cardiomyopathy, ventricular septal defect, constrictive pericarditis and left ventricular failure.

1.15 A 56-year-old man presents to the Emergency Department after a blackout. On admission, he is found to be in complete heart block. What would you expect to see in the jugular venous pressure?

- ☐ **A** Cannon a-waves
- ☐ **B** Giant v-waves
- ☐ **C** Rapid y-descent
- ☐ **D** Rise in the JVP with inspiration
- ☐ **E** Steep x-descent

1.16 A 55-year-old man presents with chest pain. His ECG shows ST depression and T wave inversion in leads II, III and aVF. His troponin-T is abnormally high at 8 h after the onset of chest pain. Occlusion of which coronary vessel is most likely to account for his symptoms?

- ☐ **A** Left anterior descending artery
- ☐ **B** Left circumflex artery
- ☐ **C** Left main stem artery
- ☐ **D** Right coronary artery
- ☐ **E** Intermediate artery

1.17 A 61-year-old man presents to the Emergency Department with features of an acute coronary syndrome. He goes on to have coronary angiography, which shows 95% ostial stenosis of the left anterior descending artery, which is amenable to angioplasty. Which of the following treatments is most likely to improve subsequent outcome when given at the time of the angioplasty?

- ☐ **A** Abciximab
- ☐ **B** Cefotaxime
- ☐ **C** Diclofenac
- ☐ **D** Streptokinase
- ☐ **E** Warfarin

A

1.15 Answer: A

The a-wave coincides with atrial contraction (hence absent in atrial fibrillation). Cannon a-waves are caused by atrial contraction against a closed tricuspid valve, and are a feature of complete heart block (randomly occurring) and nodal or junctional rhythms (occur with every heartbeat). Large a-waves are seen in tricuspid stenosis, pulmonary hypertension and pulmonary stenosis.

1.16 Answer: D

The right coronary artery and its major branches supply the (i) inferior wall of the LV, (ii) posterior wall of the LV in most people via posterior descending branch, (iii) right ventricle via right ventricular branch, and (iv) sinus and AV nodes.

1.17 Answer: A

Abciximab is beneficial in some patients, eg those with intracoronary thrombus or after insertion of multiple stents. Antiplatelet therapy and stent insertion (including drug-eluting stents) are associated with improved outcome. Streptokinase and other thrombolytics have not been shown to improve outcome.

1.18 A 48-year-old woman is referred to the Cardiology Outpatient Clinic with a history of exertional dyspnoea, orthopnoea and ankle swelling. An echocardiogram shows a dilated right and left ventricle, severe global left ventricular systolic dysfunction and mitral regurgitation. Which of the following is most likely to explain these findings?

 A Alcohol excess

 B Carcinoid syndrome

 C Loeffler's syndrome

 D Sarcoidosis

 E Previous radiotherapy

1.19 A 24-year-old man is referred to the Cardiology Clinic with a history of syncope. His brother died suddenly at 27 whilst playing football. What examination finding would most strongly suggest a diagnosis of hypertrophic cardiomyopathy?

 A Double apical impulse

 B Ejection click

 C Prominent v wave in the JVP

 D Slow rising pulse

 E Systolic murmur that increases in intensity with squatting

1.20 Which of the following would be most helpful in the initial management of a young patient with suspected hypertrophic cardiomyopathy?

 A 24-h Holter monitoring

 B Carotid Doppler

 C Exercising ECG

 D Genetic testing

 E Transthoracic echocardiogram

A

1.18   Answer: A

The history and echo findings are compatible with dilated cardiomyopathy.

The others are more likely to cause a restrictive cardiomyopathy. Other recognised causes of dilated cardiomyopathy are ischaemic, hereditary, postpartum, hypertension, thiamine deficiency, viral infection (eg HIV, coxsackievirus), primary myopathies (eg Duchenne muscular dystrophy, myotonic myopathy, Friedrich's ataxia), thyroid disease and doxorubicin.

1.19   Answer: A

Double or multiple apical impulse, and the apex beat tends to be forceful. The pulse character tends to be jerky, with a rapid carotid upstroke. Other recognised features are prominent a-wave in JVP, late ejection systolic murmur that diminished on squatting, palpable systolic thrill, fourth heart sound, and mitral regurgitation.

1.20   Answer: E

Echocardiography can detect LVH, outflow tract obstruction and abnormal mitral valve motion. Exercise stress testing can provoke syncope, chest pain or breathlessness and poor BP response to exercise indicates risk of sudden death. Holter monitoring may be useful in detecting arrhythmias in some patients.

1.21   You are asked to examine a 25-year-old woman who is 22 weeks pregnant. Which of the following statements best describes the haemodynamic alterations that can accompany pregnancy?

    ☐ **A** Cardiac output falls by 30–40%

    ☐ **B** Stroke volume falls during pregnancy

    ☐ **C** Systolic blood pressure usually increases

    ☐ **D** Systemic and pulmonary vascular resistance increase

    ☐ **E** Total blood volume increases by around 40–50%

1.22   A 55-year-old man in shock undergoes Swan–Ganz catheterisation, which shows:

    Cardiac index (normal reference):   1.7 (2.8–4.2 l/min/m²)
    Pulmonary capillary wedge pressure: 20 (6–12 mmHg)
    Systemic vascular resistance: 1850 (770–1500 dynes.s/cm²)
    Mixed venous oxygen saturation: 47% (60–75%)

    Which of the following treatments would be most appropriate in this situation?

    ☐ **A** Hydrocortisone and chlorpheniramine

    ☐ **B** Intravenous antibiotics

    ☐ **C** Intravenous diuretics

    ☐ **D** Intravenous fluids and norepinephrine

    ☐ **E** Ionotropes and intra-aortic balloon pump insertion

1.23   You are asked to review a 72-year-old woman on the Coronary Care Unit, who was admitted with an inferior MI earlier that day. She has become hypotensive (BP 85/50) and clammy, and a bedside echo shows a dilated right ventricle. Urgent Swan–Ganz catheterisation shows raised CVP, reduced PCWP and low cardiac output (CO). Which of the following initial treatments is most appropriate?

    ☐ **A** Coronary angiography and possible angioplasty

    ☐ **B** Diuretics

    ☐ **C** Norepinephrine

    ☐ **D** Rapid administration of fluids

    ☐ **E** Intravenous GTN

1.21 Answer: E

Cardiac output increases by up to 30–40%, and blood pressure falls due to a significant reduction in systemic vascular resistance. Other features are decreased pulmonary vascular resistance and increased stroke volume and heart rate.

1.22 Answer: E

Low cardiac index and high pulmonary capillary wedge pressure (PCWP) indicate cardiogenic shock. If thought due to ischaemic heart disease, coronary angiography and revascularisation should be considered.

1.23 Answer: D

The features suggest right ventricular infarction, complicating an inferoposterior MI. Intravascular volume should be expanded in order to increase RV preload and output and thereby optimise left ventricular filling pressures. Ionotropic support and possible angioplasty of an occluded right coronary artery may also be helpful. Nitrates and diuretics would be potentially hazardous.

1.24 A 52-year-old man with diabetes and hyperlipidaemia is referred to Cardiology Outpatients with exertional chest tightness and dyspnoea. An exercise tolerance test is terminated at 2 min 15 s because of chest pain associated with ST depression and T wave inversion in ECG leads V1–V4, I and AVL. Narrowing of which coronary artery is most likely to account for these features?

- [ ] A Left anterior descending artery
- [ ] B Left circumflex artery
- [ ] C Left main stem artery
- [ ] D Posterior descending artery
- [ ] E Right coronary artery

1.25 You review a 60-year-old woman with aortic stenosis in the Cardiology Outpatient Department. Which of the following is most helpful in judging the severity of aortic stenosis?

- [ ] A Displaced apex beat
- [ ] B Intense systolic murmur
- [ ] C Narrow pulse pressure
- [ ] D Presence of a diastolic murmur
- [ ] E Quiet first heart sound

1.26 A 58-year-old woman with known aortic stenosis is admitted to hospital for investigation of exertional chest tightness and breathlessness. Which of the following initial investigations would be most helpful?

- [ ] A Cardiac catheterisation studies
- [ ] B Chest X-ray
- [ ] C Exercising ECG
- [ ] D Pulmonary function tests
- [ ] E Repeat echocardiogram

1.24   Answer: A

The ECG abnormalities predominantly involve the anterior and lateral walls of the left ventricle, which are normally supplied by the LAD.

1.25   Answer: C

Other indicators of severe aortic stenosis are left ventricular failure, soft second sound or paradoxically split second sound, praecordial thrill, slow-rising pulse, prolonged murmur and left ventricular hypertrophy.

1.26   Answer: E

This would allow assessment of disease progression (gradient across the aortic valve and aortic valve area), and determine LV function.

1.27 You review a 70-year-old man with mixed aortic valve disease in clinic. What pulse character is most characteristically associated with this condition?

- A Jerky pulse
- B Low volume pulse
- C Pulsus alternans
- D Pulsus bisferiens
- E Pulsus paradoxus

1.28 A 46-year-old man complains of sharp stabbing chest pain made worse by inspiration and lying supine. Examination shows temperature 38°C, normal heart sounds and an added coarse murmur. ECG shows 1 mm ST elevation in leads I, II, aVL, aVF, V_5, V_6. What is the most likely cause?

- A Acute myocardial infarction
- B Acute pericarditis
- C Atypical angina
- D Prinzmetal's angina
- E Pulmonary thromboembolism

1.29 A 57-year-old woman is referred to the Cardiology Outpatient Department with a history of exertional chest tightness and breathlessness. A resting ECG shows normal sinus rhythm. An exercise test is terminated because of chest pain associated with significant ST depression and T wave inversion in the anteroseptal leads at 4 min 27 s. A subsequent coronary angiogram is reported as normal. What is the most likely explanation?

- A Coronary microangiopathy
- B False-positive exercise tolerance test
- C Psychogenic chest pain
- D Variant angina
- E Vincent's angina

1.27   Answer: D

This pathognomonic finding manifests as a double peak. Pulsus alternans is alternating large and small volume pulses, due to severe heart failure. Pulsus paradoxus is an exaggerated fall in pulse volume on inspiration. A jerky pulse is associated with hypertrophic cardiomyopathy.

1.28   Answer: B

Pericardial friction rub is often softly heard and can be mistaken for a murmur. The ECG in acute pericarditis typically shows diffuse ST elevation that later evolves into T-wave inversion. PR depression occurs in the early stages of pericarditis and usually involves the limb and praecordial leads.

1.29   Answer: A

Coronary syndrome X is thought due to abnormal function of perforating myocardial vessels. Symptoms attributable to ischaemia and objective ECG signs indicate ischaemia. Symptoms with no ECG changes suggest a psychogenic cause, whereas ST depression in the absence of symptoms can be associated with a false-positive test.

1.30 A 48-year-old woman is referred to the General Medical Clinic with a history of fever, malaise, weight loss, and arthralgia. Investigations show raised ESR, peripheral leukocytosis and mild haemolytic anaemia. There is a loud first heart sound and P_2, and a murmur in early diastole. One week earlier, she noticed weakness of her left face and arm, which resolved over 36 h. What is the most likely underlying diagnosis?

- A   Left atrial myxoma
- B   Mitral stenosis
- C   Pulmonary thromboembolism
- D   Subacute bacterial endocarditis
- E   Systemic vasculitis

1.31 You review a 66-year-old man with chronic atrial fibrillation in the Cardiology Clinic. He is currently taking digoxin and aspirin, and you are considering starting warfarin therapy. Which of these statements best describes its effects?

- A   Addition to aspirin does not increase bleeding risk significantly
- B   ADP receptor antagonist
- C   Selective inhibition of factor Xa
- D   Teratogenic effects are well characterised
- E   Therapy can be monitored using the APTT

1.32 You review a 66-year-old woman with persistent atrial fibrillation in the Cardiology Outpatient Department. She has previously been intolerant of warfarin due to a severe blistering rash over her torso, and you are considering the use of ximelagatran. Which of the following statements best describes the effects of this drug?

- A   Glycoprotein IIb/IIIa receptor antagonist
- B   It has a more delayed onset than warfarin
- C   Liver enzyme disturbance occurs in around 5% of patients
- D   Selective inhibition of COX-2
- E   Selective inhibition of factor Xa

1.30   Answer: A

Patients may be asymptomatic. Features may include murmurs mimicking mitral valve disease (can be postural), systemic embolisation, and constitutional symptoms of fever, malaise, weight loss and arthralgia. An early diastolic 'tumour plop' is characteristic of atrial myxoma however. Diagnosis is usually confirmed by echocardiography.

1.31   Answer: D

Warfarin is teratogenic and increases the risks of fetal and placental haemorrhage. Warfarin inhibits post-ribosomal modification of vitamin K dependent clotting factors (II, VII, IX and X).

1.32   Answer: C

Currently not licensed in the UK, but used elsewhere. Prodrug of the oral thrombin inhibitor melagatran. It has rapid onset of effect (within 1 h), wider therapeutic window than warfarin and does not require therapeutic drug monitoring. Hepatotoxicity occurs in 4–7% of patients.

1.33 A 56-year-old man from Pakistan presents with progressive abdominal and ankle swelling, fatigue and dyspnoea. Pulse is 100/min and irregular in rate. Jugular venous pressure (JVP) is elevated, rises further with inspiration. Apex beat is impalpable, and heart sounds are barely audible. Chest X-ray shows a rim of pericardial calcification. What is the most likely cause of his symptoms?

- [ ] **A** Acute myocardial infarction
- [ ] **B** Acute pericarditis
- [ ] **C** Constrictive pericarditis
- [ ] **D** Mitral stenosis
- [ ] **E** Tricuspid regurgitation

1.34 You are asked to review a 60-year-old man on the cardiothoracic ward 24 h after coronary bypass grafting. He has become breathless, and feels dizzy and faint. BP is 90/65 mmHg and pulse rate 120. His JVP is elevated, and apex beat is impalpable. On auscultation, heart sounds are softly audible and lung fields are clear. An ECG shows an alternans pattern. What is the most likely diagnosis?

- [ ] **A** Cardiac tamponade
- [ ] **B** Constrictive pericarditis
- [ ] **C** Pulmonary embolism
- [ ] **D** Right ventricular infarction
- [ ] **E** Septic shock

1.35 A 62-year-old smoker presents to the Emergency Department with a 10-h history of chest pain. An ECG shows ST elevation in the anterior and septal leads, and both troponin T and creatinine kinase concentrations are raised. Which one of the following is most likely to improve survival within the first 24 h of symptom onset?

- [ ] **A** Atenolol
- [ ] **B** Diltiazem
- [ ] **C** Glyceryl trinitrate
- [ ] **D** Lisinopril
- [ ] **E** Oxygen

1.33 Answer: C

Typically presents with ascites and peripheral oedema. JVP signs include prominent x and y descents, and Kussmaul's sign. Calcification suggests tuberculosis pericarditis. It is often difficult to distinguish clinically between constrictive pericarditis and restrictive cardiomyopathy.

1.34 Answer: A

A small amount of pericardial fluid. eg < 200 ml, can cause cardiac tamponade if it accumulates quickly, whereas up to 2 l can be accommodated if it develops slowly. Symptoms are secondary to reduced cardiac output. Symptoms include chest discomfort, cough, dysphagia, hoarseness or hiccups. Kussmaul's sign is often positive. Treatment is urgent pericardiocentesis.

1.35 Answer: D

Most of the mortality benefit conferred by ACE inhibitor treatment is derived within the first 24 h post-infarction. Therefore, treatment should not be delayed unnecessarily. Beta-blockers also improve survival by reducing arrhythmic deaths. Nitrates and opiates confer symptomatic relief only.

1.36 You review a 61-year-old woman with dilated cardiomyopathy in Cardiology Outpatient Clinic. She has severe left ventricular systolic dysfunction. Which of the following is most likely to improve long-term survival?

☐ A Angiotensin II

☐ B Digoxin

☐ C Milrinone

☐ D Prolonged bedrest

☐ E Spironolactone

1.37 A 70-year-old man with ischaemic heart disease and severe heart failure (ejection fraction 25%) presents to the Emergency Department with breathlessness and chest discomfort. His ECG shows a broad complex tachycardia. He has a short-lived arrest due to ventricular fibrillation in the Emergency Department that is reversed by resuscitation. Which of the following treatment strategies is most likely to improve his long-term survival?

☐ A Automated implantable cardiac defibrillator

☐ B Amiodarone

☐ C Flecainide

☐ D Permanent pacemaker insertion

☐ E Propafenone

1.38 You are on call for Cardiology. You are asked to review a 48-year-old man with suspected aortic dissection. Which of the following statements is most accurate with regard to thoracic aortic dissection?

☐ A Commonly associated with bicuspid aortic valve

☐ B Descending aorta is commonest site of aortic dissection

☐ C Medical treatment is sufficient for most ascending aorta dissections

☐ D Stroke is a recognised complication

☐ E Transthoracic echocardiography is the investigation of choice

1.36   Answer: E

As with many positive ionotropes, milrinone increases mortality in heart failure. ACE inhibitors, angiotensin II receptor antagonists and β-blockers improve survival in patients with severe heart failure.

1.37   Answer: A

Implantable cardiac defibrillators (ICDs) reduce mortality in heart failure patients that have had VT or VF. Biventricular pacing can improve haemodynamic symptoms in patients unresponsive to medical therapy that have broad QRS complexes on ECG. Amiodarone reduces mortality in heart failure patients who have had ventricular arrhythmias, but ICDs appear more effective. Flecainide and propafenone may precipitate arrhythmias in ischaemic heart disease.

1.38   Answer: D

Other features include spinal and coronary artery occlusion. Magnetic resonance imaging (MRI), transoesophageal echocardiography, or contrast computed tomography (CT) are more detailed than transthoracic echo. Recognised associations are: aortic stenosis, hypertension, Marfan's syndrome, cystic medial degeneration, giant cell arteritis, pregnancy, trauma, cocaine use, aortic coarctation, congenital bicuspid aortic valve, Turner's syndrome and Noonan's syndrome.

1.39 A 60-year-old man is referred by his GP with a history of breathlessness, hoarseness and dysphagia. On examination, he has a collapsing pulse and an early diastolic murmur over the left lower sternal edge. His BP is 180/70 mmHg. His chest X-ray shows a widened mediastinum. Which of the following best explains his presenting features?

- A Aortic dissection
- B Aortic regurgitation
- C Mitral stenosis
- D Oesophageal cancer
- E Thoracic aortic aneurysm

1.40 You are reviewing the biochemistry results of a newly admitted patient in the Acute Medical Admissions Unit. These show: Na^+ 134 mmol/l, K^+ 6.1 mmol/l, urea 21 mmol/l, creatinine 403 µmol/l, HCO_3^- 11 mmol/l. What corresponding abnormality is most likely to be seen on the patient's ECG?

- A Narrow QRS complexes
- B Short PR interval
- C Tall p waves
- D Tall R wave in V1
- E Tall T waves

1.41 An 18-year-old patient with newly diagnosed hypertension is referred to the Cardiovascular Risk Clinic. Her GP has suggested a diagnosis of aortic coarctation in the referral letter. Which one of the following features would most strongly support this diagnosis?

- A Anterior notching of the ribs on plain chest X-ray
- B Asthma in childhood
- C Female gender
- D Presence of ventricular septal defect
- E Systolic blood pressure higher in right legs than right arms

1.39   Answer: E

Widened mediastinum, which is a feature of aortic aneurismal enlargement (not a feature of dissection), retrosternal goitre, mediastinal lymphadenopathy and thymoma. Wide pulse pressure and murmur indicate aortic incompetence (possibly secondary). Hoarseness and dysphagia are due to mechanical compression of the recurrent laryngeal nerve and oesophagus.

1.40   Answer: E

Tall 'tented' T waves are an early feature of hyperkalaemia. Later features include prolonged PR interval, reduced p-wave amplitude and prolonged QRS duration.

1.41   Answer: D

2–5 times more common in males, accounts for 7% of congenital heart defects. Posterior rib notching is caused by increased collateral blood flow via intercostal arteries (anterior intercostal arteries do not lie in the costal grooves). Associated with bicuspid aortic valve (and aortic stenosis and aortic regurgitation), patent ductus arteriosus, ventricular septal defect (VSD), Turner's syndrome, berry aneurysms and renal abnormalities.

1.42 A 26-year-old asylum seeker presents to the Emergency Department with a history of breathlessness, fatigue and haemoptysis. On examination she has finger clubbing and is centrally cyanosed. Her JVP is raised and there is a loud P2 on auscultation and added third and fourth heart sound. A soft systolic murmur and diastolic murmur are heard over the second left intercostal space. Her ECG shows right axis deviation and peaked p-waves, and chest X-ray shows cardiomegaly, bilateral hilar enlargement and peripheral pruning of the pulmonary arteries. What is the most likely diagnosis?

☐ **A** Eisenmenger's syndrome

☐ **B** Patent ductus arteriosus (PDA)

☐ **C** Primary pulmonary hypertension

☐ **D** Severe mitral stenosis

☐ **E** Tuberculosis

1.43 A 62-year-old man with moderate mitral regurgitation attends the dentist with dental caries necessitating dental extraction. Which of the following should he receive before the procedure in addition to local anaesthesia?

☐ **A** Amoxicillin 1 g given 1 h before procedure

☐ **B** No antibiotic prophylaxis necessary

☐ **C** Flucloxacillin 1 g immediately before the procedure

☐ **D** Metronidazole 500 mg immediately before the procedure

☐ **E** Tetracycline 800 mg given 1 h before the procedure

1.44 A 68-year-old man with severe aortic stenosis is referred for consideration for aortic valve replacement. When considering the type of valve replacement, which of the following statements is most accurate?

☐ **A** Bioprosthetic valves are more durable than mechanical valves

☐ **B** Bioprosthetic valves are more suitable in patients with renal failure

☐ **C** Patients with bioprosthetic valves do not require antibiotic prophylaxis before invasive procedures

☐ **D** Patients with prosthetic valves must receive anticoagulation

☐ **E** Risk of endocarditis is similar for bioprosthetic and mechanical valves

1.42   Answer: A

Features are irreversible pulmonary hypertension accompanied by reversal of a left to right shunt. It is more commonly a complication of VSD and PDA than ASD. Eisenmenger's may be complicated by infective endocarditis, cerebral abscess, paradoxical embolisation, arrhythmias and sudden death, heart failure and pneumonia.

1.43   Answer: A

Antibiotic prophylaxis is indicated in patients with prosthetic valves, previous infective endocarditis, hypertrophic cardiomyopathy, congenital heart disease (except ASD), mitral valve prolapse with regurgitation, pacemaker and cardiac defibrillator implantations.

1.44   Answer: E

Mechanical valves are more durable, and can last up to 30 years. 10–30% of bioprostheses fail within 10–15 years. Bioprosthetic valves do not require anticoagulation, as they have a low risk of valve thrombosis and embolism, but they degenerate more rapidly in patients with renal failure or hypercalcaemia.

1.45 You review a 60-year-old man with ischaemic heart disease in the Cardiology Outpatient Department. He is concerned that his breasts have enlarged. Which of the following medications is most likely to have caused this?

- A Candesartan
- B Carvedilol
- C Furosemide
- D Spironolactone
- E Warfarin

1.46 You are doing a CCU ward round and review a new patient who had been admitted overnight. He has an intra-aortic balloon pump in place. Which of the following statements regarding this device is correct?

- A Heparin should be avoided due to risk of haemorrhage
- B Increases afterload and left ventricular work
- C Increases coronary perfusion pressure in diastole
- D Useful in the management of severe aortic regurgitation
- E Useful in type B aortic dissection

1.47 You review a 52-year-old man in the Cardiovascular Risk Clinic. He has hypertension, hyperlipidaemia and type 2 diabetes mellitus. His BMI is 34 kg/m² despite a programme of diet, exercise and behavioural modification. Which of the following drugs might be most helpful in managing his obesity?

- A Dexfenfluramine
- B Fenfluramine
- C Furosemide
- D Orlistat
- E Thyroxine

1.45   Answer: D

Other commonly recognised drug causes of gynaecomastia are digoxin, cimetidine, cyproterone acetate, oestrogens, ketoconazole, phenothiazines and cannabis use.

1.46   Answer: C

Intra-aortic balloon pump is inflated and deflated in time with the cardiac cycle, and provides haemodynamic support and improves coronary blood flow. It is indicated in cardiogenic shock and refractory unstable angina. It is contraindicated in aortic dissection, aortic aneurysm, aortic insufficiency and severe peripheral vascular disease.

1.47   Answer: D

Orlistat is a lipase inhibitor, and reduces the absorption of dietary fat. Fenfluramine and dexfenfluramine were previously marketed by Wyeth-Ayerst, but have been withdrawn due to the occurrence of pulmonary hypertension and valvular heart disease. Thyroxine, caffeine and furosemide all stimulate appetite and can increase core body weight.

1.48 A 55-year-old apparently healthy man is referred to the Cardiology Clinic. A routine insurance medical ECG shows left bundle branch block (LBBB). Which of the following would be most likely to cause this?

- [ ] **A** Aortic valve disease
- [ ] **D** Cardiomyopathy
- [ ] **C** Ischaemic heart disease
- [ ] **D** Left ventricular hypertrophy
- [ ] **E** Normal variant

1.49 You review a 72-year-old woman with mitral stenosis in the Cardiology Clinic. Which of the following most strongly indicates a diagnosis of mild mitral stenosis?

- [ ] **A** Graham–Steel murmur
- [ ] **B** Loud P_2
- [ ] **C** Right ventricular heave
- [ ] **D** Short interval between S_2 and the opening snap
- [ ] **E** Valve area > 1.5 cm²

1.50 You have decided to do some voluntary work for the Red Cross and are posted to a small hospital in India. A 15-year-old girl is referred with fever, joint pains and breathlessness. You think that she may have acute bacterial endocarditis. Which of the following features most strongly supports this diagnosis?

- [ ] **A** Choreoform movements
- [ ] **B** Erythema marginatum
- [ ] **C** Osler's nodes
- [ ] **D** Prolonged QRS duration on ECG
- [ ] **E** Raised ESR

1.51 Which of the following statements best describes the pathophysiology of acute rheumatic fever?

- [ ] **A** Caused by *Trypanosoma cruzi*
- [ ] **B** Exaggerated immune response to group A streptococcal infection
- [ ] **C** Infection on the endocardial surface of the heart
- [ ] **D** Infection with the spirochaete *Borrelia burgdorferi*
- [ ] **E** Results from cardiotoxin production by *Corynebacterium diphtheriae*

1.48   Answer: D

LBBB is never physiological; the other listed items are recognised causes, but unlikely in the absence of cardiovascular symptoms or signs. Other causes include myocarditis, valve replacement and right ventricular pacemaker.

1.49   Answer: E

The other answers are features of severe mitral stenosis. A loud P_2 and right ventricular heave indicate pulmonary hypertension, and Graham–Steel murmur indicates pulmonary regurgitation. Severe mitral stenosis is associated with a valve area < 1.0 cm² and moderate mitral stenosis with a valve area of 1.0–1.5 cm².

1.50   Answer: C

Raised ESR is non-specific, whereas the other listed features are suggestive of acute rheumatic fever.

1.51   Answer: B

Streptococcal antigens closely resemble glycoprotein in human cardiac tissue. *Borrelia burgdorferi* causes Lyme disease, *Trypanosoma cruzi* causes Chagas' disease, and *Corynebacterium diphtheriae* liberates cardiotoxin (myocarditis recognised complication of all three infections).

1.52 A 54-year-old woman presents with syncope, chest discomfort and dyspnoea. On examination her blood pressure is 85/50 mmHg, respiratory rate 24/min and pulse 120/min and regular. Oxygen saturation is 82% on air, and chest X-ray is normal. ECG shows a sinus tachycardia, right bundle branch block and right axis deviation. Arterial blood gases show a type 1 pattern of respiratory failure. What is the most likely diagnosis?

    A Acute left ventricular failure

    B Acute pneumonia

    C Cardiogenic shock

    D Pulmonary embolism

    E Septic shock

1.53 Which of the following investigations would be most helpful for confirming a diagnosis of suspected acute pulmonary thromboembolism?

    A Blood cultures

    B CT pulmonary angiography (CTPA)

    C D-dimers

    D Swan–Ganz catheterisation

    E Ventilation-perfusion (V/Q) scanning

1.54 A 58-year-old man presents to the Emergency Department with a history of flu-like symptoms, fever and right-sided weakness. On examination, temperature is 38°C, respiratory rate 18/min and pulse 92/min and regular. His JVP is not raised, there is no peripheral oedema and heart sounds are normal. An early diastolic murmur is audible at the lower left sternal edge. His chest is clear. He has a right spastic hemiparesis and dysphasia. Urinanalysis shows blood++ and protein++. Fundoscopy shows a retinal haemorrhage with a pale centre. Which of the following investigations would be most likely to establish the underlying diagnosis?

    A Carotid Doppler

    B CT scan of thorax

    C Fasting glucose

    D Repeated blood cultures

    E Urine culture

1.52   Answer: D

Often the ECG and chest X-ray are normal (> 25% for each). The most common ECG abnormality is sinus tachycardia; other features include right axis deviation, right bundle branch block and an S1-Q3-T3 morphological pattern.

1.53   Answer: B

CTPA reliably diagnoses proximal clot, although may not identify small peripheral emboli. Serum D-dimers can be useful but there is a high false-positive rate. VQ scanning is less useful in acutely unwell patients, and is easiest to interpret in the absence of lung disease.

1.54   Answer: D

The most likely unifying diagnosis is infective endocarditis, and this is best established by demonstration of bacteraemia. About 10% of patients with endocarditis have culture-negative endocarditis.

1.55 Which of the following is most characteristically found as a complication of subacute bacterial endocarditis?

☐ A Ashleaf macules

☐ B Focal proliferative glomerulonephritis

☐ C Heberden's nodes

☐ D Nail pitting

☐ E Polycythaemia

1.56 A 46-year-old man is referred to the Cardiology Clinic for investigation of an early diastolic murmur heard over the left lower sternal edge. He has a raised temperature, splinter haemorrhages in several nailbeds, and echocardiography shows two distinct vegetations on the aortic valve with moderate aortic regurgitation. A blood culture report shows growth of *Staphylococcus aureus*. What would be the most appropriate treatment?

☐ A Anticoagulation with heparin

☐ B Intravenous benzylpenicillin

☐ C Intravenous flucloxacillin

☐ D Oral co-amoxiclav

☐ E Oral flucloxacillin

1.57 You are asked for advice regarding coronary artery bypass grafting (CABG) by one of your patients in the Cardiology Outpatient Clinic. Which of these statements is most accurate with regard to the procedure?

☐ A 50% of patients report an improvement in angina symptoms

☐ B 90% of saphenous vein grafts are patent after 10 years

☐ C CABG improves prognosis in patients with left main stem or triple-vessel coronary artery disease

☐ D Long-term patency of venous grafts is superior to that of arterial grafts

☐ E Repeat CABG is associated with similar operative mortality to the first operation

1.55   Answer: B

Characterised by asymptomatic haematuria, proteinuria and renal impairment. Occasionally results in nephrotic syndrome and renal failure. Infective endocarditis may be associated with Janeway lesions, not ashleaf macules (tuberous sclerosis). Anaemia is a recognised feature.

1.56   Answer: C

Additional treatments with anti-staphylococcal activity are gentamicin and vancomycin (guided by advice from local microbiology laboratory). Urgent referral for consideration of valve repair should be considered.

1.57   Answer: C

When compared with medical therapy. It also improves long-term survival in patients with two-vessel disease that includes the left anterior descending artery. Around 50–60% of saphenous grafts and 90% of left internal mammary grafts are patent at 10 years. Redo coronary artery bypass graft (CABG) carries a 2- to 3-fold increased risk compared to the first operation.

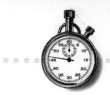

1.58 You are examining the JVP of a patient on the Cardiology Ward, and note that there are large v-waves. Which of the following statements best fits the description of v-waves?

A Coincide with atrial contraction

B May indicate tricuspid incompetence

C Occur in mitral stenosis

D Recognised feature in complete heart block

E Usually associated with a collapsing pulse character

1.59 You are supervising exercise stress tests on outpatients. Which of these statements most accurately describes the role of this investigation?

A Rise in blood pressure indicates high risk of adverse cardiac events

B Exercise-induced ST elevation indicates increased risk of sudden death

C Frequent ventricular ectopics and ventricular tachycardia can be seen in normal individuals and are of no consequence

D Helps stratifying risk in patients with left coronary artery main stem disease

E It is a useful means of assessing severity of aortic stenosis

1.60 A 52-year-old man with atypical chest pain has been referred for exercise stress testing. He is unable to exercise sufficiently (he has severe osteoarthritis of his right knee). Which of the following would be the most appropriate alternative investigation?

A Cardiac electron beam CT scanning

B Doppler echocardiography

C Multiple gated acquisition (MUGA) scan

D Myocardial perfusion scanning during pharmacological stress

E Tilt testing

1.58   Answer: B

v-waves are caused by a rise in RA pressure due to bulging of the tricuspid valve towards the atrium during systole. Giant v-waves can indicate tricuspid regurgitation, which might also be associated with pulsative hepatomegaly.

1.59   Answer: B

Can be used to assess severity and prognosis in coronary artery disease. Limited diagnostic value in patents with abnormal ECG (eg LBBB). Indicators of cardiac risk are poor exercise tolerance (< 5 METS), ≥ 2 mm ST depression at low workload, ST depression in (5 ECG leads, prolonged (> 5 min) ST depression after exercise, exercise-induced ST elevation, fall in BP during exercise, ventricular ectopics at low workload.

1.60   Answer: D

Dobutamine stress echocardiography is another means, and both modalities have equivalent sensitivity and specificity for diagnosing coronary artery disease, and assessing prognosis.

1.61 You review a 61-year-old woman in the Cardiology Outpatient Department. She has asked you for information about rimonabant because she has read that it may be a helpful treatment for obesity. Which of the following statements most accurately describes the effects of rimonabant?

- [ ] **A** Inhibits uptake of norepinephrine and serotonin
- [ ] **B** Lipase inhibitor
- [ ] **C** No better than placebo at promoting smoking cessation
- [ ] **D** Reduces HDL cholesterol
- [ ] **E** Selective cannabinoid receptor blocker

1.62 Which of the following statements is correct in relation to management of coarctation of the aorta?

- [ ] **A** Balloon angioplasty is a recognised treatment
- [ ] **B** Correction may worsen lower limb blood flow
- [ ] **C** Dacron grafts should normally be avoided
- [ ] **D** Recurrence is a rare complication of surgical repair
- [ ] **E** Site involved is usually proximal to the right common carotid artery

1.63 A 58-year-old woman is admitted for investigation of severe chest pain radiating to the back. On examination, you can hear a soft early diastolic murmur. Which of the following would be most helpful for establishing a diagnosis?

- [ ] **A** Barium swallow
- [ ] **B** Contrast CT chest
- [ ] **C** Plain chest X-ray
- [ ] **D** Right heart catheterisation studies
- [ ] **E** Transthoracic echocardiography

1.64 A 33-year-old woman presents with sharp left-sided chest pain and is found to have a pericardial rub and widespread ST segment elevation on her ECG. What treatment is most likely to be helpful?

- [ ] **A** Diuretic therapy
- [ ] **B** Ibuprofen
- [ ] **C** Pericardiocentesis
- [ ] **D** Pericardiectomy
- [ ] **E** Warfarin

1.61 Answer: E

Targets endocannabinoid receptors in brain and adipose tissue, which are thought to play a role in food cravings. Promotes weight loss in obese patients and aids smoking cessation in smokers. Associated with an increase in HDL cholesterol. (Not currently licensed in the UK.)

1.62 Answer: A

Coarctation recurs in 5–10% of cases following surgical repair. Most common site is immediately distal to the origin of the left subclavian artery, and can present with hypertension, heart failure, or intermittent claudication. Severity is assessed by echocardiography, MRI and aortography. Coarctation may be complicated by hypertension, left ventricular failure, endocarditis and aortic dissection.

1.63 Answer: B

The history and examination findings strongly suggest thoracic aortic dissection and aortic incompetence. Contrast CT chest will establish diagnosis and determine extent of any associated aneurysm (determines medical or surgical management).

1.64 Answer: B

Treatment aims to reverse any underlying cause, and to give symptomatic relief. Non-steroidal anti-inflammatory drugs are highly effective, but associated with significant adverse effects.

1.65 You are asked to give advice on a 42-year-old patient in whom the radial pulse volume feels very different between inspiration and expiration. Which of the following conditions is most likely to be associated with this physical sign?

- A Dehydration
- B Diabetes
- C Hay fever
- D Heart failure
- E Uncontrolled asthma

1.66 A 61-year-old man with known aortic valve stenosis is found to have a peak gradient of 78 mmHg by echocardiogram, and underlying left ventricular function is normal. Before undertaking aortic valve repair, invasive angiography is arranged. What information will be most likely to influence his subsequent management?

- A Aortic regurgitation
- B Aortic valve gradient
- C Co-existing mitral valve disease
- D Coronary artery stenosis
- E High right heart pressures

1.67 You are examining a 56-year-old man in the Coronary Care Unit and you notice that his JVP is slightly elevated, and rises further during deep inspiration. What is the most likely underlying cause of this physical sign?

- A Alcoholic cardiomyopathy
- B Cardiac tamponade
- C Congestive cardiac failure
- D Myocardial infarction
- E Uraemic pericarditis

1.68 Which of the following diseases is most likely to be associated with a hyperdynamic circulatory state?

- A Alcoholic cardiomyopathy
- B Beri-beri
- C Polycythaemia
- D Porphyria
- E Rhabdomyolysis

1.65   Answer: E

Pulsus paradoxus is an exaggeration of the normal fall in pulse pressure that occurs during inspiration (usually expiratory–inspiratory pressure > 20 mmHg), and is also found in constrictive pericarditis, cardiac tamponade, severe COPD, and massive pulmonary embolus.

1.66   Answer: D

In patients with significant coronary artery disease, coronary artery bypass grafting can be undertaken at the same time as aortic valve replacement. Echocardiography is a sufficient means of assessing left ventricular function and aortic valve gradient in most cases.

1.67   Answer: B

Normally, right atrial pressure falls during inspiration. Kussmaul's sign arises when the right heart chambers are unable to accommodate increased blood flow due to restriction. Other recognised causes are constrictive pericarditis and restrictive cardiomyopathy.

1.68   Answer: B

Hyperdynamic states are characterised by increased cardiac output and, typically, there is tachycardia, peripheral vasodilatation and wide pulse pressure. Other recognised causes are pregnancy, anaemia, and thyrotoxicosis.

Cardiology answers

1.69 A 68-year-old man is referred to the Cardiology Clinic by his GP, who thought he could hear a murmur. On auscultation, you hear an added fourth heart sound and no additional murmurs. What is the most likely underlying cause?

- [ ] **A** Amyloidosis
- [ ] **B** Atrial fibrillation
- [ ] **C** Hypertension
- [ ] **D** Ischaemic heart disease
- [ ] **E** Thyrotoxicosis

1.70 A 46-year-old man is brought to the Emergency Department after collapsing at home. His ECG shows a broad complex tachycardia, with heart rate around 170 per min. Which of the following characteristics most strongly suggests an underlying diagnosis of ventricular tachycardia?

- [ ] **A** Administration of adenosine restores sinus rhythm
- [ ] **B** Cardiac axis remains normal
- [ ] **C** Fusion beats are seen
- [ ] **D** Previous myocardial infarction 18 months before
- [ ] **E** QRS 106 ms

1.71 Which of the following conditions is most likely to cause prolongation of the QT interval on a resting 12-lead ECG?

- [ ] **A** Hyperkalaemia
- [ ] **B** Hypermagnesaemia
- [ ] **C** Hyperthyroidism
- [ ] **D** Hypocalcaemia
- [ ] **E** Hyponatraemia

1.72 Which of the following treatments would be most appropriate in a patient with *torsade de pointes* secondary to ischaemic heart disease?

- [ ] **A** Amiodarone
- [ ] **B** Digoxin
- [ ] **C** Epinephrine
- [ ] **D** Intravenous calcium administration
- [ ] **E** Overdrive pacing

1.69   Answer: C

A fourth heart sound is always pathological. It occurs in early diastole in association with atrial contraction (hence not a recognised feature in atrial fibrillation). Other recognised causes are left ventricular hypertrophy, hypertrophic cardiomyopathy, cardiac amyloid deposition (less common than hypertension!).

1.70   Answer: D

Ventricular tachycardia (VT) is more likely than supraventricular tachycardia (SVT) in patients with a history of ischaemic heart disease, if the QRS duration is > 140 ms, if the cardiac axis is grossly abnormal and if there is concordance of electrical activity across the ECG lateral leads.

1.71   Answer: D

Other recognised causes are ischaemic heart disease, hypokalaemia, hypomagnesaemia, hypothermia, hypothyroidism, mitral valve prolapse, and a number of different drugs.

1.72   Answer: E

Isoprenaline can be used as a temporary measure if pacing is not available. Intravenous magnesium may also be helpful.

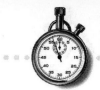

1.73   Which of the following features is most strongly associated with an underlying diagnosis of tetralogy of Fallot?

☐ A   Ejection murmur loudest on expiration

☐ B   Left ventricular hypertrophy on an ECG

☐ C   Methaemoglobinaemia

☐ D   Polycythaemia

☐ E   Pulmonary congestion

1.74   Which of the following statements is most correct with respect to atrial septal defects?

☐ A   Left to right shunt ratio should only be corrected in symptomatic patients

☐ B   Ostium primum defects are associated with leftward cardiac axis deviation

☐ C   Pulmonary oedema and congestive cardiac failure

☐ D   Risk of endocarditis is not increased

☐ E   Systemic hypertension is a recognised complication

1.73   Answer: D

Clinical features include cyanosis, finger clubbing, parasternal (right ventricular) heave, pulmonary systolic murmur (and thrill). The ECG may show right axis deviation and changes of right atrial and ventricular hypertrophy. Chest X-ray shows oligaemic lung fields. Complications include polycythaemia, thromboembolism, endocarditis, cerebral abscess and heart failure.

1.74   Answer: B

Whereas ostium secundum defects are more typically associated with right axis deviation; both are associated with right axis deviation. Recognised complications of ASD are pulmonary hypertension, right ventricular failure, tricuspid regurgitation, atrial fibrillation or flutter, stroke and (rarely) infective endocarditis. Left to right shunt ratio > 2:1 should be corrected regardless of symptoms.

2. CLINICAL PHARMACOLOGY

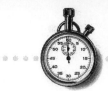

2.1   Which of the following statements regarding the mechanism of action of non-steroidal anti-inflammatory drugs (NSAIDs) is correct?

☐ **A** Can be used to treat patent foramen ovale

☐ **B** Inhibit production of prostaglandins and thromboxane

☐ **C** Inhibition of cyclo-oxygenase-1 (COX-1) is responsible for most of their anti-inflammatory effects

☐ **D** They have analgesic but not antipyretic properties

☐ **E** They may improve blood pressure response to thiazide diuretics

2.2   You review a 66-year-old man in the Outpatient Department. He has been diagnosed with metastatic prostate carcinoma, and is taking regular morphine sulphate. Recently, he has complained of increasing back pain. Which of the following statements related to opiate treatment is correct?

☐ **A** Buprenorphine has better analgesic efficacy than morphine

☐ **B** Acquired tolerance to the analgesic effects of opiates is recognised

☐ **C** Morphine half-life is typically 10–14 h

☐ **D** Oral morphine has 70–90% bioavailability

☐ **E** Renal impairment causes accumulation of morphine

2.3   Which of the following statements is true of drugs with a wide volume of distribution (V_d)?

☐ **A** Maximum V_d is around 50 l in a 70 kg man

☐ **B** Most have short plasma half-lives

☐ **C** They are subject to rapid renal clearance

☐ **D** They tend to be lipophilic

☐ **E** Typically they are largely confined to the circulating compartment

2.1   Answer: B

COX-2 is induced in presence of inflammation; inhibition responsible for some analgesic, antipyretic and anti-inflammatory properties. COX-1 inhibition causes toxic effects, especially gastrointestinal (GI). NSAIDs cause salt and water retention and limit the effectiveness of diuretic treatment.

2.2   Answer: B

Inter-individual differences in opiate sensitivity; tolerance can necessitate dose escalation. Morphine has poor oral bioavailability (10–20%), subject to hepatic metabolism, and plasma half-life of 1–2 h; active metabolite morphine-6-glucuronide accumulates in renal impairment, causing prolonged effects.

2.3   Answer: D

Drugs with a wide volume of distribution are highly bound to tissues and proteins, and circulate in low concentrations. Half-life tends to be long, and clearance low. It is a theoretical volume that can vastly exceed actual bodily volume, eg amiodarone V_d 200–300 l.

2.4 A 52-year-old woman with longstanding rheumatoid arthritis is admitted for investigation of abdominal pain, nausea and vomiting. Upper GI endoscopy shows peptic ulceration affecting the gastric pylorus and first part of the duodenum. *Helicobacter pylori* 'clostridium-like organism' test is positive and you are contemplating eradication therapy. Which of the following treatment options would be most appropriate for eradication in 1 week?

☐ **A** Lansoprazole 15 mg bd, amoxicillin 1 g bd and clarithromycin 500 mg bd

☐ **B** Lansoprazole 30 mg bd and co-amoxiclav 375 mg tid

☐ **C** NSAID treatment must be discontinued in all cases

☐ **D** Omeprazole 20 mg bd, amoxicillin 500 mg tid and metronidazole 400 mg tid

☐ **E** Ranitidine 150 mg bd, amoxicillin 1 g bd and metronidazole 400 mg tid

2.5 You review a 46-year-old man in the Medical Outpatient Department. He has a past history of ulcerative colitis, and has been taking sulfasalazine for more than 5 years. Which of the following statements regarding aminosalicylates is correct?

☐ **A** Balsalazide is contraindicated in patients with sulphonamide allergy

☐ **B** Mesalazine is not effective in treating acute exacerbations of colitis

☐ **C** Microcytic anaemia is a recognised complication of sulfasalazine treatment

☐ **D** Sulfapyridine is subject to hepatic acetylation

☐ **E** Sulfasalazine can be given by the oral route of administration only

2.6 A 47-year-old woman has returned to the UK after a 2-week holiday to Spain with her family. She has been suffering crampy abdominal pain for 3 days, associated with fever and profuse watery diarrhoea. Which of the following statements is correct regarding infective diarrhoea?

☐ **A** Antispasmodic treatment is particularly effective in children

☐ **B** Ciprofloxacin will shorten duration of symptoms in most cases

☐ **C** Loperamide has 80–90% oral bioavailability

☐ **D** Paralytic ileus is a recognised adverse effect of codeine phosphate

☐ **E** Yoghurt containing lactobacilli prevents gastroenteritis

2.4   Answer: D

NSAIDs may be needed in patients with severe inflammatory disease, and healing doses of proton pump inhibitor should be continued for more than 1 week. Consideration should be given to a more potent and efficacious PPI, for example, esomeprazole.

2.5   Answer: D

Sulfasalazine is a combination of sulfapyridine and 5-aminosalicylic acid (5-ASA), given orally or rectally. Mesalazine (5-ASA), balsalazide (5-ASA prodrug) and olsalazine (5-ASA dimer) avoid sulphonamide adverse effects, which include megaloblastic anaemia, hypersensitivity reactions and Stevens–Johnson syndrome.

2.6   Answer: D

Antispasmodics and antiemetics are rarely effective in children, but may be useful adjuncts in adults. Most simple gastroenteritis is viral, and antibiotics are reserved for bacterial gastroenteritis with systemic features. Lactobacillus preparations have not been shown to prevent gastroenteritis. Loperamide has poor oral bioavailability, and its anti-motility action is a local effect on gut opiate receptors. Codeine phosphate has a predominantly central effect.

2.7 A 33-year-old woman attends the Medical Outpatient Department with a 9-month history of intermittent left iliac fossa pain and occasional diarrhoea. Routine haematology and biochemistry investigations are normal, and sigmoidoscopy and barium enema investigations show normal bowel appearance. She is diagnosed with irritable bowel syndrome (IBS), and you are contemplating possible treatments. Which of the following statements is correct?

☐ **A** GI symptoms usually respond to treatment with amitriptyline

☐ **B** Ispaghula husk should be avoided in patients with diarrhoea

☐ **C** Loperamide should be avoided in IBS patients

☐ **D** Mebeverine reduces smooth muscle spasm and relieves pain

☐ **E** Mesalazine gives symptomatic relief in most patients

2.8 You are asked to review a 68-year-old man in the Outpatient Department. Three months ago, he developed a painful vesicular rash over the right side of his lower chest wall. The rash completely resolved more than 6 weeks ago, but he is still suffering pain and the area is extremely sensitive to minimal stimulation. You suspect that he has developed post-herpetic neuralgia. Which of the following is true regarding this condition?

☐ **A** Aciclovir treatment reduces the risk of neuralgia after herpes zoster

☐ **B** Around 50% of patients develop neuralgia after herpes zoster

☐ **C** Corticosteroids can reduce the duration of post-herpetic neuralgia

☐ **D** Post-herpetic neuralgia persists for several years in most patients

☐ **E** Simple analgesics are adequate after neuralgia is established

2.9 A 64-year-old man is taking multiple medications. He attends his GP with sudden onset of pain and inflammation affecting the first metatarsophalangeal joint of his right foot. The GP suspects acute gout. Which of the following is most likely to precipitate acute gout?

☐ **A** Atenolol

☐ **B** Hydrocortisone

☐ **C** Lisinopril

☐ **D** Low dose aspirin

☐ **E** Triamterene

2.7 **Answer: D**

Bulking agents are more effective in patients with constipation, but can improve stool consistency and lessen diarrhoea. Loperamide can be useful for control of diarrhoea, and causes less central effects/dependency than codeine. Mesalazine is reserved for inflammatory bowel disease. Many patients have underlying psychological stressors, but routine antidepressant use is not recommended.

2.8 **Answer: C**

10% of patients develop neuralgia after herpes zoster, which can last for several months to years. Aciclovir and valaciclovir do not reduce risk of neuralgia but reduce duration of symptoms. Simple analgesia is usually ineffective, and low-dose amitriptyline, gabapentin and TENS may be helpful.

2.9 **Answer: D**

Low dose aspirin inhibits renal tubular secretion of urate, so overall urate clearance is lower. Angiotensin converting enzyme (ACE) inhibitors and angiotensin II receptor antagonists are uricosuric. Triamterene is a potassium sparing diuretic and has little effect on urate. Thiazides reduce urate clearance, and loop diuretics cause a small increase in urate due to haemoconcentration.

2.10 A 56-year-old woman attends the Medical Outpatient Department with a 1-week history of dizziness, unsteadiness and vertigo, and she had suffered flu-like symptoms 10 days before. You suspect viral labyrinthitis affecting the left side, and prescribe a short course of cinnarizine. Which of the following properties regarding cinnarizine is true?

- [ ] **A** Highly effective in patients with Parkinson's disease
- [ ] **B** Histamine H_1 agonist properties
- [ ] **C** Potent peripheral vasoconstrictor
- [ ] **D** Reduces nystagmus after rotational stimulation of the vestibular apparatus
- [ ] **E** Stimulates calcium channel activation

2.11 You see a 24-year-old woman, who is referred to the Outpatient Department for investigation of an urticarial rash. She has a history of mild asthma and seasonal hay fever. Which of the following statements regarding possible treatments is correct?

- [ ] **A** Drowsiness may not become apparent for 48–72 h after treatment
- [ ] **B** Most antihistamines have additional anti-nicotinic properties
- [ ] **C** Non-sedating antihistamines do not interact with alcohol
- [ ] **D** Oral corticosteroids are the treatment of choice
- [ ] **E** Sedating antihistamines relieve itch more effectively than non-sedating ones

2.12 A 28-year-old woman is brought to the Emergency Department after a suspected drug overdose. The ambulance crew brought two empty amitriptyline packets that were found at the scene. On examination, she smells strongly of alcohol and has reduced conscious level. Which of the following features would most strongly suggest that an alternative or additional drug had been ingested?

- [ ] **A** Dry mucous membranes
- [ ] **B** Extensor plantar responses
- [ ] **C** Miosis
- [ ] **D** Prolonged QRS duration on an electrocardiogram (ECG)
- [ ] **E** Sinus tachycardia

2.10 Answer: D

Reduces peripheral and central vestibular responses. Blocks peripheral calcium channels, improves cerebral and peripheral blood flow, and is used to treat peripheral vascular disease. Also has H_1 antagonist properties. Can impair mobility in parkinsonism.

2.11 Answer: E

Drowsiness can diminish after several days' treatment. Alcohol may interact with both sedative and non-sedative antihistamines. Most have additional anti-muscarinic properties. Sedation appears to aid relief from itch.

2.12 Answer: C

Tricyclic overdose typically causes tachycardia, mydriasis, abnormal neurology, (can be hyperreflexia, extensor plantars or absent reflexes), and dry mouth due to anti-muscarinic effects. Prolonged QRS duration indicates increased risk of arrhythmia or seizure. Miosis suggests opiate ingestion.

Clinical pharmacology answers

2.13 A 47-year-old man presents to the Emergency Department alleging to have taken 28 × 500 mg paracetamol tablets 10 h earlier. He is complaining of vague abdominal pain and nausea. Which of the following statements regarding his clinical management is most appropriate?

☐ A Acute alcohol intake increases risk of paracetamol-induced liver toxicity

☐ B Cimetidine increases the risk of paracetamol-induced liver toxicity

☐ C Measure paracetamol level immediately to determine need for N-acetylcysteine treatment

☐ D Measure paracetamol level in 4 h time to determine treatment

☐ E Start N-acetylcysteine immediately and await paracetamol level

2.14 A 64-year-old man is admitted to hospital for investigation of an acutely tender, swollen right knee. Joint aspiration of the affected joint reveals urate crystals and moderate numbers of lymphocytes. He is suspected of suffering from acute gout. Which of the following statements is correct regarding treatment of acute gout?

☐ A Allopurinol increases renal tubular secretion of urate

☐ B Cephalosporin treatment should be given empirically

☐ C Colchicine prevents phagocytosis of urate crystals

☐ D High dose aspirin dramatically lowers serum urate concentrations

☐ E Ibuprofen reduces joint pain and inflammation

2.15 A 31-year-old female is brought to the Emergency Department late at night by a friend who was worried that she may have taken a deliberate drug overdose. On examination, she is drowsy but rousable and smells strongly of alcohol. Pupils are widely dilated and eye movements appear normal. Heart rate is 112 bpm, blood pressure 108/76 mmHg, reflexes are brisk and symmetrical and there is sustained ankle clonus. Ingestion of which of the following drugs is most likely to account for these features?

☐ A Doxazosin

☐ B Ecstasy

☐ C Imipramine

☐ D Metamphetamine

☐ E Temazepam

2.13   Answer: E

Potentially fatal paracetamol ingestion (> 12 g in previously healthy adult) more than 8 h earlier necessitates immediate NAC while awaiting paracetamol concentrations. Acute alcohol ingestion may be protective, whereas chronic alcohol intake increases risk through up-regulation of P450 enzyme activity. Cimetidine is a P450 enzyme inhibitor.

2.14   Answer: E

Allopurinol inhibits xanthine oxidase. Acute gout can mimic septic arthritis, but routine antibiotic use is not helpful. Colchicine inhibits production of a pro-inflammatory glycoprotein by neutrophils. NSAIDs and high dose aspirin reduce pain, swelling and inflammation and are the treatment of choice.

2.15   Answer: C

Doxazosin is unlikely to alter conscious level directly. Ecstasy and amphetamines might also cause hyperreflexia and tachycardia, but they are characteristically associated with agitation and arousal.

2.16   Isoniazid undergoes hepatic acetylation, which is subject to genetic variation. Which of the following statements regarding isoniazid metabolism is correct?

☐ **A**   Around 5% of the UK population are rapid acetylators

☐ **B**   Rapid acetylators are more prone to neuropathy

☐ **C**   Rapid acetylators need careful dose reduction to avoid adverse effects

☐ **D**   Slow acetylators are more prone to hepatitis

☐ **E**   Slow acetylators show greater therapeutic response

2.17   A 27-year-old man presents to the Emergency Department alleging to have taken a mixed overdose of his own medications. He has had anxiety and depression for 3 years, and is normally treated with temazepam 10 mg nocte and venlafaxine 75 mg bd. Which one of the following findings would be in keeping with overdose of these agents?

☐ **A**   High alanine transaminase

☐ **B**   Miosis

☐ **C**   Prolonged PR interval on ECG

☐ **D**   Raised creatinine kinase

☐ **E**   Tachypnoea

2.18   Genetic polymorphism is a major determinant of drug metabolism in humans. Metabolism of which of the following drugs is *not* significantly influenced by genetic polymorphism?

☐ **A**   Hydralazine

☐ **B**   Isoniazid

☐ **C**   Norfloxacin

☐ **D**   Procainamide

☐ **E**   Sulfasalazine

2.16   Answer: E

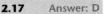

Around 50% of the UK population are rapid acetylators: low isoniazid levels, poor response to treatment and tuberculosis (TB) relapses. Slow acetylators: higher isoniazid levels and greater risk of neuropathy. Hepatitis is due to a metabolite, and is more common in rapid acetylators.

2.17   Answer: D

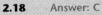

Benzodiazepine overdose may cause reduced conscious level, respiratory depression and diminished reflexes. Venlafaxine is highly toxic in overdose and may cause tachycardia, mydriasis, hyperreflexia, prolonged QT interval, serotonergic syndrome, seizures, coma and death.

2.18   Answer: C

The others are metabolised by acetylation, including the sulfapyridine component of sulfasalazine.

2.19   A 47-year-old female patient presents to the Emergency Department alleging to have taken a drug overdose. She has reduced conscious level, gross ataxia and there is bruising over all of her limbs. There is coarse nystagmus on left and right lateral gaze. Overdose of which of the following drugs might account for her clinical condition?

A   Atenolol

B   Carbamazepine

C   Digoxin

D   Furosemide

E   Sertraline

2.20   A 23-year-old woman attends her GP and describes a number of allergic episodes that have followed ingestion of peanuts. These had been characterised by facial flushing, headache, wheeze and nausea. Which of the following statements is correct in relation to treatment of allergy?

A   Bronchospasm usually develops 3–4 h after allergen exposure

B   Desensitisation to foodstuff allergens is generally effective

C   Diagnosis is typically established using skin tests

D   Patients with asthma have greater likelihood of anaphylaxis

E   Pollen extract desensitisation is usually effective in allergic hay fever

2.21   A patient is taking multiple medications, and presents to the Emergency Department with reduced conscious level. The ambulance crew found a number of empty medicine packets at the scene, and a drug overdose is suspected. For which of the following drugs would measurement of plasma drug concentrations be most useful?

A   Amlodipine

B   Digoxin

C   Furosemide

D   Gabapentin

E   Isoniazid

2.19   Answer: B

Carbamazepine and phenytoin overdose cause prominent cerebellar toxicity, often mistaken for alcohol intoxication. Repeated doses of activated charcoal should be considered, ECG monitoring and correction of electrolyte abnormalities.

2.20   Answer: D

Bee and wasp allergen and grass and tree pollen extracts can be used for desensitisation, but carry a risk of anaphylaxis. Used in patients who do not respond to antihistamines. Desensitisation to foodstuffs and animal dander is ineffective. Diagnosis depends on detailed history, skin tests may be unreliable.

2.21   Answer: B

Levels can guide the need for antidote or inform prognosis. For monitoring to be useful there should be a close relationship between plasma concentration and drug effects or toxicity. Digoxin concentrations determine the need for Fab antibody antidote.

2.22 A 56-year-old woman with a long history of bipolar disorder is admitted to the Medical Assessment Unit with a 48 h history of progressive confusion and slurred speech. On examination, she has reduced conscious level, and initial investigations show Na^+ 123 mmol/l, K^+ 3.6 mmol/l, urea 3.4 mmol/l and creatinine 108 µmol/l. Serum osmolality is 236 mOsm/kg and urinary osmolality 261 mOsm/kg. Which of the following is most likely to account for these abnormalities?

- A Carbamazepine-induced hyponatraemia
- B Carbamazepine-induced syndrome of inappropriate ADH
- C Diuretic abuse
- D Lithium-induced diabetes insipidus
- E Psychogenic polydipsia

2.23 A 74-year-old lady with dementia is brought to the Emergency Department by her care assistant, concerned that she has accidentally taken an overdose of 8 × 100 µg thyroxine tablets. Which of the following is true regarding thyroxine overdose?

- A A normal TSH concentration excludes a significant overdose
- B It is more common amongst younger adults
- C Myocardial infarction is a recognised complication
- D Ophthalmoplegia indicates thyroxine toxicity
- E Symptoms can be delayed for several days after ingestion

2.24 A 37-year-old woman attends the medical Outpatient Department after experiencing a number of short-lived episodes of anxiety, associated with palpitations, sweating, choking sensation and numbness of both upper limb extremities. Physical examination and routine investigations are normal. You diagnose panic attacks as the underlying cause of her symptoms. Which of the following is true regarding pharmacological treatment of this condition?

- A 5–10% of patients relapse within 12 months of drug discontinuation
- B Diazepam use can lead to dependence
- C Only a short-term course of treatment is necessary in most patients
- D Paroxetine rapidly relieves panic with agoraphobia
- E Tricyclic antidepressants are of no benefit in this condition

2.22 Answer: B

Carbamazepine is a recognised cause of syndrome of inappropriate antidiuretic hormone (SIADH) due to excess ADH secretion, while chlorpropamide and rifampicin increase renal tubular sensitivity to ADH. Hyponatraemia does not explain low serum osmolality and inappropriately high urine osmolality.

2.23 Answer: E

Thyroxine (T_4) is metabolised to the more active tri-iodothyronine (T_3), and tachycardia, sweating and tremor can be delayed. Sinus tachycardia and atrial fibrillation are recognised complications. Thyroid function tests should be measured; high T_4 concentrations indicate risk of toxicity.

2.24 Answer: B

Benzodiazepines have rapid onset, but should be reserved for short-term treatment to avoid dependence and tolerance. Selective serotonin reuptake inhibitors (SSRIs) and tricyclic antidepressants (TCAs) have slower onset of action and exacerbate symptoms. 30–75% of patients relapse within 6–12 months of drug discontinuation, and long-term treatment may be needed.

2.25 You are on-call overnight, and called to review a 56-year-old man with a past history of schizophrenia. During the past 4 h, he has become increasingly agitated, and he is becoming impulsive and violent towards the ward staff. Which of the following would be the most appropriate initial sedative treatment in this emergency situation?

- ☐ **A** High dose intramuscular chlorpromazine
- ☐ **B** High dose rectal diazepam
- ☐ **C** Intramuscular haloperidol in high doses
- ☐ **D** Intravenous haloperidol and lorazepam in standard doses
- ☐ **E** Oral risperidone

2.26 Which one of the following statements regarding the treatment of chronic schizophrenia is correct?

- ☐ **A** Around 10% of patients taking oral antipsychotics relapse in 3 years
- ☐ **B** Olanzapine causes parkinsonism more frequently than chlorpromazine
- ☐ **C** Relapse rate is lower in patients taking atypical antipsychotics
- ☐ **D** Therapeutic effects are due to cerebellar D_2 receptor blockade
- ☐ **E** Withdrawal characteristically complicates antipsychotic discontinuation

2.27 You see a 46-year-old man in the Medical Outpatient Department for investigation of an infected leg ulcer. He has a past history of alcohol excess, and is currently taking disulfiram 100 mg daily. Which of the following drugs is most likely to adversely interact with disulfiram and should be avoided?

- ☐ **A** Atenolol
- ☐ **B** Captopril
- ☐ **C** Metformin
- ☐ **D** Theophylline
- ☐ **E** Valsartan

2.25   Answer: D

Combination of intravenous (iv) or intramuscular (im) haloperidol (or oral risperidone) with iv or im lorazepam (or rectal diazepam) has a synergistic effect. Intravenous administration allows rapid onset of effect, but the im route may be less hazardous in the acute situation.

2.26   Answer: C

Relapse within 3 years occurs in 80% of untreated patients, 50% taking oral antipsychotics, and 20% receiving depot preparations. Relapse less common with atypical antipsychotics (eg clozapine). Pharmacological effects in part due to mesolimbic D_2 blockade; parkinsonism is less common with clozapine and olanzapine than others.

2.27   Answer: D

Disulfiram inhibits hepatic aldehyde-NAD reductase, causing accumulation of acetaldehyde after ethanol ingestion: flushing, nausea and vomiting. A similar reaction occurs due to interaction with metronidazole. Disulfiram causes non-specific P450 inhibition so phenytoin and theophylline toxicity are more likely.

2.28 A 64-year-old woman attends the Medical Outpatient Department complaining of recurrent cough. She is taking a number of medications, which you feel might be responsible. Which of the following drugs is most likely to cause a cough that resolves after drug withdrawl?

- A Amiodarone
- B Bleomycin
- C Methotrexate
- D Perindopril
- E Sulfasalazine

2.29 A 30-year-old woman with essential hypertension presents to the Antenatal Clinic at 6 weeks after conception. She is currently taking nifedipine MR 10 mg daily, and her blood pressure is consistently high, averaging 168/104 mmHg. Which of the following additional anti-hypertensive medications would be most appropriate for controlling her blood pressure?

- A Atenolol
- B Bendroflumethiazide
- C Lisinopril
- D Methyldopa
- E Valsartan

2.30 A 24-year-old man presents with agitation and central chest pain, and alleges to have used cocaine earlier in the evening. On examination, his pulse rate is 104 bpm and blood pressure 170/112 mmHg. Which one of the following features is most consistent with cocaine toxicity?

- A Hypercalcaemia
- B Hyperkalaemia
- C Hyperthermia
- D Hyponatraemia
- E Hypothermia

2.28   Answer: E

ACE inhibitors are associated with cough in up to 30%. This is reversible in > 80% of cases, and in the remainder is likely to have been present before treatment. The other drugs listed are characteristically associated with pulmonary fibrosis.

2.29   Answer: D

Methyldopa is not known to be harmful in pregnancy. Beta-blockers can cause intrauterine growth retardation. ACE inhibitors (and probably angiotensin II receptor antagonists) are teratogenic, whilst thiazides can cause neonatal thrombocytopenia.

2.30   Answer: C

Other complications include tachyarrhythmia, myocardial ischaemia and stroke. Hyponatraemia is a less common occurrence, due to pressure natriuresis in the context of elevated blood pressure.

2.31 You review a 48-year-old man with a renal transplant who has been taking several medications for immunosuppression and blood pressure control. His renal function is normal, but his serum potassium has risen to 6.4 mmol/l. Which one of the following drugs is *least* likely to have caused hyperkalaemia?

☐ A Candesartan
☐ B Ciclosporin A
☐ C Nifedipine
☐ D Ramipril
☐ E Sirolimus

2.32 A 72-year-old woman is receiving long-term warfarin treatment for chronic atrial fibrillation. Her International Normalised Ratio (INR), which had been stable for 9 months at 2.2–2.6 is now found to be 1.4. Which of the following drugs is most likely to account for this fall in her INR?

☐ A Amiodarone
☐ B Carbamazepine
☐ C Cimetidine
☐ D Co-proxamol (paracetamol + dextropropoxyphene)
☐ E Glipizide

2.33 A 45-year-old man presents to the Emergency Department within 1 h of ingesting 40 tablets of slow release theophylline. Which of the following statements regarding treatment of this patient is correct?

☐ A Alkaline diuresis reduces theophylline toxicity
☐ B Ipecacuanha is the best method to reduce gut absorption
☐ C Metabolic alkalosis indicates a poor prognosis
☐ D Oral activated charcoal is ineffective in reducing gut absorption
☐ E The degree of hypokalaemia is a marker of severity of poisoning

2.31   Answer: C

Hyperkalaemia is a particular problem when renal function has declined and serum concentrations of ciclosporin, tacrolimus or sirolimus have increased. Therapeutic drug monitoring is required to prevent nephrotoxicity and hyperkalaemia.

2.32   Answer: B

Carbamazepine is a powerful enzyme inducer, so that metabolism of warfarin will be increased. Other enzyme inducers are rifampicin, phenytoin and chronic alcohol excess. Cimetidine is an enzyme inhibitor, so that INR and bleeding risk would be expected to increase.

2.33   Answer: E

Theophylline toxicity causes hypokalaemia, metabolic acidosis, arrhythmia and seizures. Oral activated charcoal is particularly useful and repeated treatment may be needed to enhance elimination. Haemodialysis can be used to assist clearance in severe toxicity. Ipecacuanha is now redundant in most overdose situations.

2.34 A 22-year-old man is brought to the Emergency Department having been found convulsing in the street at 4 am. He is agitated, has dilated pupils, heart rate is 132 bpm and blood pressure 178/112 mmHg. Which of the following is the most likely to account for these clinical features?

- [ ] **A** Amitriptyline
- [ ] **B** Chlorpromazine
- [ ] **C** Cocaine
- [ ] **D** Co-codamol (paracetamol + codeine)
- [ ] **E** Methadone

2.35 You are asked to review a 21-year-old university student in the Medical Outpatient Department. She has suffered recurrent migraine attacks over the past 3 years, which render her unable to concentrate on her studies for several days each time. Which of the following statements is correct regarding migraine prophylaxis?

- [ ] **A** Amitriptyline prevents migraine but is commonly associated with antimuscarinic effects
- [ ] **B** Pizotifen is commonly associated with agitation and weight loss
- [ ] **C** Prophylactic therapy avoids the need for symptomatic treatment
- [ ] **D** Prophylaxis should be used if migraine occurs at least every 6 months
- [ ] **E** Propranolol is preferred to atenolol due to lack of cardioselectivity

2.36 When considering the use of haemodialysis to assist drug elimination in a patient with chronic renal impairment, which of the following properties of the drug would make haemodialysis most effective?

- [ ] **A** High drug-receptor affinity
- [ ] **B** Highly lipophilic drug
- [ ] **C** Large volume of distribution
- [ ] **D** Low degree of plasma protein binding
- [ ] **E** Short drug elimination half-life

2.34   Answer: C

Amitriptyline is associated with tachycardia and dilated pupils, and conscious level tends to be reduced. Chlorpromazine, codeine and methadone tend to be sedative, and reduce conscious level.

2.35   Answer: A

Pizotifen can cause drowsiness and weight gain. Prophylaxis reduces migraine frequency and severity, and is used when more than one or two attacks per month. Propranolol is lipid soluble, and therefore has better CNS penetration.

2.36   Answer: D

Haemodialysis is most effective in clearing drugs with low volume of distribution, ie confined largely to the circulating component. These tend to be water-soluble drugs that are not highly bound to tissue proteins. Dialysis is most useful where half-life would ordinarily be long.

2.37 A case report is published describing fulminant hepatic failure in a patient exposed to an oral anti-diabetic drug launched on the market 2 years previously. The case shows a temporal relationship, suggesting a causal link. Which of the following is the most appropriate step by the regulatory authorities in investigating this association?

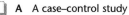

- [ ] **A** A case–control study
- [ ] **B** A prospective cohort study
- [ ] **C** A randomised controlled trial
- [ ] **D** Review of all existing spontaneous adverse reports
- [ ] **E** Withdraw the drug from clinical use

2.38 A 64-year-old woman presents to hospital 12 h after ingestion of 6 g quinine sulphate. Which of the following would be expected as a feature of drug toxicity?

- [ ] **A** Flaccid hemiparesis
- [ ] **B** Hyperacusis
- [ ] **C** Horizontal nystagmus
- [ ] **D** Intractable vomiting
- [ ] **E** Thrombocytosis

2.39 You are asked to review the prescription chart of a 56-year-old woman in the High Dependency Unit, who suffered a pathological fracture of her left neck of femur 3 days ago. She is complaining of severe hip and groin pain, and headache. Which of the following statements is correct in relation to analgesic therapy?

- [ ] **A** Bisphosphonates can relieve bone pain due to metastases
- [ ] **B** Carbamazepine is effective in treating acute bony pain
- [ ] **C** Corticosteroids worsen headache in raised intracranial pressure due to fluid retention
- [ ] **D** NSAIDs should be avoided due to bleeding risk at the injury site
- [ ] **E** Slow-release morphine should be initiated

2.37 Answer: D

The frequency and severity of adverse events determine the safety profile of any drug. The decision to withdraw a drug from clinical use depends on drug safety profile, its efficacy and the availability of alternative treatments for particular diseases.

2.38 Answer: C

Quinine causes nausea, vomiting, tremor, tinnitus and deafness. Blurred vision may progress to blindness within a few hours. Tachycardia, arrhythmias, hypotension, intravascular haemolysis and acute renal failure, seizures and coma are also recognised features.

2.39 Answer: A

Carbamazepine and gabapentin can be effective for neuropathic pain; corticosteroids can relieve pain due to neuropathy, raised intracranial pressure and bony metastases. NSAIDs are effective for inflammatory bone pain, although risk of GI bleeding is increased. Opiates may be needed, and initiated with short-acting preparations.

2.40 A 30-year-old male with a history of rheumatoid arthritis is being investigated for infertility, and is keen to avoid taking any medications that would reduce his sperm count. Which of the following drugs is most likely to cause oligospermia?

- [ ] **A** Gold
- [ ] **B** Hydroxycobalamin
- [ ] **C** Penicillamine
- [ ] **D** Prednisolone
- [ ] **E** Sulfasalazine

2.41 A 65-year-old man is brought to the Emergency Department having been found unconscious in the street at 2 am. On examination, he is localising to painful stimuli, and there is no evidence of head injury or meningism. Initial investigations showed Na$^+$ 145 mmol/l, K$^+$ 3.4 mmol/l, venous bicarbonate 16 mmol/l, urea 10.4 mmol/l, creatinine 142 µmol/l, glucose 5.4 mmol/l and serum osmolality 318 mOsm/kg. Which of the following is most likely to account for these initial findings?

- [ ] **A** Ethylene glycol ingestion
- [ ] **B** Lactic acidosis
- [ ] **C** Longstanding sleep apnoea
- [ ] **D** Rhabdomyolysis
- [ ] **E** Diclofenac toxicity

2.42 A 58-year-old non-diabetic woman was found to have blood pressure 168/94 mmHg, proteinuria +++, and serum creatinine 172 µmol/l. Renal biopsy revealed membranous glomerulonephritis, and treatment with lisinopril is started. Which of the following changes is most likely to occur as a result of this treatment?

- [ ] **A** Increased serum low density lipoprotein (LDL) cholesterol concentration
- [ ] **B** Increased serum magnesium concentration
- [ ] **C** Reduced serum creatinine concentration
- [ ] **D** Reduced serum potassium concentration
- [ ] **E** Reduced urinary protein excretion

2.40   Answer: E

Sulfasalazine causes oligospermia, reduced sperm motility and increased sperm morphological abnormalities. The effects are mediated at a late stage in sperm maturation, and are usually reversible on drug withdrawal. The sulphapyridine moiety is thought responsible.

2.41   Answer: B

The data suggest a metabolic acidosis; lactate should be measured. NSAID ingestion and rhabdomyolysis are typically associated with hyperkalaemia. Calculated osmolality is close to the actual measured osmolality, excluding significant circulating concentrations of ethylene glycol, methanol or alcohol. Longstanding type-2 respiratory failure can cause a metabolic alkalosis.

2.42   Answer: E

ACE inhibitor treatment will improve blood pressure and reduce the decline in GFR, but creatinine is unlikely to fall. Serum potassium may increase, particularly if there is renovascular insufficiency.

2.43 A 67-year-old woman was taking a number of regular medications for chronic back pain. One week earlier, she developed a urinary tract infection and her renal function was found to be impaired, having previously been normal. She is now admitted to hospital, having become increasingly drowsy over the past week. Which of her usual medications is most likely to account for this change in her mental state?

- ☐ **A** Aspirin
- ☐ **B** Carbamazepine
- ☐ **C** Diazepam
- ☐ **D** Morphine
- ☐ **E** Paracetamol

2.44 A 46-year-old farm worker attended the Emergency Department after a deliberate overdose of organophosphate pesticide. He was treated initially with atropine. Which one of the following clinical features can most reliably be used to assess his response to atropine?

- ☐ **A** Bronchorrhoea
- ☐ **B** Heart rate
- ☐ **C** Peripheral pulse volume
- ☐ **D** Pupil size
- ☐ **E** Systolic blood pressure

2.45 A 32-year-old woman presented to the Emergency Department 6 h after taking 30 g of paracetamol. Which one of the following factors most strongly predicts an increased risk of paracetamol-induced hepatotoxicity?

- ☐ **A** Anorexia nervosa
- ☐ **B** Cimetidine ingestion with the paracetamol
- ☐ **C** Gilbert's disease
- ☐ **D** Recreational cannabis use
- ☐ **E** Regularly smoking 20 cigarettes per day

2.43   Answer: D

Morphine has a comparatively short half-life; the duration of one of its active metabolites (morphine-6-glucuronide) is significantly prolonged in renal impairment and it accumulates. The dose and timing of morphine administration require careful adjustment in patients with renal impairment.

2.44   Answer: A

Organophosphates and nerve agents bind to acetylcholinesterase, thereby exaggerating the effects of acetylcholine (ACh) at nicotinic and muscarinic synapses. Classically, patients will have excess salivation and lacrimation, bronchorrhoea, and miosis, but effects on pupil size, heart rate and blood pressure are highly variable.

2.45   Answer: A

Anorexia, chronic alcohol excess and HIV infection are associated with malnourishment and glutathione depletion; hepatic enzyme induction (eg chronic alcohol intake, carbamazepine, phenytoin and rifampicin) is associated with more rapid formation of toxic metabolites. Chronic cigarette smoking has a weak hepatic enzyme-inducing effect.

2.46 A 26-year-old woman presented 9 h after a mixed overdose of paracetamol, diazepam and ethanol. She was drowsy, mildly dehydrated, and complaining of mild nausea. Treatment with iv N-acetylcysteine was started and, 20 min later, she developed breathlessness, facial flushing and developed a tachycardia of 140 bpm. What is the most likely explanation for this reaction?

A Acute left ventricular failure

B Allergic reaction to paracetamol

C Anaphylactoid reaction to N-acetylcysteine

D Overdose of N-acetylcysteine has been administered

E The patient has received N-acetylcysteine previously

2.47 You review the analgesia prescription for a 69-year-old woman with breast carcinoma and painful bony metastases. She has been taking regular oral modified-release morphine, and has required additional morphine solution for breakthrough pain. Which of the following pharmacokinetic factors is most important in deciding the dose and frequency of morphine to be administered?

A Half-life

B Patient body mass index

C Serum creatinine concentration

D The extent of first pass metabolism

E Volume of distribution

2.48 A 42-year-old man is diagnosed as having rheumatoid arthritis, and you are considering starting treatment with the disease modifying anti-rheumatic drug, sulfasalazine. A history of allergy to which one of the following drugs would be a contraindication to the use of sulfasalazine?

A Amiodarone

B Co-trimoxazole

C Lisinopril

D Penicillin

E Valaciclovir

2.46 Answer: C

Anaphylactoid reactions occur in around 15% of patients treated with NAC, and are usually self-limiting. Infusion should be temporarily discontinued, and treatment administered if needed (antihistamine, corticosteroids). NAC treatment can be recommenced in most cases.

2.47 Answer: A

Short acting preparations should be used initially, and then modified release preparations introduced after analgesic requirements are established. The other factors listed can be indicative of half-life, but are less important.

2.48 Answer: B

Co-trimoxazole (trimethoprim and sulfamethoxazole). Allergic reactions to sulphonamide are more likely than to trimethoprim, and suggests a high risk of allergic reaction to the sulfapyridine component of sulfasalazine. Therefore, an alternative amino-salicylic acid preparation should be used.

2.49 A 22-year-old woman with poorly controlled asthma presented to the Emergency Department with wheeze and breathlessness. Peak flow rate was 150 l/min, and she was treated with intravenous hydrocortisone and nebulised salbutamol. Her clinical condition improved within 20 min. Which one of the following statements regarding her therapy is correct?

A   Hydrocortisone inhibits adenosine release

B   Hydrocortisone up-regulates β_2 receptors in the lung

C   Increased heart rate after salbutamol is due to its β_1 agonist effects

D   Rapid response is due to additive effect of hydrocortisone and salbutamol

E   Pharmacological effects of hydrocortisone take at least 6 h

2.50 Exposure to which one of the following agents is most likely to cause significant toxic effects within 1 h?

A   Amitriptyline

B   Glue solvents

C   Lithium

D   Paracetamol

E   Warfarin

2.51 Compared with naproxen, which statement regarding celcoxib is true?

A   Anti-inflammatory effects are greater

B   Concomitant diuretic treatment can be given more safely

C   It acts by inhibiting a different enzyme pathway

D   It has a lower level of antiplatelet activity

E   There is a lower risk of hepatic adverse effects

2.49   Answer: E

The anti-inflammatory effects of corticosteroids do not manifest for several hours after administration, but should be given early in severe exacerbations of chronic obstructive pulmonary disease (COPD) or asthma. Salbutamol is a pure β_2 agonist. Tachycardia is due to functional crossover between β_1 and β_2 receptors, and due to peripheral vaodilatation.

2.50   Answer: B

Solvents (eg toluene) are readily absorbed through skin or by inhalation, leading to rapid onset of airway irritation, bronchospasm and asphyxiation. Systemic effects include nausea, reduced conscious level, and arrhythmia. Toxic effects of lithium are characteristically delayed whilst the drug accumulates intracellularly.

2.51   Answer: D

Antiplatelet activity is thought to be mediated predominantly through blockade of the COX-1 pathway.

2.52 A 60-year-old man describes a history of chest pain on exertion, and is diagnosed with angina. He is prescribed sublingual glyceryl trinitrate (GTN) as required. Which one of the following is *not* a mechanism by which GTN gives symptomatic relief?

- ☐ A Activation of guanylate cyclase
- ☐ B Dilatation of collateral coronary vessels
- ☐ C Dilatation of major peripheral veins
- ☐ D Formation of nitric oxide
- ☐ E Inhibition of calcium channels

2.53 You are asked to review a 24-year-old woman in the Medical Outpatient Department. She had attended the Emergency Department several weeks earlier complaining of anxiety symptoms, restlessness and poor concentration. Physical examination, routine blood tests, including thyroid function tests, and a resting ECG were normal, and she was given a short-term supply of diazepam. Which of the following is correct with regard to drug treatment of generalised anxiety disorder?

- ☐ A β-blockers are useful for controlling somatic symptoms of anxiety
- ☐ B Benzodiazepines should be avoided in chronic anxiety
- ☐ C Buspirone has anxiolytic properties mediated by the benzodiazepine receptor
- ☐ D Restlessness and disturbed sleep usually respond well to propranolol
- ☐ E Short-acting benzodiazepines do not increase the risk of falls in elderly patients

2.54 A 72-year-old woman presents to the Emergency Department having been thought to have accidentally taken an overdose of her normal medications. BM glucose is 1.8 mmol/l. Which of the following is most likely to cause hypoglycaemia in overdose?

- ☐ A Digoxin
- ☐ B Enalapril
- ☐ C Furosemide
- ☐ D Metoprolol
- ☐ E Paracetamol

2.52   Answer: E

GTN is metabolised by endothelium to liberate nitric oxide (NO). NO is rapidly degraded, so its effects are mediated close to its site of formation. It acts on vascular smooth muscle to cause relaxation and vasodilatation.

2.53   Answer: A

Benzodiazepines are useful for short-term control of anxiety but carry a risk of dependence and withdrawal phenomena. Sedative effects are enhanced by alcohol. Buspirone is an anxiolytic with longer duration of onset than benzodiazepines, and withdrawal is less likely to occur. Somatic symptoms (eg tachycardia) may respond well to β-blockers.

2.54   Answer: E

Hypoglycaemia is a recognised feature of paracetamol overdose, thought due to impaired glycogenolysis. A low BM recording should always be confirmed by a laboratory venous glucose measurement.

2.55 A 22-year-old male student is admitted via the Emergency Department having been found unconscious by his flatmate. Initial investigations show serum Na^+ 140 mmol/l, K^+ 4.0 mmol/l, Ca^{2+} 1.8 mmol/l, bicarbonate 12 mmol/l, and albumin 42 mmol/l. Ingestion of which of the following drugs is most likely to have caused these laboratory findings?

A Amitriptyline

B Ecstasy (MDMA)

C Ethylene glycol

D Heroin

E Paracetamol

2.56 A 72-year-old man with disseminated prostatic carcinoma is taking regular modified release oral morphine and regular paracetamol, with standard-release morphine for breakthrough pain. He is complaining of worsening rib and thoracic spine pain, associated with severe nausea, and you wish to adjust his drug regimen. Which of the following interventions would be most appropriate?

A Add carbamazepine and reduce the dose of morphine

B Add dexamethasone and reduce the dose of morphine

C Add ibuprofen and reduce the dose of morphine

D Substitute a once-daily morphine formulation

E Substitute diamorphine given by continuous subcutaneous infusion

2.57 Which of the following is a recognised feature of cyclophosphamide treatment?

A Absorbed poorly from the gut

B Dermal photosensitivity

C Haemorrhagic cystitis

D Hirsutism

E Inhibition of folic acid

2.55 Answer: C
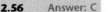

Ethylene glycol ingestion is associated with severe metabolic acidosis, hypocalcaemia, renal failure, seizures, arrhythmia and coma. Treatment is with ethanol (to compete for metabolism and reduce toxic metabolite formation) and haemodialysis to assist elimination of ethylene glycol and its metabolites.

2.56 Answer: C

NSAID treatment is effective for inflammatory bone pain. More flexible pain control can be achieved by combined long and short-acting oral morphine preparations than continuous administration (bioavailability also more predictable). Carbamazepine can be effective in neuropathic pain, and dexamethasone is useful for headache associated with raised intracranial pressure (ICP).

2.57 Answer: C

Acrolein, a metabolite, causes this serious adverse effect. Mesna reacts with the metabolite, and prevents urothelial toxicity. Methotrexate exerts a folate antagonist effect, which can be avoided by administration of folinic acid.

2.58 You see a 48-year-old man in the Medical Outpatient Department and note that he is receiving flupentixol as a depot preparation. Which one of the following statements regarding depot antipsychotic medications is correct?

A Are associated with poorer bioavailability than oral preparations

B Around 20% of patients with schizophrenia receive depot preparations

C Can easily be titrated to control adverse effects

D Drug release can be delayed by up to several months

E They allow a greater remission rate than oral preparations

2.59 A 42-year-old woman reports progressive weight gain of around 8 kg in the past 6 months, having started a new antidepressant therapy at that time. She is upset by the weight gain, and wishes to discontinue treatment. Which of the following treatments is *least* likely to cause significant weight gain?

A Amitriptyline

B Carbamazepine

C Lithium

D Mirtazapine

E Venlafaxine

2.60 You see a 46-year-old in the Emergency Department on a Saturday night. He smells strongly of alcohol, and has slurred speech and unsteady gait. He is uncooperative with physical examination but there are no abnormal cardiac, respiratory or abdominal findings, and an ECG and chest X-ray are normal. You suspect from his demeanour that he regularly drinks alcohol to excess, and are concerned about the possibility of alcohol withdrawal syndrome (AWS). Which of the following is most accurate regarding AWS?

A Alpha-blockers are useful in reducing symptom severity

B Chlordiazepoxide is anxiolytic but does not reduce risk of seizure

C Oral thiamine is recommended to prevent neuropathy

D Suicidal ideation is a recognised feature

E Wernicke's encephalopathy can occur due to pyridoxine deficiency

2.58 Answer: E

Depot preparations are associated with high remission rates and assured compliance (used in 60% of patients in Europe). A disadvantage is the inability to down-titrate dose in the event of adverse effects. Drug release can be delayed by up to several weeks.

2.59 Answer: E

Tricyclics can cause weight gain, typically between 1 and 6 kg in 6 months. Weight gain is less common with SSRIs and trazodone. Mirtazapine increases appetite and weight, and some patients experience carbohydrate craving. Lithium commonly causes thirst, hunger and weight gain. Venlafaxine is less likely to cause weight gain but carries a significant risk of cardiotoxicity.

2.60 Answer: D

Thiamine is a co-factor for carbohydrate metabolism, and deficiency can be precipitated by dextrose administration (iv pabrinex should be administered to prevent this). Diazepam and chlordiazepoxide are effective in symptom control in reducing courses, and reduce seizure risk.

2.61   A 34-year-old man presents 36 h after an intentional overdose of paracetamol, alcohol and fluoxetine. Which of the following tests would be most helpful in determining prognosis?

- A   Platelet count
- B   Prothrombin time
- C   Serum alanine transaminase
- D   Serum alkaline phosphatase
- E   Serum creatinine

2.62   You are asked to see a 28-year-old woman who is pregnant. She has been complaining of cough and fever for 3 days, and on respiratory examination is found to have crackles at the left lung base. You decide to prescribe a short course of antibiotics. Which of the following should be avoided?

- A   Cefotaxime
- B   Co-amoxiclav
- C   Co-trimoxazole
- D   Erythromycin
- E   Metronidazole

2.63   A 34-year-old woman has developed cellulitis, 2 weeks after giving birth to a healthy baby girl. There is marked erythema and tenderness of skin overlying the medial aspect of her left breast, and you wish to prescribe a course of antibiotics. She is breast-feeding her child. Which of the following drugs would be most important to avoid?

- A   Co-amoxiclav
- B   Erythromycin
- C   Flucloxacillin
- D   Metronidazole
- E   Trimethoprim

2.61   Answer: B

At 36 h after ingestion, it is unlikely that there will be a significant risk due to fluoxetine. Prothrombin time and alanine transaminase (ALT) are indicative of hepatocellular damage after paracetamol ingestion. Platelet count, ALT, renal function and lactate influence clinical management, but do not reliably inform prognosis.

2.62   Answer: C

Co-trimoxazole is potentially teratogenic, due to anti-folate effects of trimethoprim. Sulphonamides confer a risk of neonatal haemolysis and methaemoglobinaemia. The others, including penicillin, are regarded as safe. Metronidazole is teratogenic in animals, but appears safe in humans.

2.63   Answer: D

Significant amounts of metronidazole are secreted in breast milk, which can alter neonatal gut flora to cause significant diarrhoea. Clarithromycin should be avoided, but erythromycin is only secreted in small amounts and appears safe. Penicillins and trimethoprim are secreted in breast milk in small amounts but appear safe.

2.64 Which one of the following drugs taken by a mother poses the greatest risk to her breast-fed infant?

   A Aspirin

   B Diclofenac

   C Dipyridamole

   D Heparin

   E Warfarin

2.65 A 59-year-old woman presented to hospital 4 h after an alleged drug overdose. Initial investigations showed serum Na$^+$ 139 mmol/l, K$^+$ 6.3 mmol/l and urea 6.2 mmol/l. Ingestion of which one of the following drugs is most likely to have caused this metabolic abnormality?

   A Amitriptyline

   B Digoxin

   C Salbutamol

   D Theophylline

   E Verapamil

2.66 Which of the following poses the greatest risks to the developing fetus when taken by the mother in therapeutic doses?

   A Carbidopa

   B Carbimazole

   C Cefalexin

   D Cimetidine

   E Ciprofloxacin

2.67 A 32-year-old woman has had epilepsy for 9 years, which is well controlled with phenytoin 100 mg bd. She is now pregnant, and presents seeking advice regarding her treatment. Which of the following would be the most appropriate course of action?

   A Continue current treatment and indicate the risks of teratogenicity

   B Discontinue phenytoin and substitute carbamazepine

   C Discontinue phenytoin and substitute lamotrigine

   D Stop phenytoin and use diazepam as required for seizure control

   E Suggest termination of pregnancy

2.64   Answer: A

Aspirin poses the risk of Reye's syndrome; high maternal doses of aspirin can impair neonatal platelet function (greater sensitivity). Dipyridamole is present in small amounts in breast milk, and requires some caution. The others are generally regarded as safe.

2.65   Answer: B

Other features include nausea, vomiting, xanthopsia, arrhythmia, seizures and coma. Toxic features (particularly arrhythmia) are more likely in the presence of hypokalaemia. Theophylline toxicity is associated with hypokalaemia and metabolic acidosis, and salbutamol causes dose-dependent hypokalaemia.

2.66   Answer: B

Risks of neonatal goitre and hypothyroidism. Ciprofloxacin and other quinalones usually avoided because animal studies have shown arthropathy.

2.67   Answer: A

Most anti-epileptic drugs are known to be teratogenic, and the mother should be counselled. Benefits of continuing treatment outweigh the potential adverse consequences (to mother and fetus) of seizures associated with treatment discontinuation.

2.68 A 34-year-old woman is undergoing ante-natal screening and found to have consistently high blood pressure, averaging 164/82 mmHg. You wish to commence antihypertensive treatment. Which of the following is regarded as most safe?

- A Bendroflumethiazide
- B Bisoprolol
- C Methyldopa
- D Nifedipine
- E Perindopril

2.69 Which of the following drugs should be used with particular caution in very elderly patients?

- A Amoxicillin
- B Enalapril
- C Low dose aspirin
- D Quinine
- E Ranitidine

2.70 Which one of the following drugs is significantly more likely to cause adverse effects in elderly rather than young adults, when used in normal therapeutic doses?

- A Co-amoxiclav
- B Erythromycin
- C Omeprazole
- D Temazepam
- E Thyroxine

2.71 You see a 72-year-old man in the Outpatient Department for assessment of high blood pressure. Despite lifestyle interventions over the past 3 months, his blood pressure remains elevated at around 172/88 mmHg. Which of the following statements regarding antihypertensive treatment in elderly patients is correct?

- A Bendroflumethiazide is generally ineffective
- B β-blockers are contraindicated beyond age 65 years
- C Doxazosin is an ideal first-line treatment
- D Lisinopril is an optimal first-line treatment
- E Nifedipine is an appropriate first-line treatment

2.68   Answer: C

Thiazide diuretics can cause neonatal thrombocytopenia, whereas β-blockers cause intrauterine growth retardation. Calcium channel blockers may inhibit labour, and are teratogenic in animals. ACE inhibitors and angiotensin 2 receptor antagonists are associated with oligohydramnios.

2.69   Answer: B

In older patients with impaired renal blood flow, NSAIDs, ACE inhibitors and AT receptor antagonists reduce efferent arteriolar tone and can cause a dramatic reduction in glomerular filtration.

2.70   Answer: D

Drugs with sedative properties are likely to cause greater effects in elderly patients, and caution is required, eg benzodiazepines, antidepressants, antipsychotics, due to inefficiency of the blood–brain barrier and cerebral atrophy.

2.71   Answer: E

Elderly patients respond better to thiazides and calcium channel blockers, whereas patients < 65 years respond better to ACE inhibitors and β-blockers. β-blockers are useful if co-existent angina. α-blockers are reserved for third-line use or if there is concomitant prostatism (may increase risk of heart failure).

2.72 A 64-year-old man is referred to the Outpatient Clinic for investigation of falls. On examination, he has features suggesting Parkinson's disease. Which of the following would be most effective as a potential treatment?

- [ ] A Carbidopa
- [ ] B Dopamine
- [ ] C Lithium
- [ ] D Methyldopa
- [ ] E Selegeline

2.73 You see a 76-year-old woman in the Outpatient Department. She has had parkinsonism for a number of years, successfully treated with co-beneldopa (L-dopa and benserazide), one capsule 3 times daily. However, she has recently noticed that her mobility has become progressively worse just before each dose. Which of the following changes to her medications would be most appropriate?

- [ ] A Add bromocriptine
- [ ] B Discontinue co-beneldopa and commence L-dopa
- [ ] C Discontinue co-beneldopa and commence selegeline
- [ ] D Increase dose to two capsules 3 times per day
- [ ] E Maintain usual daily amount but switch to modified-release preparation

2.74 You review an 81-year-old man in the Medical Outpatient Department. He has been suffering from recurrent falls, and reduced mobility. He had been started on L-dopa by his GP 4 weeks ago for suspected Parkinson's disease, but had not noted any significant improvement. On examination, his seated blood pressure was 148/84 mmHg, and 116/80 mmHg on standing. Which of the following statements is correct?

- [ ] A Bromocriptine is a more appropriate treatment than L-dopa
- [ ] B Fludrocortisone treatment should be introduced
- [ ] C His blood pressure drop on standing indicates autonomic neuropathy
- [ ] D Lack of response to L-dopa excludes Parkinson's disease
- [ ] E L-Dopa should be combined with an extra-cerebral decarboxylase inhibitor

2.72   Answer: E

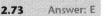

Selegeline can be used as monotherapy or in addition to L-dopa. Carbidopa is a peripheral dopa decarboxylase inhibitor that is ineffective in the absence of L-dopa. Dopamine is broken down before crossing the blood–brain barrier, whereas methyldopa is primarily an antihypertensive.

2.73   Answer: E

'End of dose deterioration' can be addressed by switching to long-acting formulations, or adding adjunctive treatment, eg entacapone. This avoids potential adverse effects of increasing the total daily dose.

2.74   Answer: E

Dopamine agonists (eg bromocriptine, cabergoline, ropinirole) are less appropriate in elderly patients due to potential neuropsychiatric adverse effects. Postural hypotension is a common adverse effect of L-dopa, which is less common in combination with a peripheral dopa decarboxylase inhibitor.

2.75 Which of the following drugs should be avoided, where possible, in patients with severe renal impairment?

☐ **A** Amoxicillin

☐ **B** Metformin

☐ **C** Omeprazole

☐ **D** Paracetamol

☐ **E** Simvastatin

2.76 A 74-year-old woman is referred to the Medical Outpatient Department for investigation of renal impairment. Urea was found to be 12.0 mmol/l and creatinine 167 µmol/l. She is taking multiple medications; which one of the following is most likely to account for her renal impairment?

☐ **A** Bendroflumethiazide

☐ **B** Ciprofloxacin

☐ **C** Digoxin

☐ **D** Ibuprofen

☐ **E** Morphine sulphate

2.77 A 46-year-old woman is admitted to hospital for treatment of severe gastroenteritis and dehydration. Which one of the following drugs would be most likely to account for a sudden deterioration in her renal function?

☐ **A** Ceftriaxone

☐ **B** Ciprofloxacin

☐ **C** Erythromycin

☐ **D** Metronidazole

☐ **E** Oral vancomycin

2.75 Answer: B

Metformin can cause lactic acidosis, especially in patients with renal impairment. The adverse effects of simvastatin (hepatitis and myositis) are more likely in patients with renal impairment, and it should be used with caution.

2.76 Answer: D

All NSAIDs are capable of impairing renal function. The dose of ciprofloxacin, digoxin and morphine should be reduced to avoid adverse effects caused by drug/metabolite accumulation in renal failure. A benzodiazepine is generally ineffective in the absence of normal renal function.

2.77 Answer: B

Severe dehydration increases the risk of ciprofloxacin-induced crystalluria, especially where high doses are used.

2.78 A 56-year-old man has been receiving warfarin for recurrent deep venous thrombosis, and his INR has been stable at 2.4–2.8 for the past 8 months. He presents to the Emergency Department pale, hypotensive and tachycardic after suffering abdominal pain and melaena. He had been started on antibiotic therapy 5 days earlier for a suspected respiratory tract infection. Which of the following drugs is most likely to have increased his risk of bleeding?

   ☐ **A** Amoxycillin

   ☐ **B** Ciprofloxacin

   ☐ **C** Metronidazole

   ☐ **D** Oxytetracycline

   ☐ **E** Rifampicin

2.79 A 32-year-old man attends his GP with a 48-h history of severe, pulsating left-sided headache associated with nausea. He is suspected of suffering an acute migraine attack. Which of the following statements regarding treatment of migraine is correct?

   ☐ **A** Dopaminergic agonists should be avoided in acute attacks

   ☐ **B** Ergotamine can worsen headache due to peripheral vasodilatation

   ☐ **C** Oral drug absorption is often impaired during an acute attack

   ☐ **D** Simple analgesics are rarely effective even if taken early in the attack

   ☐ **E** Sumatriptan is ineffective after headache is established

2.80 A 42-year-old woman is admitted to the Emergency Department with severe colicky abdominal pain, nausea and vomiting. You diagnose left-sided ureteric colic and possible pyelonephritis. Which of the following is correct regarding symptomatic treatment?

   ☐ **A** Azapropazone causes less GI irritation than ibuprofen

   ☐ **B** Diclofenac is associated with 10-fold increased risk of aplastic anaemia

   ☐ **C** Meptazinol causes greater respiratory depression than morphine

   ☐ **D** Morphine provides rapid relief of pain and nausea

   ☐ **E** Pethidine is associated with tachycardia and hypertension

2.78   Answer: B

Ciprofloxacin is an enzyme inhibitor, so INR and bleeding risk will increase. Metronidazole has weak hepatic enzyme inhibiting properties. Other important enzyme inhibitors are erythromycin, cimetidine and allopurinol. Rifampicin is an enzyme inducer that is likely to cause a fall in INR.

2.79   Answer: C

Simple analgesia (paracetamol, NSAIDs) often effective if taken early. Gastroparesis reduces drug absorption, hence prokinetics (eg metoclopramide) can be helpful. Ergots must be given early, and carry risk of peripheral vasospasm. 5-HT$_1$ agonists effective once headache established, but more effective if given early.

2.80   Answer: B

Azapropazone appears to give greatest risk of GI irritation, and ibuprofen lowest risk amongst NSAIDS. Meptazinol is a partial agonist, thought to cause less respiratory depression. Opiates give effective pain relief, but cause nausea and haemodynamic effects (tachycardia and hypotension) partly due to histamine release.

2.81 You are asked to review a 56-year-old woman who was admitted 3 days earlier for treatment of severe community-acquired pneumonia. Her liver biochemistry tests were normal on admission to hospital, but now show: bilirubin 58 µmol/l, alanine transaminase 52 IU/l, alkaline phosphatase 256 IU/l, γ-glutamyl transpeptidase (GGT) 54 IU/l and albumin 41 g/l. Which one of the following drugs is most likely to have caused these abnormalities?

☐ **A** Amoxicillin

☐ **B** Ciprofloxacin

☐ **C** Clarithromycin

☐ **D** Co-amoxiclav

☐ **E** Trimethoprim

2.82 A 45-year-old businesswoman has returned to the UK from a 6-month business trip to Pakistan. Two weeks earlier, she had suffered fever, breathlessness and cough, and was commenced on treatment. Her blood tests show: bilirubin 52 µmol/l, alanine transaminase 196 IU/l, alkaline phosphatase 76 IU/l, GGT 64 IU/l and albumin 37 g/l. Which one of the following drugs is most likely to have caused these abnormalities?

☐ **A** Ciprofloxacin

☐ **B** Co-amoxiclav

☐ **C** Erythromycin

☐ **D** Ethambutol

☐ **E** Rifampicin

2.83 A 17-year-old woman presented to the Emergency Department 2 h after deliberately taking a paracetamol overdose. A 4-h serum paracetamol level was 260 mg/l and intravenous N-acetylcysteine (NAC) administration was commenced. One hour later, she became nauseated, and was found to have facial flushing and an urticarial rash over her trunk and back. You suspect an anaphylactoid reaction to the NAC treatment. Which of the following statements is correct?

☐ **A** Anaphylactoid reactions occur in 2–5% of patients treated with NAC

☐ **B** Antihistamines must be administered early

☐ **C** Corticosteroid treatment should routinely be administered

☐ **D** NAC treatment should be discontinued and not re-introduced

☐ **E** Nebulised salbutamol can improve clinical condition

2.81   Answer: D

The pattern of biochemical abnormalities is consistent with biliary obstruction or cholestatic jaundice. Also recognised as an adverse effect of erythromycin and, rarely, ciprofloxacin.

2.82   Answer: E

The biochemical abnormalities are consistent with hepatitis. Rifampicin, isoniazid, pyrazinamide and rifabutin can all cause hepatotoxicity. Ethambutol can cause visual disturbances, especially in patients with renal impairment.

2.83   Answer: E

Stopping the infusion is often all that is required. Antihistamine may be necessary, and corticosteroids are indicated only if reaction is severe. Nebulised bronchodilators should be used if bronchospasm is significant. NAC can often be recommenced at a lower rate.

Clinical pharmacology answers

2.84 A 25-year-old man presents to the Emergency Department 36 h after ingesting a large quantity of paracetamol tablets. He is complaining of nausea, anorexia and abdominal pain, which are thought due to his recent overdose. Which of the following would most strongly suggest an alternative cause for his symptoms?

☐ A Hypocalcaemia

☐ B Hypoglycaemia

☐ C Metabolic acidosis

☐ D Raised alanine transferase

☐ E Raised serum lactate

2.85 A 56-year-old man has been treated for asthma for 8 years, and is taking regular theophylline and inhaled beclomethasone, and salbutamol when required. Four days ago, he suffered increased cough and fever, and was commenced on an antibiotic. He is now complaining of severe nausea and headache, and plasma theophylline concentration is found to be 186 µmol/l (therapeutic range 55–110 µmol/l). Which of the following drugs is most likely to have precipitated theophylline toxicity?

☐ A Amoxicillin

☐ B Ciprofloxacin

☐ C Co-amoxiclav

☐ D Metronidazole

☐ E Penicillin V

2.86 Which of the following statements is correct regarding the development of potential new drugs?

☐ A Further development is abandoned if no therapeutic effects are seen in phase I studies

☐ B Head-to-head comparison to existing therapy occurs only in phase IV studies

☐ C Oral bioavailability can be examined in phase I studies

☐ D Phase I studies typically involve 100–500 patients

☐ E Phase IV studies must be completed before a marketing licence is given

2.84   Answer: A

Hypocalcaemia is not a recognised feature of paracetamol overdose. This might suggest acute pancreatitis, an uncommon complication. Hypokalaemia and hypoglycaemia are commonly recognised. Metabolic acidosis and raised lactate concentrations are late features.

2.85   Answer: B

Theophylline is metabolised by the liver, and has a narrow therapeutic range. Ciprofloxacin is an enzyme inhibitor, so that theophylline metabolism is delayed and clearance reduced. Others include erythromycin, allopurinol and omeprazole.

2.86   Answer: C

Phase I studies (including 'first in human') determine safety, and usually involves healthy volunteers. Data from single and multiple administration dose-escalation studies can be used to determine pharmacokinetics. Efficacy is determined in phases II and III, often against a comparator. Phase IV studies are often undertaken post-marketing.

2.87 You are approached by a pharmaceutical sales representative who tells you that their new antihypertensive 'dropolol' is better than atenolol, which is the existing hospital choice of β-blocker. She shows you data indicating that dropolol 5 mg daily causes a similar blood pressure reduction to atenolol 50 mg daily but is 20% cheaper. Which of the following statements is correct regarding the new treatment?

- A It has greater efficacy
- B It is likely to have fewer adverse effects
- C It is more cost-effective
- D It is more potent
- E It should be adopted into clinical practice

2.88 You are involved in the conduct of a study to investigate the effects of a new treatment for septic shock in patients admitted to ITU. Which of the following statements is correct regarding the conduct of such a study?

- A A double-blind randomised placebo-controlled design must be used
- B Consent need not be sought because most patients will be unconscious
- C If suitability for inclusion is in doubt then patients should be enrolled to increase statistical power
- D It is usually acceptable to withhold standard care during a clinical trial
- E Next of kin can provide consent on behalf of the patient

2.89 You are supervising a single ascending dose phase I study in healthy subjects. On reviewing the safety data after the second dose tier, you note that one of eight subjects had an elevated alanine transaminase (145 IU/l) at 24 h after dose administration. Which of the following statements is correct?

- A Development of the drug should be abandoned
- B Further dose escalation should be halted
- C Interpretation depends on clinical and laboratory safety variables and pharmacokinetic data
- D The study blinding code must be broken
- E The subject in question must have received active drug

2.87   Answer: D

The similar drop in BP suggests both drugs have equal antihypertensive efficacy. Potency is a measure of efficacy that takes account of drug dose, and is less relevant to clinical practice. Effectiveness cannot be assessed without knowledge of its adverse effects profile and impact on long-term outcomes, eg myocardial infarction. Costs of the drug might be offset by costs of increased monitoring for adverse effects and more information is required.

2.88   Answer: E

Where possible, informed consent should be sought. If appropriate, this can be obtained from the next of kin or appointed guardian, and an independent arbitrator can oversee in cases of doubt. It would be exceptional for standard therapy to be withheld, particularly in a critical care environment.

2.89   Answer: C

It is not uncommon for abnormal liver function tests to occur, sometimes > 2× upper limit of normal, even after placebo administration (hence need for placebo arm in early phase I). The study code need only be broken if the adverse effect is regarded as serious and possibly study drug-related.

2.90 A 62-year-old woman has been taking the same dose of digoxin for 8 years for chronic atrial fibrillation. She attends the Emergency Department with a short history of nausea, vomiting and visual disturbance, and is found to have a serum digoxin level of 3.4 nmol/ml (therapeutic range 1.1–2.5 nmol/l). Introduction of which of the following drugs is most likely to have precipitated digoxin toxicity?

   ☐ **A** Atenolol

   ☐ **B** Doxazosin

   ☐ **C** Omeprazole

   ☐ **D** Ramipril

   ☐ **E** Verapamil

2.91 A 52-year-old man attends the Medical Outpatient Department for investigation of anaemia. Initial investigations show bilirubin 58 μmol/l, haemoglobin 8.7 g/dl and mean cell volume 101 fl. Which of the following drugs is most likely to account for these abnormalities?

   ☐ **A** Amiodarone

   ☐ **B** Hydralazine

   ☐ **C** Methyldopa

   ☐ **D** Methotrexate

   ☐ **E** Thyroxine

2.92 You are reviewing data regarding development of a novel compound for the treatment of asthma. Drug 'A' is a more potent bronchodilator than drug 'B'. Which of the following statements regarding drug 'A' is correct?

   ☐ **A** Causes the same response as drug 'B' at any given dose

   ☐ **B** It causes a greater clinical response

   ☐ **C** It is more efficacious

   ☐ **D** It is associated with fewer adverse effects

   ☐ **E** Lower concentrations can cause the same effects as drug 'B'

2.90   Answer: E

Verapamil and nifedipine impair renal clearance of digoxin.
Verapamil, diltiazem and β-blockers enhance AV nodal blockade but
do not significantly increase digoxin concentrations.

2.91   Answer: C

The investigations indicate anaemia, mild macrocytosis and
hyperbilirubinaemia, which strongly suggest haemolysis.
Urobilinogen on urinalysis is also recognised. Methyldopa and
penicillin cause antibody-mediated warm autoimmune haemolytic
anaemia (WAHA).

2.92   Answer: E

Potency is an expression of drug efficacy with regard to the
administered dose/tissue concentration. Both drugs might be equally
efficacious, and no comment can be made regarding clinical utility.

2.93 A 13-year-old girl presents with a history of severe headache and nausea. She undergoes a lumbar puncture examination, and cerebrospinal fluid (CSF) microscopy is strongly suggestive of viral meningitis. You are asked to prescribe analgesia in view of her persisting headache. Which of the following statements is correct?

A Combined codeine–paracetamol preparations are more effective than paracetamol alone

B High dose aspirin would be a suitable treatment

C Non-steroidal anti-inflammatory drugs are effective

D Paracetamol should be avoided in this condition

E Short-acting opiate treatment is preferred

2.94 A 34-year-old woman attends the Emergency Department having suffered intermittent and severe left-sided headaches over the past 10 days. She suffered similar symptoms around 3 years ago and was investigated at another hospital. You suspect that she is suffering from cluster headaches. Which of the following is true regarding the pharmacological treatment of cluster headache?

A Alcohol excess can increase the risk of a further headache cluster

B Inhalation of 100% oxygen can abort headache

C Oral ergotamine treatment is highly effective

D Prophylactic treatment has no clear role in management

E Symptoms do not respond to NSAIDs

2.95 You are reviewing the clinical trial literature regarding tamoxifen, a partial oestrogen agonist. Which of the following statements regarding partial agonists is correct?

A Higher doses are needed to achieve the same response as a pure receptor agonist

B They competitively antagonise the effects of pure receptor antagonists

C They do not exhibit any dose–response relationship

D They have a lower E_{max} than pure receptor agonists

E They show binding affinity but no intrinsic efficacy

2.93   Answer: A

Combinations of codeine or dihydrocodeine with paracetamol have marginally greater analgesic efficacy than paracetamol alone. Aspirin has better anti-inflammatory effects but is contraindicated in patients < 16 years of age, due to risk of Reye's syndrome. Opiates increase nausea, hence use sparingly.

2.94   Answer: B

Oral ergotamine is too slow-acting, and access to 100% oxygen is limited. Parenteral dihydroergotamine or serotonin-1 ($5\text{-}HT_1$) agonists have rapid onset. Alcohol precipitates headache during cluster, but does not evoke clusters when in remission. Prophylactic treatment includes lithium, verapamil and pizotifen. Chronic paroxysmal hemicrania variant responds well to indomethacin.

2.95   Answer: D

Agonists, antagonists and partial agonists all exhibit binding affinity. Agonists have full intrinsic efficacy, antagonists have none, and partial agonists are intermediate. Partial agonists will have lower E_{max} than agonists, regardless of whether the dose can competitively inhibit the effects of a full agonist.

2.96 Which of the following is *most* likely to be a feature of buprenophine treatment?

☐ **A** Causes greater respiratory depression in overdose than morphine

☐ **B** Effects are not reversed by naloxone

☐ **C** It has a lower potential for dependence than morphine

☐ **D** It is < 5% bound to plasma proteins

☐ **E** Plasma half-life is around 18 hours

2.97 Which of the following statements best describes the role of local Drug and Therapeutics Committees?

☐ **A** Cheaper drugs are always recommended as first-line treatments

☐ **B** Decide optimum treatment on basis of monthly prescription cost

☐ **C** Determine the safety and efficacy of new drugs

☐ **D** Evaluate the clinical and cost-effectiveness of drugs

☐ **E** Primarily ration delivery of effective treatments

2.98 Adverse drug effects and drug interactions place individual patients at risk, and add an additional healthcare burden to the NHS. What proportion of patients is admitted to acute medical units in the United Kingdom wholly or partly as a result of adverse drug effects?

☐ **A** 0.01%

☐ **B** 0.3%

☐ **C** 3%

☐ **D** 15%

☐ **E** 40%

2.96   Answer: C

Buprenorphine is a mixed agonist–antagonist that behaves as an opiate partial agonist. It is less effectively reversed by naxolone. It has less potential for dependence and withdrawal syndromes and can be a useful adjunct in opiate withdrawal programmes. Plasma protein binding is >95%, and half-life is 2–3 hours.

2.97   Answer: D

Regulatory authorities (eg MHRA) determine quality and safety of new drugs. Drug and Therapeutics Committees are interested in ensuring that clinically effective and cost-effective treatments are used appropriately in clinical practice.

2.98   Answer: C

The proportion is significantly higher, although acute hospital attendances directly attributable to adverse effects of medications is thought to be 2–12%.

2.99 One of your patients asks for some general advice regarding laxative treatment for simple constipation. Which one of the following statements is correct regarding treatment of simple constipation?

☐ **A** Bisocodyl acts as a faecal softener

☐ **B** Ispaghula husk should be avoided in patients with diverticular disease

☐ **C** Lactulose is a disaccharide that is not absorbed from the gut

☐ **D** Magnesium salts act as stool bulking agents

☐ **E** Senna typically takes 48–72 h to take effect

2.100 Which of the following recreational drugs is likely to present with features of agitation and hyponatraemia?

☐ **A** Benzodiazepines

☐ **B** Cannabis

☐ **C** Cocaine

☐ **D** Ecstasy

☐ **E** Heroin

2.99   Answer: C

Stimulant laxatives, eg bisacodyl and senna, act within 6–12 h. Bulking agents, such as ispaghula husk, can take 48–72 h to take effect, and are useful in patients with stomata, diverticulosis and irritable bowel sydrome. Osmotic laxatives increase water in the large bowel, including phosphate enemas, magnesium and sodium salts, and lactulose.

2.100   Answer: D

This may be one of the mechanisms by which ecstasy increases the risk of seizures. Other characteristic effects include euphoria or dysphoria, restlessness, hyperthermia, coma and multi-organ failure.

3. CLINICAL SCIENCES

3.1 Which of the following statements is most accurate with respect to hepcidin?

- A   High levels cause iron overload in haemochromatosis
- B   It increases iron absorption from the gut
- C   It is a 55 kDa glycoprotein
- D   Levels are increased in anaemia of chronic disease
- E   Most circulating hepcidin is of dietary origin in people

3.2 A patient presents to you with a painful knee joint which has been swollen for some time now. The patient is concerned that the knee is giving way when weight-bearing. What is the most likely underlying cause?

- A   Amyloidosis
- B   Diabetes insipidus
- C   Lead toxicity
- D   Syringomyelia
- E   Vitamin B_{12} deficiency

3.3 Which of the following is the most commonly recognised feature of relapsing polychondritis?

- A   Airway compromise from tracheolaryngeal disease is an important cause of mortality
- B   Co exisiting auto-immune or connective tissue disease is rare
- C   It is usually inherited in an autosomal dominant pattern
- D   Non-cartilaginous tissue is the predominant site of involvement
- E   Treatment is with long-term antibiotics

3.4 Which of the following features is the most commonly associated with nephrotic syndrome?

- A   High serum calcium concentration
- B   Hypogammaglobulinaemia
- C   Hypertriglyceridaemia
- D   Raised APPT and PTR
- E   Reduced urinary albumin

3.1 Answer: D

Involved in iron metabolism: enterocyte iron absorption and macrophage iron cycling. High levels associated with anaemia of chronic disease, low levels associated with iron overload (eg in haemochromatosis).

3.2 Answer: D

Charcot's joint is a rapidly destructive arthritis associated with neurological disease. Common causes are diabetic neuropathy, leprosy and tabes dorsalis.

3.3 Answer: A

Cartilage is classically affected resulting in collapse of nasal bridge, cardiac valve dysfunction and hearing loss. Diagnosis is via auricular cartilage biopsy. Treatment is with high dose steroids and cytotoxic agents.

3.4 Answer: B

Recognised features are hypogammaglobulinaemia, hypercholesterolaemia, hypercoagulability and low serum calcium (normal corrected calcium). Hypogammaglobulinaemia due to non-selective loss of proteins increases risk of infections, particularly by capsulated organisms such as pneumococcus.

3.5 Which of the following statements best describes the long-term management of the nephrotic syndrome?

☐ **A** Antibiotics are required routinely

☐ **B** Anticoagulation is not required routinely

☐ **C** Diuretics should be avoided

☐ **D** Lipid-lowering drugs are ineffective in this disorder

☐ **E** Salt restriction is an important measure

3.6 Von Willebrand factor (vWF) is an important protein in maintaining cardiovascular integrity. Which of the following best describes the features of von Willebrand's disease?

☐ **A** Bleeding time is prolonged, vWF is increased, factor VIII is reduced

☐ **B** Bleeding time is prolonged, vWF is reduced, factor VIII is reduced

☐ **C** Bleeding time is prolonged, vWF is reduced, factor VIII is increased

☐ **D** Bleeding time is reduced, vWF is reduced, factor VIII is increased

☐ **E** Bleeding time is reduced, vWF is reduced, factor VIII is reduced

3.7 A GP refers a patient with α-galactosidase A deficiency to the Medical Outpatients Department for investigation of renal impairment. Which of the following is most accurate with regards to this condition?

☐ **A** Corneal microdeposits suggest an alternative diagnosis

☐ **B** Diagnosis is confirmed by skin biopsy

☐ **C** End stage renal failure is a rare complication

☐ **D** Inheritance is autosomal dominant

☐ **E** Treatment involves administration of α-galactosidase

3.8 A Turkish man presents to the Emergency Department with a painful genital ulcer. On examination, he also has conjunctival injection and you consider a diagnosis of Behçet's disease. Which of the following is most strongly supportive of this diagnosis?

☐ **A** Anterior uveitis

☐ **B** Erythema nodosum

☐ **C** HLA B51 positive

☐ **D** Positive pathergy test

☐ **E** Recurrent genital and oral ulceration

3.5 Answer: E

Salt restriction is important in managing oedema. In severe oedema, low sodium diet and large doses of combination diuretics may be required.

3.6 Answer: B

vWF is a carrier protein for factor VIII, and forms bridges between platelets and collagen, so allowing platelets to adhere to damaged vessel walls. Bleeding is often superficial brusing or mucosal bleeds (epistaxis/gastrointestinal/menorrhagia).

3.7 Answer: E

Renal failure is often apparent by the fifth decade. There is deposition of glycospinolipids in liver, kidney, nerve cells and blood cells, and inheritance is X-linked recessive.

3.8 Answer: C

There is a strong association with HLA B51, although not essential for the diagnosis. Note that pathergy is a hypersensitivity reaction at the site of minor trauma.

3.9 Which one of the following features is least likely to be found in Werner's syndrome (MEN I) and might suggest an alternative diagnosis?

- A Autosomal dominant inheritance pattern
- B Gastrinoma
- C Medullary carcinoma thyroid
- D Pituitary tumours
- E Primary hyperparathyroidism

3.10 Which of the following most strongly suggests a diagnosis of Sipple's syndrome (MEN II) in a patient with high serum calcium?

- A Autosomal recessive inheritance pattern
- B Marfanoid habitus
- C Multinodular goitre
- D Pancreatic cyst on CT scan
- E Primary hyperparathyroidism

3.11 A 53-year-old television presenter comes to you in clinic with a history of painful right eye, diarrhoea and weight loss. On examination, he has diffuse hyperpigmentation of his skin. Which of the following diagnoses is most likely?

- A Addison's disease
- B Coeliac disease
- C Cushing's syndrome
- D Reiter's disease
- E Whipple's disease

3.12 Which of the following features most strongly suggests a diagnosis of Wilson's disease?

- A Autosomal dominant pattern of inheritance
- B Cerebellar incoordination
- C Lens dislocation
- D Serum copper levels are increased
- E Urinary copper levels are reduced

3.9   Answer: C

MEN I: primary hyperparathyroidism, pituitary tumours, pancreatic tumours.

3.10   Answer: B

Other features include medullary carcinoma of the thyroid, mucosal neuromata, phaeochromocytoma and primary hyperparathyroidism (the latter is too common to support a MEN syndrome in the absence of other abnormalities).

3.11   Answer: E

Features include CNS involvement (dementia, ophthalmoplegia and facial myoclonus). The causative organism is *Trophyrema whippelii*, and the condition can be diagnosed by the appearance of macrophages containing PAS positive glycoprotein granules on jejunal biopsy. Treatment is with antibiotics and may be prolonged.

3.12   Answer: D

Defect in synthesis of caeruloplasmin prevents excretion of copper through bile (normal route). Therefore, increased serum copper/urine copper and hepatic copper content. Reduced serum caeruloplasmin levels.

3.13   Which of the following conditions is most likely to be a feature of
Wilson's disease in adults?

  A   Alcoholic liver disease

  B   Hypercalcaemia

  C   Low serum bicarbonate

  D   Raised reticulocyte count

  E   Wilms' tumor

3.14   A young man presents to you with dysdiadochokinesia and an ataxic
gait. There is no vertigo or hearing loss. Which one of the following
is most likely?

  A   Acoustic neuroma

  B   Myasthenia gravis

  C   Neurofibromatosis type II

  D   Von Hippel–Lindau syndrome

  E   Von Recklinghausen's disease

3.15   Which one of the following statements regarding neurofibromatosis
is correct?

  A   Gene abnormality located on chromosome 17 in type 2

  B   Gene abnormality located on chromosome 22 in type 1

  C   Lisch nodules present in neurofibromatosis type I

  D   Type 1 typically presents with bilateral acoustic neuromas

  E   Von Recklinghausen's disease results from malignant transformation

3.16   Tuberous sclerosis is rare neurological condition with a number of
clinical manifestations. Which of the following is most likely to be a
feature of the condition?

  A   Acne vulgaris

  B   Hypertension

  C   Marfanoid body habitus

  D   Peri-ungual fibroma

  E   Torticollis

3.13   Answer: D

Recognised features are haemolysis, hepatocellular carcinoma, parkinsonism and renal tubular acidosis. Wilms' tumor or nephroblastoma is a childhood urological malignancy and not related to Wilson's disease.

3.14   Answer: D

Autosomal dominant inheritance. A combination of retinal and intra-cranial haemangioblastomas, typically cerebellar.

3.15   Answer: C

NF I (chromosome 17), also known as Von Recklinghausen's, is the peripheral form, presents with cutaneous manifestations, including iris fibromas (Lisch nodules). NF II (chromosome 22) presents with bilateral acoustic neuromas. Malignant change can occur in NF I or II.

3.16   Answer: D

Tuberous sclerosis is a classic triad of mental retardation, epilepsy and cutaneous manifestations (shagreen patches/ash leaf macules/peri/sub-ungual fibromas/adenoma sebaceum). Peripheral calcification of cerebral tissue can occasionally be seen on plain skull X-ray.

3.17 Which of the following is *least* likely to be a feature of the Peutz–Jeghers syndrome?

⬜ **A** Autosomal dominant pattern of inheritance

⬜ **B** Bowel obstruction due to intussusception

⬜ **C** Malignant transformation of gastrointestinal polyps

⬜ **D** Peri-oral mucocutaneous pigmentation

⬜ **E** Vitamin B_{12} deficiency

3.18 A 38-year-old man presents with diarrhoea and evidence of malabsorption. There is no history of travel abroad and you suspect coeliac disease, and you arrange a jejunal biopsy. Which of the following findings most strongly supports this diagnosis?

⬜ **A** CLO test positive

⬜ **B** Granulomata

⬜ **C** Inclusion bodies seen after silver staining

⬜ **D** Lymphocyte infiltration of the sub-villous margin

⬜ **E** Sub-total villous atrophy on microscopy

3.19 Which of the following disorders is correctly paired with the corresponding genetic abnormality responsible?

⬜ **A** Down's syndrome – trisomy 12

⬜ **B** Fragile X syndrome – 46 XYY

⬜ **C** Klinefelter's syndrome – 46 XXY

⬜ **D** Testicular feminisation syndrome – 46 XXY

⬜ **F** Turner's syndrome – 45 XO

3.20 Which of the following disorders is most likely to be associated with hyperkalaemia?

⬜ **A** Addison's disease

⬜ **B** Anorexia nervosa

⬜ **C** Bartter's syndrome

⬜ **D** Conn's syndrome

⬜ **E** Cushing's syndrome

3.17   Answer: E

GI tract involvement includes polyps which may undergo malignant change, and regular review is required, with polypectomy where necessary.

3.18   Answer: E

Sub-total villous atrophy on jejunal biopsy, is also seen with viral gastroenteritis, giardiasis, hypogammaglobulinaemia, and soya milk and cow milk protein intolerance.

3.19   Answer: C

Fragile X is a trinucleotide disorder, where CGG repeats at least 30 times over. XYY syndrome results in males who tend to be more aggressive and antisocial.

3.20   Answer: A

Addison's presents with hyperkalaemia, hyponatraemia, hypoglycaemia, and mild metabolic acidosis. The other listed disorders are associated with hypokalaemia.

3.21 Which of the following statements best describes the role of mast cells?

   A Activated by complement but not physical injury

   B Derived from eosinophils

   C Do not contain lytic enzymes

   D Release histamine

   E Stimulate IgG-mediated responses

3.22 Which of the following features is most commonly recognised as a manifestation of immune thrombocytopenic purpura?

   A Diarrhoea

   B Hypothermia

   C Liver failure

   D Neurological involvement

   E Raised white cell count

3.23 Which of the following disorders is most likely to show genetic anticipation?

   A Charcot–Marie–Tooth

   B Duchenne muscular dystrophy

   C Friedreich's ataxia

   D Hereditary spherocytosis

   E Wilson's disease

3.24 Which of the following statements Is most correct with respect to the process of apoptosis?

   A Apoptosis is a random process

   B Caspases are proteases involved in apoptosis

   C It is a pro-inflammatory event

   D Macrophages play an important early role

   E There is local lymphocyte infiltration

3.21   Answer: D

Mast cells are basophilic cells that express IgE, and can be stimulated by a number of triggers to cause inflammatory and immune responses.

3.22   Answer: D

Classical features are fever, microangiopathic haemolytic anaemia, neurological involvement and renal failure. Diarrhoea is a common feature.

3.23   Answer: C

Genetic anticipation is a phenomenon where successive generations develop disease earlier and severity increases. Other examples are Huntington's disease, myotonic dystrophy and spinocerebellar ataxia.

3.24   Answer: B

In contrast to necrosis, where there is cell destruction, apoptosis is not an inflammatory process. Cells undergo compaction of chromatin and cytoplasmic budding forming apoptotic bodies, which eventually undergo phagocytosis. *P53* is a tumour suppressor gene that causes apoptosis.

3.25   Which of the following conditions would *not* be expected to cause macrocytosis, suggesting an alternative diagnosis?

☐ A   Alcohol abuse

☐ B   Hypothyroidism

☐ C   Pregnancy

☐ D   Reticulocytosis

☐ E   Turner's syndrome

3.26   Which of the following disorders is most likely to cause the appearance of macrocytes on a peripheral blood film?

☐ A   Anaemia of chronic disease

☐ B   Iron deficiency anaemia

☐ C   Lead poisoning

☐ D   Sideroblastic anaemia

☐ E   Thalassaemia trait

3.27   Which of the following appearances on a peripheral blood film most strongly suggests a diagnosis of vitamin B_{12} deficiency?

☐ A   Bite cells

☐ B   Foam cells

☐ C   Howell–Jolly bodies

☐ D   Hypersegmented neutrophils

☐ E   Smear cells

3.28   Regarding auto-immune diseases, which of the following disorders is likely to involve multiple systems?

☐ A   Graves' disease

☐ B   Hashimoto's thyroiditis

☐ C   Insulin-dependent diabetes

☐ D   Pernicious anaemia

☐ E   Rheumatoid arthritis

3.25 Answer: E

Pregnancy is a physiological cause of macrocytosis.

3.26 Answer: A

Anaemia of chronic disease is usually associated with a normal MCV, and the appearance of normocytes, microcytes and macrocytes on a blood film.

3.27 Answer: D

Bite cells suggest G6PD deficiency, foam cells suggest Gaucher's disease, Howell–Jolly bodies suggest hyposplenism, and smear cells suggest chronic lymphocytic leukaemia.

3.28 Answer: E

Rheumatoid arthritis affects various organs, and non-organ-specific autoantibodies are often present. Graves' disease can have ophthalmological and dermatological involvement.

3.29 Which of the following mechanisms is believed to be most important in the development of SLE?

- [ ] A Hypogammaglobulinaemia
- [ ] B Immune complex formation
- [ ] C Mast cell degranulation
- [ ] D Suppression of cytokine release
- [ ] E T-cell autoantibody production

3.30 Which of the following metabolic effects is most likely due to the effects of PTH?

- [ ] A Increased bone osteoblast activity
- [ ] B Increased intestinal calcium absorption
- [ ] C Renal reabsorption of phosphate
- [ ] D Renal tubular calcium secretion
- [ ] E Suppression of 1,25-dihydroxy vitamin D_3 formation

3.31 Which one of the following statements best describes the features of pseudohypoparathyroidism?

- [ ] A A syndrome of end organ resistance to parathyroid hormone
- [ ] B Di George's syndrome is a congenital form
- [ ] C Grand mal convulsions secondary to basal calcification
- [ ] D McCune–Albright syndrome affects only men
- [ ] E Parathyroid failure may be due to infective causes

3.32 Which of the following is most likely to be a feature of Di George's syndrome?

- [ ] A Chromosome 24 defect
- [ ] B Intussusception common
- [ ] C Maldevelopment arising from second and third branchial arches
- [ ] D Thymic hypoplasia
- [ ] E Transient hypermagnesemia

3.29   Answer: B

B-cell activation results in autoantibody formation and hypergammaglobulinaemia. T-cell regulation of immune responses is also disrupted.

3.30   Answer: B

PTH activity serves to increase circulating calcium concentrations, including increased bone breakdown (osteoclast activity) and increased renal reabsorption.

3.31   Answer: A

Pseudohypoparathyroidism is due to resistance rather than parathyroid failure. Albright's hereditary osteodystrophy is the typical phenotype (short stature, short metacarpals, low IQ). Grand mal convulsions occur secondary to hypocalcaemia.

3.32   Answer: D

Mnemonic 'CATCH 22':

C – Cleft palate and other facial anomalies (micrognathia, abnormal ears)
A – Antibody responses impaired (IgA/IgG)
T – Thymic hypoplasia – third and fourth branchial arches = T cell deficiency
C – Congenital cardiac defects
H – Hypocalcaemic tetany
22 – Located on chromosome 22

3.33 A 58-year-old man presents with bitemporal hemianopia, prompting suspicion of a chiasmal lesion. Which one of the following hormones is most likely to be preserved in the setting of a compressive lesion arising from the anterior pituitary?

- ☐ A Antidiuretic hormone
- ☐ B ACTH
- ☐ C Growth hormone
- ☐ D Gonadotrophins
- ☐ E TSH

3.34 Which of the following is *least* likely to be involved by a lesion affecting the cavernous sinus?

- ☐ A Cranial nerve VI
- ☐ B Internal carotid artery
- ☐ C Occulomotor nerve
- ☐ D Trigeminal nerve
- ☐ E Trochlear nerve

3.35 A 31-year-old male presents with arthritis and back pain. Examination reveals pigmentation of the ear cartilage, and a plain X ray spine shows intervertebral disc calcification. Which of the following is most correct regarding the underlying diagnosis?

- ☐ A Autosomal recessive inheritance pattern
- ☐ B Maple syrup odour from urine
- ☐ C Neuropsychiatric manifestations common
- ☐ D Overproduction of homogentisic acid oxidase
- ☐ E Sub-periostial bone resorption is a recognised feature

3.36 Which of the following features is most characteristic of porphyria cutanea tarda?

- ☐ A Autosomal dominant
- ☐ B Photosensitivity with rash and bullae are common findings
- ☐ C Reduced phorobilinogen deaminase activity
- ☐ D Responds well to phenytoin
- ☐ E Urine turns dark orange on standing

3.33 Answer: A

ADH (vasopressin) and oxytocin are released from the posterior pituitary. The others (and dopamine) are produced by the anterior pituitary.

3.34 Answer: A

The sixth cranial nerve (abducens) lies just outside the cavernous sinus and is particularly vulnerable to compression in the setting of raised intracranial pressure.

3.35 Answer: A

Alkaptonuria (ochronosis) is a deficiency of enzyme homogentisic acid oxidase, resulting in deposition of alkapton in cartilaginous tissues. Urine turns brown/black on standing. Maple syrup urine is an independent inborn error of amino acid metabolism.

3.36 Answer: B

Porphyria cutanea tarda is caused by reduced porphobilinogen decarboxylase activity. Urine colour is normal. Inheritance is genetic but the pattern is variable. Treatment is with venesection and chloroquine.

3.37 Which one of the following would most often be expected in acute intermittent porphyria?

☐ **A** Autosomal recessive inheritance pattern

☐ **B** Good response to high protein diet

☐ **C** Increased porphobilinogen deaminase activity

☐ **D** Male predominance

☐ **E** Neuropsychiatric involvement

3.38 Deficiency of which of the following enzymes is thought responsible for phenylketonuria?

☐ **A** Alanine transaminase

☐ **B** Cystathionine β synthase

☐ **C** Homogentisic acid oxidase

☐ **D** Phenylalanine hydroxylase

☐ **E** Tyrosine hydroxylase

3.39 A 49-year-old lady presents to you with a calcium concentration of 3.8 mmol/l, and you commence treatment with intravenous saline whilst trying to determine the underlying cause. Which of the following medications is most likely to contribute to hypercalcaemia?

☐ **A** Aspirin

☐ **B** Atenolol

☐ **C** Bendroflumethiazide

☐ **D** Gliclazide

☐ **E** Theophylline

3.40 A 29-year-old business man presents to the Emergency Department with a fractured ankle after a fall whilst playing football. Incidentally you find that he has abnormal pigmentation and hepatosplenomegaly. A full blood count reveals a normochromic anaemia with mild renal impairment. Which of the following diagnoses most fully explains these abnormalities?

☐ **A** Acute lymphocytic leukaemia

☐ **B** Aymloidosis

☐ **C** Gaucher's disease

☐ **D** Hyperparathyroidism

☐ **E** Tuberculosis

3.37   Answer: E

Treatment is supportive including high carbohydrate diet. Gonadotrophin releasing hormones may prevent attacks, and antidepressants can be effective in some cases.

3.38   Answer: D

Alkaptonuria results from homogentisic acid oxidase deficiency, and homocystinuria results from cystathionine β synthase deficiency.

3.39   Answer: C

Theophylline is a recognised cause of hypercalcaemia, but less important.

3.40   Answer: C

Lysosomal storage disease characterised by deficiency of β-glucosidose. Results in Gaucher's cells infiltrating the bone marrow, and pathological fractures are a recognised feature.

3.41 Which one of the following is most characteristically associated with the biological actions of complement?

  A Apoptosis

  B Chemotaxis

  C Necrosis

  D Neoplastic transformation

  E Plasma cell death

3.42 Which of the following complement deficiencies is most commonly associated with SLE?

  A C1 esterase deficiency

  B C5–C9 deficiency

  C Deficiency of classical pathway

  D Deficiency of factor H

  E Isolated C3 deficiency

3.43 Which of the following statements is most accurate with regard to immunoglobulins?

  A IgA normally activates the classical complement pathway

  B IgE expressed by both mast cells and basophils

  C IgG does not cross the placenta

  D IgM concentrations are high at birth and decay during first year of life

  E IgM deficiency affects 10–15% of all adults

3.44 A number of hormone and endocrine peptides are believed to play a contributory role in the development of obesity. Which of the following statements is correct with regards to the physiological role of leptin?

  A Adequate leptin levels are required for normal physiological function

  B Circulating leptin levels are directly proportional to fat mass

  C Leptin is a steroid molecule released from adipocytes

  D Leptin levels rise in starvation

  E Obese individuals have high levels of leptin

3.41   Answer: B

Other classical features include cell lysis, opsonisation and inflammation. Membrane attack complex (C5–C9) punctures cell surface. Apoptosis is not a recognised feature.

3.42   Answer: C

Of note, deficiency of factor H (decay accelerating factor) and membrane inhibitor of reactive lysis results in paroxysmal nocturnal haemoglobinuria. An acquired defect with spontaneous lysis of red cells.

3.43   Answer: B

IgM is very effective against bacteria and is the main immunoglobulin of the primary immune system. It is undetectable at birth, adult levels attained by 12 months.

3.44   Answer: B

Adequate leptin levels are required for onset of puberty, but are not regarded as essential in adult physiology (comparatively little information is currently available).

3.45 A 51-year-old man presents to the General Medical Outpatient Clinic with blurred vision. He has facial muscle atrophy, frontal balding and distal limb muscle weakness, and he tells you there is a genetic predisposition to muscle weakness in his family. What is the most likely underlying diagnosis?

☐ A Duchenne muscular dystrophy

☐ B Fascio–scapulo–humeral dystrophy

☐ C Huntington's disease

☐ D Myasthenia gravis

☐ E Myotonic dystrophy

3.46 A 15-year-old boy walks into the clinic accompanied by his mother. He is generally performing well at school, except that he has been unable to cope with sports activities. He has required help when standing from the floor on a number of occasions, and has been seen to use his hands to climb up his legs. On examination, there is marked proximal muscle wasting, particularly in the lower extremities, accompanied by hypertrophy of his calf muscles. Resting ECG is normal. What is the most likely diagnosis?

☐ A Becker's muscular dystrophy

☐ B Duchenne's muscular dystrophy

☐ C Fascio–scapular–humeral dystrophy

☐ D Limb girdle dystrophy

☐ E Thomsen's disease

3.47 A 27-year-old man attends clinic complaining of severe cramp whilst trying to exercise, usually after only a few moments. There is no evidence of muscle wasting and neurological examination is normal. Full blood count and routine electrolytes including lactate are normal. Urine dipstick shows myoglobinuria, and no protein or glucose. What is the most likely diagnosis?

☐ A Hypokalaemic periodic paralysis

☐ B Lambert–Eaton syndrome

☐ C McArdle's syndrome

☐ D MELAS

☐ E Rhabdomyolysis

3.45 Answer: E

Inherited as an autosomal dominant disorder associated with CTG trinucleotide repeat, and displaying genetic anticipation. Affects males and females equally, cardiac involvement includes heart block, and congenital myotonic dystrophy is a recognised cause of respiratory arrest. Subcapsular cataracts are a common long-term complication.

3.46 Answer: A

X-linked recessive, resulting in dystrophin deficiency. Scenario describes characteristic 'Gower's sign' whilst attempting to stand. The fact he has walked in to clinic effectively excludes Duchenne's, where disability is severe by age 10.

3.47 Answer: C

Autosomal recessive disorder, lack of skeletal muscle myophosphorylase, causing easy fatiguability. A characteristic finding is the lack of lactate rise with exercise.

3.48 A 17-year-old thin male, who has been wearing a plaster cast after an ankle fracture, presents with foot drop after the cast is removed. Which of the following features most strongly suggest a common peroneal nerve palsy?

   A Absent sensation over dorsum of foot, foot drop, lack of eversion

   B Absent sensation over dorsum of foot, foot drop, lack of inversion

   C Absent sensation over dorsum of foot, foot drop, peroneal muscle wasting

   D Normal sensation over dorsum of foot, foot drop, lack of eversion

   E Normal sensation over dorsum of foot, foot drop, lack of inversion

3.49 A 49-year-old man of Mediterranean origin presents to the Emergency Department with mild jaundice. His initial investigations show Hb 91 g/l. Which of the following findings most strongly suggest an underlying diagnosis of glucose-6-phosphate dehydrogenase deficiency?

   A Coomb's test positive

   B Deranged liver biochemistry

   C Family history in a second-degree relative

   D Haemolysis after exposure to aspirin

   E Smear cells on blood film

3.50 A 48-year-old woman presents with symptoms of nasal regurgitation, especially after taking fluids. Her voice has a nasal intonation. On examination there is evidence of lower limb muscle wasting, increased tone in the upper limbs and a wasted fibrillating tongue. What is the most likely diagnosis?

   A Alzheimer's disease

   B Motor neurone disease

   C Parkinsonism

   D Spastic paraparesis

   E Vascular dementia

3.48   Answer: A

On the other hand, lack of ankle inversion is caused by L5 nerve root lesions.

3.49   Answer: D

Exposure to fava beans or drugs (aspirin, dapsone, quinolones) may cause haemolysis in G6PD. Heinz bodies are a characteristic feature. Positive Coomb's test suggests autoimmune haemolytic anaemia.

3.50   Answer: B

There are features of lower and upper motor neurone degeneration. Progressive bulbar palsy involves lower cranial nerves resulting in dysarthria, dysphagia and nasal regurgitation of fluids. Cerebellar signs, extrapyramidal signs, dementia and sphincter involvement are rare.

3.51   An overweight lady presents to you with symptoms of nocturnal pain in her left hand. On examination there is wasting of the left thenar eminence and Tinel's sign positive. Which of the following is most likely to predispose to this condition?

- [ ] **A**   Acromegaly
- [ ] **B**   Diabetes insipidus
- [ ] **C**   Hyperthyroidism
- [ ] **D**   Ochronosis
- [ ] **E**   Osteoarthritis

3.52   Which of the following tissue staining methods would be most appropriate in confirming the presence of *Cryptococcus* sp. in CSF in a patient presenting with features of meningitis?

- [ ] **A**   Congo red
- [ ] **B**   Perl's stain
- [ ] **C**   Rubeonic stain
- [ ] **D**   Silver stain
- [ ] **E**   Ziehl–Nielsen

3.53   Which one of the following clinical characteristics is most likely to be found in a patient with congenital syphilis?

- [ ] **A**   Accessory nipple
- [ ] **B**   Cataracts
- [ ] **C**   Cleft palate
- [ ] **D**   Interstitial keratitis
- [ ] **E**   Phaecomyelia

3.54   A mother with longstanding well-controlled SLE gives birth to a baby with complete heart block. Which of the following antibody tests is most likely to be positive in the newborn?

- [ ] **A**   ANA
- [ ] **B**   Anti-double-stranded DNA
- [ ] **C**   Anti-La antibodies
- [ ] **D**   Anti-Ro antibodies
- [ ] **E**   Anti-RNP antibodies

3.51   Answer: A

The features suggest carpal tunnel syndrome, causing compression of the median nerve. Other recognised associations are diabetes insipidus, hypothyroidism, pregnancy and simple obesity.

3.52   Answer: D

Congo red for amyloidosis, Perl's stain for iron deposition (haemochromatosis), Ziehl–Nielsen for *Mycobacterium tuberculosis*. Silver stain can also be used to identify *Pneumocystis carinii*.

3.53   Answer: D

Other features include inner ear deafness and saddle nose deformity. Cataracts are a feature of galactosemia and intrauterine measles, but not congenital syphilis. Hutchinson's triad consists of cataracts, cleft palate, interstitial keratitis, and Hutchinson's pointed teeth.

3.54   Answer: D

ANA is increased in drug-induced lupus, anti-ds DNA is a feature of SLE, and anti-RNP is a feature of mixed connective tissue disease (overlap syndromes).

3.55 Which of the following organisms is most commonly associated with development of gas gangrene?

- A *Clostridium botulinum*
- B *Clostridium novyi*
- C *Clostridium perfringens*
- D *Clostridium septicum*
- E *Clostridium tetani*

3.56 Which of the following features is most strongly suggestive of hypertrophic obstructive cardiomyopathy?

- A Asymmetrical septal hypertrophy
- B Dilated left ventricle
- C Left ventricular aneurysm
- D Right ventricular dilatation
- E Right ventricular hypertrophy

3.57 Which of the following disorders is most likely to occur as a complication of chronic hypertriglyceridaemia?

- A Acute cholecystitis
- B Diabetes mellitus
- C Hypothyroidism
- D Nephrotic syndrome
- E Xanthelasmata

3.58 A 22-year-old man presents with progressive ataxia. Examination shows bilateral pes cavus, scoliosis, absent ankle reflexes with extensor plantars. What is the most likely underlying diagnosis?

- A Cervical spondylosis
- B Friedreich's ataxia
- C Motor neurone disease
- D Multiple sclerosis
- E Tabes dorsalis

3.55   Answer: C

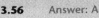

Also known as *Clostridium welchii*; less common causes are *Clostridium septicum* and *Clostridium novyi*.

3.56   Answer: A

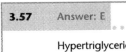

There is left ventricular hypertrophy and septal hypertrophy causing almost complete obliteration of the left ventricle, dilatation is not generally recognised.

3.57   Answer: E

Hypertriglyceridaemia is a recognised feature of diabetes mellitus, hypothyroidism and nephrotic syndrome (hypercholesterolaemia more common in the latter).

3.58   Answer: B

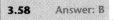

A trinucleotide repeat disorder of autosomal recessive inheritance. Characterised by spinocerebellar tract degeneration, and cardiomyopathy.

3.59   Which of the following statements most correctly describes the features of *Pseudomonas* sp.?

- A   Capsulated bacteria
- B   Gentamycin resistance is common
- C   Gram-positive bacillus
- D   Greenish-blue pigmentation in culture
- E   Route of transmission is normally by direct inoculation

3.60   Which of the following disorders is least likely to be caused by production of an auto-antibody (ie autoimmune disease)?

- A   Addison's disease
- B   Cryptogenic fibrosing alveolitis
- C   Graves' disease
- D   Hashimoto's disease
- E   Myasthenia gravis

3.61   Which of the following disorders is most likely to be encountered as a complication of streptococcal skin infection?

- A   Amyloidosis
- B   Glomerulonephritis
- C   Liver failure
- D   Rheumatic fever
- E   Toxic shock syndrome

3.62   Which of the following disorders is a characteristic feature of Still's disease?

- A   Foot drop
- B   Heart block
- C   Lymphadenopathy
- D   Parotid swelling
- E   Polycythaemia

3.59 Answer: D

This is a Gram-negative bacillus, normally sensitive to gentamicin and quinolone antibiotics. Burns victims and patients with interstitial lung disease and cystic fibrosis are at greatest risk.

3.60 Answer: B

The exact aetiology is unclear. The other disorders are all mediated by auto-antibodies, and there is often clustering of multiple autoimmune conditions, eg vitiligo, Addison's disease and autoimmune thyroid disease.

3.61 Answer: B

Rheumatic fever is now much less common as a result of more effective treatment of the primary infection. Toxic shock syndrome is due to *Staphylococcus aureus* enterotoxin.

3.62 Answer: C

Other features also include pyrexia, splenomegaly and serositis.

3.63 'Saturday night palsy' resulting in wrist drop, is characteristically caused by a lesion affecting which nerve?

☐ A Axillary

☐ B Median

☐ C Nerve to serratus anterior

☐ D Radial

☐ E Ulnar

3.64 Which of the following disorders is most likely to be associated with a raised concentration of α-fetoprotein?

☐ A Choriocarcinoma

☐ B Hepatoma

☐ C Pregnancy

☐ D Seminoma

☐ E Teratoma

3.65 Which one of the following hormones belongs to the amine group?

☐ A Aldosterone

☐ B Cortisol

☐ C Catecholamine

☐ D Retinoic acid

☐ E Testosterone

3.66 Which of the following best describes the action of corticosteroids?

☐ A Act on DNA to alter gene expression

☐ B Bind to extracellular cytosolic receptors

☐ C Close relationship between plasma levels and intracellular effects

☐ D Stimulate cGMP secondary messengers

☐ E Trigger intracellular cAMP

3.63 Answer: D

Usually caused by compression of the radial nerve at the level of the upper humerus. Usually reversible, but palsy can be permanent if the period of compression is prolonged.

3.64 Answer: B

Beta HCG is produced from trophoblast layer of non-germ cell tumours, and is characteristically raised in the other disorders listed (A, C, D, E).

3.65 Answer: C

The remainder are steroids.

3.66 Answer: A

Bind to intracellular receptors to exert effects on DNA transcription without triggering an intracellular cascade of second messengers. cAMP, cGMP and IP3 second messengers are important for hormones that bind to extracellular receptors.

3.67 Which of the following disorders is thought to be mediated via a G-protein defect?

☐ A Graves' disease

☐ B Hypoparathyroidism

☐ C Osteoporosis

☐ D Relapsing polychondritis

☐ E Vitamin D resistant rickets

3.68 Investigations show Na^+ 145 mmol/l, K^+ 5.0 mmol/l, creatinine 178 µmol/l, urea 9.0 mmol/l, bicarbonate 20 mmol/l, chloride 100 mmol/l and glucose 11 mmol/l. Based on these blood results, what is the calculated anion gap?

☐ A 15

☐ B 20

☐ C 25

☐ D 30

☐ E 35

3.69 Investigations in an apparently healthy 20-year-old man show Na^+ 136 mmol/l, K^+ 4.0 mmol/l, creatinine 156 µmol/l, urea 6.0 mmol/l, bicarbonate 18 mmol/l, chloride 102 mmol/l and glucose 10 mmol/l. What is the calculated serum osmolarity?

☐ A 156

☐ B 172

☐ C 296

☐ D 302

☐ E 312

3.70 The chromosomes associated with a large number of genetic disorders are known. Which of the following chromosomes is thought to contain the gene responsible for Edwards' syndrome?

☐ A 7

☐ B 13

☐ C 18

☐ D 21

☐ E 22

3.67   Answer: B

Others include acromegaly and night-blindness.

3.68   Answer: D

Anion gap = [(Na + K) – (HCO$_3$ + Cl)], normal range = 10–18 mmol/l.

3.69   Answer: C

Calculated plasma osmolarity: [2 × (Na + K) + urea + glucose]. A significantly higher result from measured osmolality suggests the presence of an unmeasured osmotic agent, eg ethylene glycol. Normal = 275–295 mOsm/kg.

3.70   Answer: C

Williams syndrome is associated with chromosome 7, Patau syndrome with chromosome 13, Di George syndrome with chromosome 22 and Down's syndrome with chromosome 21.

3.71 Which of the following disorders is believed to be inherited in an autosomal dominant manner?

☐ A   Criggler–Najjar severe form

☐ B   Dubin–Johnson syndrome

☐ C   Gilbert's disease

☐ D   Rotor syndrome

☐ E   Wilson's disease

3.72 Which of the following features is most strongly suggestive of cholesterol atheroembolism in a patient with a vasculitic skin rash overlying both feet?

☐ A   Acute renal failure

☐ B   Eosinophilia

☐ C   Livedo reticularis

☐ D   Raised ESR

☐ E   Recent angiography procedure

3.73 Which one of the following disorders is most likely to be associated with a negative anti-neutrophil cytoplasmic antibody (ANCA) test?

☐ A   Churg–Strauss

☐ B   Goodpasture's

☐ C   Henoch–Schonlein purpura

☐ D   Microscopic polyangiitis

☐ E   Wegener's granulomatosis

3.74 Which one of the following microscopic findings is most likely to be present in a healthy individual with no renal disease?

☐ A   Granular casts

☐ B   Hyaline casts

☐ C   Red cell casts

☐ D   Tubular casts

☐ E   White cell casts

3.71   Answer: C

Of the congenital hyperbilirubinaemias, double-barrel syndromes tend to be inherited in an autosomal recessive manner (eg Dubin–Johnson and Criggler–Najjar severe form), whereas Rotor syndrome and Gilbert's syndrome are autosomal dominant.

3.72   Answer: E

The other items are recognised features. Spontaneous atheroembolism is comparatively rare, whereas it usually follows some invasive vascular procedure.

3.73   Answer: C

ANCA titres correlate with disease activity in the other conditions.

3.74   Answer: B

Tamm–Horsfall protein (hyaline casts) is not pathological. Red cell casts are found in glomerulonephritis, granular casts suggest haemoglobin traversing the glomerular membrane, white cell casts suggest acute pyelonephritis, and tubular casts are found in ATN.

3.75 Which of the following is most likely to cause nephrolithiasis when found in increased urine concentrations?

- [ ] A Calcium
- [ ] B Cystine
- [ ] C Magnesium
- [ ] D Potassium
- [ ] E Xylose

3.76 Which of the following is most commonly associated with amyloidosis?

- [ ] A Alzheimer's disease is not associated with true amyloid deposits
- [ ] B Amyloid A protein is seen in familial Mediterranean fever
- [ ] C Beta-2 microglobin is found in lymphoma-associated amyloidosis
- [ ] D Congo red stain shows amyloid as a charcoal-black appearance
- [ ] E Serum amyloid P is unhelpful in clinical practice

3.77 A 43-year-old woman is referred to the General Medical Clinic for assessment of weakness affecting elbow flexion in her left arm. On examination, there is grade 4 power of left elbow flexion. Reflexes in the upper limbs are normal and symmetrical. What is the likely cause?

- [ ] A Biceps muscle injury
- [ ] B Brachial plexus injury
- [ ] C C5, 6 nerve root compression
- [ ] D Cervical radiculopathy
- [ ] E Radial nerve contusion

3.78 A 32-year-old man fell down a flight of stairs 2 days ago whilst intoxicated. He did not report any loss of consciousness. Since that time, he has been aware of difficulty moving his left shoulder. On examination, there is profound weakness of left shoulder abduction. What is the most likely cause for these findings?

- [ ] A Atlanto-axial subluxation
- [ ] B Axillary nerve compression
- [ ] C C4, 5 nerve root compression
- [ ] D C6, 7 nerve root compression
- [ ] E Deltoid muscle contusion

3.75 Answer: B

Calcium alone does not cause urinary crystals. Other common causes include increased concentrations of oxalate, phosphate and urate.

3.76 Answer: B

SAP scan allows quantification of disease progression. Congo red staining shows apple green appearance of amyloid deposits under polarised light. Beta-2 microglobin amyloid is found in dialysis-dependent patients.

3.77 Answer: A

Preservation of normal reflexes excludes significant upper or lower motor neurone involvement, and local muscle pathology is most likely.

3.78 Answer: C

Shoulder abduction is served by the deltoid muscle, which is subserved predominantly by C5 fibres carried by the axillary nerve.

3.79 A 36-year-old woman with longstanding severe rheumatoid arthritis has noticed increasing difficulty with dressing. On examination, she is found to have significant weakness of left elbow supination. Which of the following explanations is most appropriate?

- ☐ **A** Axillary nerve lesion
- ☐ **B** C5, 6 nerve root lesion
- ☐ **C** C8 nerve root lesion
- ☐ **D** Median nerve lesion
- ☐ **E** Ulnar nerve lesion

3.80 A 43-year-old labourer presents to the Emergency Department with low back pain. He is found to have weakness of hip flexion on the left side. What is the most likely explanation?

- ☐ **A** Disc prolapse and L2, 3 nerve root compression
- ☐ **B** Disc prolapse and S1, 2 nerve root compression
- ☐ **C** Dissecting abdominal aneurysm
- ☐ **D** Metastatic lumbar spine involvement
- ☐ **E** Paraneoplastic neuropathy

3.81 A 67-year-old man has experienced progressive difficulty with mobility, and is found to have significant weakness of left knee extension, associated with diminished knee jerk reflex on the left. What is the most likely explanation?

- ☐ **A** Generalised myositis secondary to statin therapy
- ☐ **B** L3, 4 nerve root compression
- ☐ **C** Lead toxicity
- ☐ **D** Quadriceps wasting
- ☐ **E** Thoracic spine compression

3.82 A 42-year-old man attends the Emergency Department and is found to have weakness of pronation of the left forearm, and reduced power on testing wrist flexion on the same side. What is the most likely explanation for these findings?

- ☐ **A** Brachial plexus lesion
- ☐ **B** Injury to the median nerve at the elbow
- ☐ **C** Median nerve damage at the wrist
- ☐ **D** Radial nerve palsy
- ☐ **E** Ulnar nerve lesion at the elbow

3.79   Answer: B

For example, an isolated motor neuropathy or part of a mononeuritis multiplex secondary to rheumatoid arthritis. Supply biceps and brachioradialis muscles via musculoskeletal and radial nerves, respectively.

3.80   Answer: A

Hip flexion usually mediated by iliopsoas muscle, supplied by nerve roots L1–L3.

3.81   Answer: B

Reduced power associated with diminished reflexes indicates a lower motor lesion. An alternative explanation is femoral nerve entrapment.

3.82   Answer: B

Causes include trauma, heavy metal poisoning and mononeuritis multiplex.

3.83 A 23-year-old cyclist is rushed to the Emergency Department after being knocked off his bicycle by a motorist. He is found to have weakness of the small muscles of his right hand, which is held in a clawed posture. There is loss of sensation overlying the medial border of the right forearm and hand. What is the most likely cause?

- A Intracranial haemorrhage
- B Radial nerve compression in the upper limb
- C Stroke
- D T1 nerve root lesion
- E Ulnar nerve contusion at the elbow

3.84 A 34-year-old woman attends the Emergency Department with sudden onset of speech impairment. On examination, she is found to have a severe expressive dysphasia. Which area of the brain is likely to be affected?

- A Left parietal lobe
- B Left temporal lobe
- C Occipital lobe
- D Right parietal lobe
- E Right temporal lobe

3.85 A 26-year-old man presents to the Emergency Department following an injury to his left leg. On examination he is found to have impaired sensation over the medial aspect of the dorsum of his left foot and lower leg. There is weakness of left ankle dorsiflexion and footdrop. Injury to which motor nerve is most likely to be responsible?

- A Common peroneal nerve
- B Femoral nerve
- C Lateral cutaneous nerve
- D Median popliteal nerve
- E Sacroiliac nerve

3.83   Answer: D

The features suggest a brachial plexus injury with features of T1 damage (Klumpke's paralysis). This can also be associated with ipsilateral Horner's syndrome.

3.84   Answer: A

Speech motor cortex is located in Broca's area of the dominant parietal lobe, whereas receptive dysphasia is more likely to result from a lesion affecting Wernicke's area in the dominant temporal lobe.

3.85   Answer: A

Most commonly, this nerve is damaged at the site where it wraps around the upper part of the fibula, just below the fibular head.

3.86 A 36-year-old man with diplopia is referred to the Ophthalmology Outpatient Department by his GP. On examination, the left eye looks down and out during forward gaze. Damage to which of the following nerves is most likely to be responsible?

- A Abducent nerve
- B Ciliary nerve
- C Cranial nerve II
- D Cranial nerve III
- E Trochlear nerve

3.87 A 45-year-old woman presents to the Emergency Department with impaired vision. She is found to have a left superior homonymous quadrantanopia. What is the most likely anatomical site of the lesion?

- A Right occipital lobe
- B Right optic nerve
- C Right optic tract
- D Right parietal lobe
- E Right temporal lobe

3.88 Which of the following muscles normally serves to abduct the larynx?

- A Cricothyroid
- B Lateral cricoarytenoid
- C Oblique arytenoid
- D Posterior cricoarytenoid
- E Transverse arytenoid

3.89 A 45-year-old man is referred to the Acute Medical Assessment Unit with left-sided facial weakness that started suddenly that day. Which of the following features most strongly suggests a diagnosis of Bell's palsy rather than acute stroke?

- A Impaired sensation over the left side of the face
- B Inability to fully close left eye
- C Increased chin jerk reflex
- D Loss of left frontalis muscle activity
- E Unable to close lips together

3.86   Answer: C

Occulomotor nerve, which supplies all the extraocular muscles except for lateral rectus (abducent nerve) and superior oblique (trochlear nerve).

3.87   Answer: E

Temporal lobe supplies fibres of the lower retina (upper visual field), whereas parietal lobe supplies fibres of the upper retina (lower visual field).

3.88   Answer: D

The others all cause adduction; the cricothyroid muscle also lengthens the larynx.

3.89   Answer: D

Due to complete loss of innervation. In stroke (UMN lesion) there is preservation of frontalis due to cross-innervation of upper motor neurone fibres. Impaired sensation is more in keeping with acute stroke.

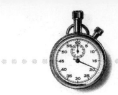

3.90 Which the following statements best describes the physiological role of gastrin?

☐ A Gastric distension inhibits its release

☐ B It is a high-molecular weight glycopeptide

☐ C Its release is diminished in the presence of hypercalcaemia

☐ D Released from pancreatic β-islet cells

☐ E Stimulates intrinsic factor secretion

3.91 A number of locally secreted peptides and molecules are important in regulation of small intestinal motility. Which one of the following is most likely to decrease small intestinal motility?

☐ A Cholecystokinin

☐ B Gastrin

☐ C Motilin

☐ D Secretin

☐ E Serotonin

3.92 A number of different factors can influence the rate of gastric emptying. Which of the following is most likely to increase the rate of gastric emptying?

☐ A Amino acids in the duodenum

☐ B Emotional distress

☐ C Free fatty acids in the stomach

☐ D Gastrin

☐ E Secretin

3.93 Interactions between central nervous system neurotransmitters is believed to play an important role in epilepsy. Which of the following statements best describes GABA metabolism in the CNS?

☐ A GABA is a powerful stimulatory neurotransmitter

☐ B GABA is normally metabolised to glutamate

☐ C Gabapentin and vigabatrin potentiate effects of GABA

☐ D Glutamate is an inhibitory neurotransmitter

☐ E Lamotrigine stimulates release of glutamate

3.90   Answer: E

Its release from G-cells in the gastric antrum is stimulated by hypercalcaemia, amino acids in the antrum, gastric distension and vagal stimulation. It also stimulates gastric acid and pepsin release.

3.91   Answer: D

Other factors include increased adrenergic agents and sympathetic autonomic activity. The agents listed above (A, B, C, E) increase intestinal motility, along with parasympathetic activity and prostaglandins.

3.92   Answer: D

Gastrin and distension of the stomach wall stimulate gastric emptying, whereas pain, headache, stress, fatty acids, secretin and low pH in the duodenum reduce gastric emptying.

3.93   Answer: C

Glutamate (stimulatory) is metabolised to GABA (inhibitory) by glutamic acid decarboxylase. Lamotrigine inhibits glutamate effects in the CNS. Note that gabapentin is a GABA pentamer.

3.94 Which of the following statements best describes the role of nitric oxide (NO) in human physiology?

☐ A cAMP mediates vascular relaxation responses to NO

☐ B NO increases platelet adhesiveness

☐ C Inducible NO synthase normally regulates vascular tone

☐ D Platelets generate and release NO in vivo

☐ E Serves an endocrine role in regulating vascular tone

3.95 A number of local factors are involved in the neurohumoral regulation of vascular tone, and may play an important role in the development of hypertension. Which of the following derangements is most likely to cause a rise in systemic blood pressure?

☐ A Angiotensin-1

☐ B Endothelin-1

☐ C L-Arginine

☐ D Nitric oxide

☐ E Prostacyclin

3.96 A 45-year-old man is being treated for severe pneumonia and sepsis in the Intensive Care Unit. His blood pressure has been difficult to maintain despite adequate fluid administration and large quantities of intravenous norepinephrine. Which of the following agents is most likely to allow restoration of normal blood pressure?

☐ A Angiotensin I infusion

☐ B Endothelin antagonist

☐ C Interleukin-1

☐ D Nitric oxide synthase (NOS) inhibitor

☐ E NSAID

3.97 A number of potentially important inflammatory mediators have been studied in order to determine their role in human diseases. Which of the following statements is most correct with respect to interleukin-1 (IL-1)?

☐ A Alpha-subtype is formed predominantly by lymphocytes

☐ B Administration prevents fever in patients with sepsis

☐ C Beta-subtype is increased after strenuous physical exercise

☐ D Oxidised LDL uptake inhibits vascular IL-1 expression

☐ E Stimulates release of vasoconstrictor molecules

3.94 Answer: D

Endothelium-derived NO is expressed constitutively by eNOS, and serves an autocrine/paracrine role in regulating vascular tone by stimulating vascular smooth muscle cGMP formation. It is rapidly broken down (hence not endocrine effects), inhibits leukocyte and platelet adhesion to endothelium.

3.95 Answer: B

Endothelin-1 is an endogenous peptide that is released from the endothelium and causes constriction of underlying vascular smooth muscle. NO and prostacyclin are powerful vasodilators. L-Arginine, a precursor to NO, appears to cause weak vasodilatation (mechanism unclear).

3.96 Answer: D

A number of arginine analogues, eg L-N-monomethylarginine, inhibit NOS in vivo, and small studies have shown them to be effective in sepsis. None are licensed for treatment, but this supports the view that inducible NOS contributes to hypotension in sepsis.

3.97 Answer: C

Also sepsis, acute exacerbations of rheumatoid arthritis and other inflammatory states. Oxidised LDL stimulates endothelial IL-1 expression, which might contribute to plaque formation. IL-1 is formed predominantly by macrophages.

3.98 Paracetamol has been shown to reduce fever, in addition to its analgesic properties. What is the most likely mechanism for this effect?

☐ **A** Bacteriostatic effects on Gram-positive organisms

☐ **B** Blockade of the TNFα receptor site

☐ **C** Cyclo-oxygenase (COX) inhibition

☐ **D** Decreased interleukin-1 formation

☐ **E** Enhanced nitric oxide release

3.99 Which of the following statements most accurately describes the role of tumour necrosis factor (TNF)?

☐ **A** Causes powerful anti-inflammatory effects in vivo

☐ **B** Effective treatment for wide range of solid tumours

☐ **C** Inhibits monocyte and macrophage migration

☐ **D** TNFα inhibits monocyte production of interleukin-1

☐ **E** TNFβ synthesised by activated T-lymphocytes

3.100 Which of the following statements is true regarding the role of antioxidants in human disease?

☐ **A** Co-enzyme Q10 treatment reduces vascular oxidative stress

☐ **B** Combined antioxidant supplements reduce risk of stroke

☐ **C** Glutathione supplementation reduces the risk of colonic cancer

☐ **D** Vitamin C is the most abundant circulating antioxidant

☐ **E** Vitamin E reduces oxidation of low density lipoprotein

3.101 Central dopamine deficiency is believed to play an important role in the pathogenesis of Parkinson's disease. Which of the following statements is correct with regard to dopamine metabolism?

☐ **A** Dopa decarboxylase is found only in the CNS

☐ **B** Dopamine is metabolised to norepinephrine by dopamine hydroxylase

☐ **C** L-Dopa is formed by the action of dopa decarboxylase on tyrosine

☐ **D** Peripheral effects of dopa include vasoconstriction

☐ **E** Tyrosine is an essential dietary precursor of L-dopa

3.98   Answer: D

Hypothalamic effect to reset thermoregulation. Mechanism unclear, but IL-1 concentrations reduced. A number of studies have found inhibition of COX enzymes, but not consistent.

3.99   Answer: E

TNFα secreted by macrophages, eosinophils and NK cells. Anti-cancer effects of TNF disappointingly poor, and high level of serious adverse effects. TNF stimulates monocyte and macrophage activity (including IL-1 release). TNF and IL-1 have a synergistic pro-inflammatory effect, eg in rheumatoid arthritis.

3.100   Answer: E

Epidemiological studies show an inverse correlation between dietary antioxidant intake and risk of cancer and cardiovascular disease. However, supplementation of various antioxidants, alone or in combination, has been disappointing in prospective trials. The most abundant circulating antioxidant is urate.

3.101   Answer: B

Phenylalanine is an essential amino acid that is metabolised to tyrosine, which is in turn metabolised to dopa. Dopa is converted to dopamine by dopa decarboxylase; peripheral dopa decarboxylase inhibitors allow greater amounts of L-dopa to cross the blood–brain barrier in treatment of parkinsonism.

3.102 A number of factors are necessary for normal physiology, but that cannot be synthesised by human metabolism. Which of the following is an essential dietary amino acid?

- [ ] A Alanine
- [ ] B Cysteine
- [ ] C Glutamic acid
- [ ] D Phenylalanine
- [ ] E Tyrosine

3.103 A 51-year-old man is admitted to hospital with breathlessness, fever and tachycardia. A chest X-ray shows diffuse pulmonary consolidation throughout the right lower zones, and investigations show serum bicarbonate 14 mmol/l and lactate 7.2 mmol/l. Which of the following statements best explains his abnormal blood tests?

- [ ] A Decreased tissue oxygenation
- [ ] B Excess build-up of tissue carbon dioxide
- [ ] C Increased anaerobic glycolysis by peripheral tissues
- [ ] D Increased glycolysis
- [ ] E Reduced hepatic glycogenolysis

3.104 A 45-year-old man is admitted for elective repair of an inguinal hernia. Shortly before being taken to theatre, one of the nursing staff reports that his urine is strongly positive for ketones. What is the most appropriate course of action?

- [ ] A Check an arterial blood gas analysis
- [ ] B Immediate insulin administration
- [ ] C Initiate intravenous dextrose
- [ ] D No immediate action required
- [ ] E Perform laboratory measurement of plasma and urine glucose

3.102   Answer: D

Phenylalanine is an essential precursor to tyrosine, which is subsequently incorporated in the synthesis of dopa and thyroid hormones. The other amino acids listed can all be synthesised in vivo.

3.103   Answer: C

Normally, aerobic metabolism supplies energy via the glucose-6-phosphate and TCA pathways. Anaerobic metabolism is increased when (i) oxygen availability is reduced, (ii) lactate utilisation is impaired (eg metformin), or (iii) both (eg sepsis). Glucose → Lactate + 2 H⁺.

3.104   Answer: D

Ketones are the end-product of lipid metabolism. In the setting of fasting or starvation, insulin secretion is suppressed, and 'ketogenic' hormones mobilise lipids to provide free fatty acids as metabolic substrate.

3.105 Factors that influence oxygen binding capacity of haemoglobin play an important role in determining oxygen transport and delivery in the human circulation. Which of the following is most likely to be associated with high oxygen binding affinity of haemoglobin?

- [ ] **A** Diabetes mellitus
- [ ] **B** High $PaCO_2$
- [ ] **C** High pH
- [ ] **D** High temperature
- [ ] **E** Raised 2,3-diphosphoglycerate (2,3-DPG)

3.106 Which of the following statements is correct with regard to normal oxygen carriage in a healthy individual breathing room air at rest?

- [ ] **A** 1 g haemoglobin carries 1.5 ml oxygen
- [ ] **B** 1 g haemoglobin carries 30 ml oxygen
- [ ] **C** 100 ml blood carries 0.1 ml oxygen
- [ ] **D** 100 ml plasma carries 10 ml oxygen
- [ ] **E** 100 ml plasma carries 100 ml oxygen

3.107 On reviewing the results of a 56-year-old woman attending clinic for investigation of headaches, you see that a paraprotein band was found. What does this signify?

- [ ] **A** A homogeneous band of one particular immunoglobulin
- [ ] **B** Abnormally high globulin concentrations
- [ ] **C** IgA overproduction
- [ ] **D** IgG overproduction
- [ ] **E** IgM overproduction

3.108 A 34-year-old woman has been attending the General Medical Outpatient Clinic for assessment of severe Raynaud's disease. You wish to check for the presence of cryoglobulins. How should the sample be handled?

- [ ] **A** Assay needs to be performed within 1 h of sample collection
- [ ] **B** Sample kept at 37°C then cooled to –20°C for separation
- [ ] **C** Separated immediately, then stored at –20°C before assay
- [ ] **D** Transported and separated at 37°C
- [ ] **E** Whole blood sample chilled to –20°C immediately after collection

3.105 Answer: C

Low temperature, reduced 2,3-DPG and low $PaCO_2$ are associated with high oxygen binding affinity (eg stored blood) so that oxygen delivery to tissues may be impaired.

3.106 Answer: A

Haemoglobin is an efficient means of oxygen carriage, whereas comparatively smaller amounts are dissolved in plasma. Around 0.5 ml oxygen will be dissolved in 100 ml plasma.

3.107 Answer: A

This is usually due to overproduction of IgA, IgG or IgM but not in all cases. It will often result in an abnormally high total protein concentration whilst albumin is unaffected (the 'globulin gap'). Suppression of normal Ig concentrations (immune paresis) is a recognised feature.

3.108 Answer: D

Cryoglobulins precipitate at cool temperatures, around 4°C, so that the sample must be kept at 37°C before separation so that these are not lost from the supernatant.

3.109 A 37-year-old woman is referred to the Outpatient Department for investigation of a skin rash overlying the bridge of her nose that is tender on palpation. She is found to have a white cell count of 12.2 $\times 10^9/l$ and raised C3 and C4 complement concentrations. What is the most likely diagnosis?

A Glomerulonephritis

B Infectious endocarditis

C Streptococcal skin infection

D Systemic lupus erythematosus

E Systemic sclerosis

3.110 A 32-year-old woman attends the General Medical Outpatient Department for investigation of recurrent episodes of fever, abdominal pain associated with nausea and vomiting. Physical examination is normal. Each episode lasts for around 3–4 days, and have occurred 3 times in the past 8 months. Investigations show low levels of C3, but other complement components are normal. What is the most likely explanation?

A Bacterial endocarditis

B Hereditary isolated C3 deficiency

C Recurrent pyelonephritis

D Recurrent ureteric calculus formation

E Systemic lupus erythematosus

3.111 A 21-year-old man with a history of asthma is brought into the Emergency Department with wheeze and circulatory collapse around 1 h after being stung by a wasp. You suspect an anaphylactic reaction. What is the most appropriate initial management?

A 5 ml of 1 in 10,000 epinephrine intravenously

B 0.5 ml of 1 in 1000 epinephrine intramuscularly

C 100 mg of intravenous hydrocortisone

D Intravenous chlorpheniramine 4 mg

E Intravenous saline at 500 ml/h

3.109   Answer: C

Raised complement levels are a non-specific marker of inflammation. Low levels are seen in SLE, post-streptococcal glomerulonephritis, serum sickness and septicaemia, and can correlate with disease severity.

3.110   Answer: C

Low C3 levels may occur with recurrent bacterial infections. Although infective endocarditis is a recognised cause, this is less likely in the absence of any other physical signs.

3.111   Answer: B

Potentially life-threatening condition; priority is to secure airway, support ventilation, and administer epinephrine to support circulation. Additional treatment includes antihistamine administration, and consideration of corticosteroid treatment (effects may be delayed for several hours).

3.112 Which of the following skin tests is best for determining a tendency to type IV hypersensitivity reactions?

☐ **A** Corticosteroid challenge

☐ **B** Intradermal injection

☐ **C** Intradermal injection after oral antihistamine administration

☐ **D** Patch test

☐ **E** Skin prick test

3.113 A young woman with well-controlled asthma is undergoing tests for suspected chronic urticaria. A skin prick test shows the development of wheal and flare within 15 min, that gradually resolves within the next 45 min. What does this test indicate?

☐ **A** False positive due to inhaled corticosteroids

☐ **B** Type I hypersensitivity

☐ **C** Type II hypersensitivity

☐ **D** Type III hypersensitivity

☐ **E** Type IV hypersensitivity

3.114 Which of the following conditions is an example of type III hypersensitivity?

☐ **A** Anaphylaxis after a bee sting

☐ **B** GVHD

☐ **C** Methyldopa-induced haemolysis

☐ **D** Phenytoin-induced gum hypertrophy

☐ **E** Tuberculin skin reaction

3.115 A 47-year-old man has longstanding hepatitis C, acquired through previous intravenous drug use. During a follow-up appointment he is found to have lost a significant amount of weight over the past 6 months, and he has become jaundiced. Which of the following tumour markers most strongly suggests the development of hepatocellular carcinoma?

☐ **A** 5-Hydroxyindoleacetic acid

☐ **B** Alpha-fetoprotein

☐ **C** Carcinoembryonic antigen

☐ **D** Human chorionic gonadotrophin

☐ **E** Vanillyl mandelic acid

3.112   Answer: E

This can provoke development of an indurated, mildly erythematous lesion after 2–4 days provocation, that resolves over 3–5 days. Intradermal injection can also be used (eg tuberculin test) but is best for examining type III hypersensitivity over 4–6 h. Skin prick test causes signs of urticaria within 20 min in type I hypersensitivity.

3.113   Answer: B

The antigen reacts with pre-formed IgE bound to the surface of mast cells to cause mast cell degranulation and local release of vasoactive substances. Type I hypersensitivity is more common in patients with asthma, eczema and allergic rhinitis.

3.114   Answer: C

Complement-dependent immune complex disease. This includes serum sickness, drug-induced haemolysis (also caused by penicillin), post-streptococcal glomerulonephritis, cryoglobulinaemia, SLE and rheumatoid arthritis.

3.115   Answer: B

Elevated concentrations are also seen in acute viral hepatitis, cirrhosis or with liver metastases. High maternal concentration can indicate twins or neural tube defect in the developing fetus.

3.116 Which of the following is most likely to account for a modestly elevated prostate specific antigen concentration in an otherwise healthy 48-year-old man?

- ☐ **A** Ciprofloxacin treatment
- ☐ **B** Digital rectal examination
- ☐ **C** Impaired renal function
- ☐ **D** Metastatic involvement of the prostate gland
- ☐ **E** Uncomplicated bacterial cystitis

3.117 Which hepatic enzyme is principally involved in detoxifying cyanates in human physiology?

- ☐ **A** Aromatase
- ☐ **B** Lactate dehydrogenase
- ☐ **C** P450 oxidative metabolism
- ☐ **D** Rhodanese
- ☐ **E** Urate oxidase

3.118 A 46-year-old woman is undergoing investigation of recurrent headaches. Which of the following disorders is most likely to be responsible for the appearance of a monoclonal immunoglobulin band in the CSF?

- ☐ **A** Lymphoma
- ☐ **B** Multiple sclerosis
- ☐ **C** Sarcoidosis
- ☐ **D** Systemic lupus erythematosus
- ☐ **E** Tuberculosis

3.119 Which one of the following disorders is most likely to cause increased urinary calcium excretion?

- ☐ **A** Coeliac disease
- ☐ **B** Hyperthyroidism
- ☐ **C** Hypoparathyroidism
- ☐ **D** Vitamin D deficiency
- ☐ **E** Thiazide diuretic treatment

3.116   Answer: B

Other causes include acute and chronic prostatitis and prostatic carcinoma. The prostate is rarely affected by metastases from elsewhere.

3.117   Answer: D

Small quantities of cyanide are ingested in foodstuffs, and inhaled due to atmospheric pollutants. Cigarette smoke contains significant quantities of cyanide, and smokers have up-regulated rhodanese activity. The enzyme is readily saturated by exposure to significant cyanide amounts, eg after smoke inhalation.

3.118   Answer: A

Multiple sclerosis, sarcoidosis and SLE are associated with raised CSF protein and oligoclonal bands, and TB associated with high total protein concentration. Benign paraproteinaemia is another recognised cause of monoclonal CSF bands.

3.119   Answer: E

The others are recognised causes of reduced urinary calcium excretion. Thiazide diuretics lower urinary calcium clearance and can reduce the frequency of urinary calcium stone formation; they are a recognised cause of hypercalcaemia.

3.120 A 43-year-old hospital inpatient is noted to have very dark urine. Laboratory examination confirms the presence of urinary haemoglobin. What is the most likely underlying cause?

   A Crush injury

   B Haemolytic anaemia

   C Nephrotic syndrome

   D Polymyositis

   E Severe myositis secondary to statin therapy

3.121 Which pattern of inheritance best describes the genetic transmission of Huntington's chorea?

   A Autosomal dominant with anticipation

   B Autosomal dominant with incomplete penetrance

   C Autosomal recessive

   D Spontaneous genetic mutation

   E X-linked recessive

3.122 Which of the following best describes the features associated with inheritance of neurofibromatosis?

   A Males affected more than females

   B Genetic testing by DNA analysis is available

   C Heterozygotes are phenotypically normal

   D Most cases arise from spontaneous genetic mutation

   E Skips generations

3.123 You are examining the family history of an index case in order to better understand the transmission of a particular disease. It appears that only men have been affected by the disease over the past three generations. What is the most likely inheritance pattern?

   A Autosomal dominant with incomplete expression

   B Autosomal recessive

   C Frequent single gene mutations

   D X-linked recessive

   E X-linked dominant

3.120   Answer: B

Haemoglobinuria can occur with severe haemolysis, eg transfusion reaction, paroxysmal nocturnal haemoglobinuria and burns injuries. Crush injuries and muscle damage result in myoglobinuria. Nephrotic syndrome is characterised by heavy proteinuria.

3.121   Answer: A

Both sexes affected equally. Complete penetration. Age at onset of disease becomes progressively earlier with successive generations (anticipation).

3.122   Answer: B

Typically inherited in an autosomal dominant pattern, therefore men and women equally affected, and manifests in every generation.

3.123   Answer: D

X-linked recessive disorders are carried by phenotypically normal women. Men who inherit the abnormality on their single X chromosome express the disease; men who are phenotypically normal have inherited the normal X-chromosome. Women who express X-linked disorders indicates an X-linked dominant pattern of disease inheritance.

3.124 Which one of the following disorders is characteristically inherited in an autosomal recessive manner?

☐ A Becker's muscular dystrophy

☐ B Cystic fibrosis

☐ C Gardner's syndrome

☐ D Glucose-6-phosphate dehydrogenase deficiency

☐ E Red–green colour blindness

3.125 Which of the following medications is most likely to cause bronchospasm in a patient with well-controlled asthma?

☐ A Inhaled disodium cromoglycate

☐ B Inhaled ipratropium bromide

☐ C Montelukast sodium

☐ D Oral salbutamol

☐ E Theophylline

3.124   Answer: B

Gardner's syndrome is inherited in an autosomal dominant manner, and the others are inherited in an X-linked manner.

3.125   Answer: A

Can prevent asthma, particularly in young patients, and is comparatively free of systemic adverse effects. However, particulate size is bigger than aerosolised medications and can irritate respiratory tract causing cough and bronchospasm.

4. DERMATOLOGY

4.1   A 23-year-old man self-presents to the Emergency Department with
a skin infection overlying his left cheek. He says that the infection
started shortly after a graze injury to the skin while playing rugby a
few days earlier. The appearance is strongly suggestive of impetigo.
What treatment would be most appropriate?

◻ **A** Oral amoxicillin

◻ **B** Oral erythromycin

◻ **C** Oral flucloxacillin

◻ **D** Regular irrigation with sterile saline

◻ **E** Topical iodine

4.2   A 32-year-old woman is referred to the Dermatology Clinic due to
development of unusual freckles over her face over the past few
weeks. The patient denies any significant sun exposure and is taking
no regular medications apart from the oral contraceptive pill. On
examination there are raised pigmented papules over the cheeks,
chin and forehead. Which of the following offers the most likely
explanation?

◻ **A** Acne vulgaris

◻ **B** Addison's disease

◻ **C** Chloasma

◻ **D** Melanoma

◻ **E** Vitiligo

4.3   You see a 45-year-old woman in the Hypertension Clinic and note a
number of discrete areas of hypopigmentation overlying her hands
and forearms. Which of the following is the most likely explanation
for this appearance?

◻ **A** Addison's disease

◻ **B** Diabetes mellitus

◻ **C** Neurofibromatosis

◻ **D** Post-scarring hypopigmentation

◻ **E** Vitiligo

4.1   Answer: C

The vast majority of cases are caused by *S. aureus* infection and should be treated with topical fusidic acid or oral flucloxacillin.

4.2   Answer: C

Usually symmetrical, more common in women and associated with the oral contraceptive pill and pregnancy. Benign condition.

4.3   Answer: E

Common site, also involves face and genitalia. Probable autoimmune aetiology, and can be associated with other autoimmune diseases. No satisfactory treatment, although repigmentation can occur spontaneously.

4.4 You are asked to review a 31-year-old man in the Medical Outpatient Department, and you note from his records that he has previously been diagnosed with Peutz–Jegher syndrome. Which one of these statements is correct regarding this diagnosis?

☐ A *BRCA1* is the responsible gene

☐ B Inherited in X-linked manner

☐ C Often occurs as part of a multiple endocrine neoplasia

☐ D Pigmentation of the lips is due to melanin deposition

☐ E There is a substantially increased risk of colonic carcinoma

4.5 Which of the following factors most strongly predicts the development of keloid scarring as a postoperative complication?

☐ A Advanced age

☐ B Asian origin

☐ C Female gender

☐ D Incision site over the upper back

☐ E Use of synthetic suture materials for wound closure

4.6 A 47-year-old woman had been referred to the Dermatology Outpatient Department for investigation of a widespread rash. Skin biopsy shows features of vasculitis with necrosis, particularly affecting the arterioles. What is the most likely diagnosis?

☐ A Allergic vasculitis

☐ B Polyarteritis nodosa

☐ C Henoch–Schönlein purpura

☐ D Systemic lupus erythematosus

☐ E Urticarial vasculitis

4.7 You are asked to review a 28-year-old woman who reports easy bruising after comparatively minor trauma. Which of the following features most strongly suggests a diagnosis of Ehlers–Danlos syndrome?

☐ A Delayed recoil of skin after stretching

☐ B Hyperextensible joints

☐ C Keloid scarring after trauma

☐ D Poor dentition

☐ E Skin hyperextensible over lower limbs only

4.4   Answer: D

Inherited in autosomal dominant manner due to the *LKB1* gene. Gastrointestinal polyposis, not associated with malignant transformation.

4.5   Answer: D

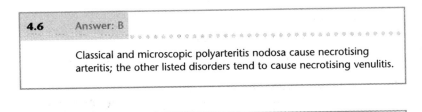

Other sites include chin, shoulder area, chest and around the earlobes. Black Afro-Caribbean patients are at greatest risk. Treatment is with local triamcinolone injections.

4.6   Answer: B

Classical and microscopic polyarteritis nodosa cause necrotising arteritis; the other listed disorders tend to cause necrotising venulitis.

4.7   Answer: B

Skin generally hyperextensible, with normal elastic recoil. After injury, scars tend to be thin and paper-like.

4.8   You review a 28-year-old man in the Outpatient Department who is very tall and has hyperextensible skin with delayed elastic recoil, which is most pronounced around his face and eyes. His past history includes two previous hospital admissions for investigation of suspected gastrointestinal bleeding. Which of the following best explains these features?

- [ ] **A** Ehlers–Danlos syndrome
- [ ] **B** Kleinfelter's syndrome
- [ ] **C** Marfan's syndrome
- [ ] **D** Pseudoxanthoma elasticum
- [ ] **E** Zollinger–Ellison syndrome

4.9   A 42-year-old man with Marfan's syndrome is under regular review in the Outpatient Department. Which of the following statements is correct regarding the aetiology of this disorder?

- [ ] **A** Inherited in an X-linked pattern
- [ ] **B** Mutation in the *MFS1* gene is responsible
- [ ] **C** There is excessive production of matrix glycoprotein fibrillin 1 (FBN-1)
- [ ] **D** There is high genetic homogeneity
- [ ] **E** Women manifest no features or very mild features only

4.10   You are examining a 73-year-old man admitted to the Acute Medical Admissions Unit earlier in the day, and note the appearance of multiple raised plaques overlying his back. These vary in colour from pale to dark brown, and are flat with irregular margins. What is the most likely explanation for these skin abnormalities?

- [ ] **A** Adenocarcinoma
- [ ] **B** Basal cell papilloma
- [ ] **C** Keratoacanthoma
- [ ] **D** Melanocytic naevi
- [ ] **E** Neurofibroma

4.8   Answer: D

Skin features are usually most notable around the neck, and the condition is associated with gastrointestinal bleeding, and myocardial infarction at a young age.

4.9   Answer: B

Therefore, defective expression of FBN-1. Inherited in autosomal dominant manner, but with considerable genetic heterogeneity; around 25% of patients are affected by a new mutation.

4.10   Answer: B

Also known as seborrhoeic warts, these are common in elderly patients and entirely benign.

4.11 A 62-year-old man is referred to the Dermatology Outpatient Department for assessment of a blistering rash overlying both of his shins. The legs appear modestly erythematous with overlying scratch marks, and there are large fluid-filled bullae. What is the most likely diagnosis?

☐ A   Bacterial cellulitis

☐ B   Bullous pemphigoid

☐ C   Chronic lymphoedema

☐ D   Pemphigus vulgaris

☐ E   Porphyria

4.12 A 38-year-old woman is being investigated for iron-deficiency anaemia, and is noted to have multiple small blisters overlying both forearms, associated with overlying scratch marks. Which of the following features is most strongly suggestive of dermatitis herpetiformis?

☐ A   Family history of the condition

☐ B   Papillary IgA deposition seen by immunofluorescence of unaffected skin

☐ C   Recent herpes simplex infection of her lower lip

☐ D   Regional lymphadenopathy

☐ E   Skin biopsy confirms blisters are intraepidermal

4.13 Which of the following is best recognised as a feature of dermatitis herpetiformis?

☐ A   Anti-endomysial antibody is normally negative

☐ B   Associated with HLA B8 and DR3 in 5–10% of patients

☐ C   Associated with increased risk of small bowel lymphoma

☐ D   Relapse after treatment is uncommon

☐ E   Treatment with dapsone should be for around 2–4 weeks

4.11   Answer: B

Typically the legs are very itchy. Treatment is with high-dose corticosteroids, and steroid-sparing agents (eg azathioprine) may be required.

4.12   Answer: B

IgA deposition also seen along the basement membrane. Rare blistering disorder with intensely itchy rash treated with dapsone.

4.13   Answer: C

As with coeliac disease; other common features between the disorders include HLA associations in 75%, good response to gluten-free diet, and positive antibodies to endomysium and gliadin.

4.14 A 35-year-old woman is referred to the Dermatology Outpatient Department for assessment of excess hair growth. She has become increasingly distressed by excessive hair growth, particularly over her face and forearms. Which of the following is most likely to be responsible?

- [ ] **A** Diabetes mellitus
- [ ] **B** Hyperthyroidism
- [ ] **C** Oral contraceptive pill use
- [ ] **D** Peripheral neuropathy
- [ ] **E** Phenytoin treatment

4.15 A 55-year-old man is referred to the Dermatology Outpatient Department for investigation of an erythematous rash overlying his face and neck, forearms and hands. What is the most likely underlying cause?

- [ ] **A** Chloasma
- [ ] **B** Discoid lupus erythematosus
- [ ] **C** Eczema
- [ ] **D** Furosemide treatment
- [ ] **E** Psoriasis

4.16 A 28-year-old man with type 1 diabetes complains of a rash overlying his lower limbs during a routine clinic appointment. He is noted to have a number of dark purple lesions overlying both shins, which are tender on palpation. What is the most likely explanation?

- [ ] **A** Lipoatrophy
- [ ] **B** Necrobiosis lipoidica
- [ ] **C** Pyoderma gangrenosum
- [ ] **D** Sarcoidosis
- [ ] **E** Urticarial vasculitis

4.14 Answer: E

Other effects include facial coarseness, acne vulgaris and gum hyperplasia. As a result, it is rarely used as first-line treatment in young patients with epilepsy.

4.15 Answer: B

Rash distribution suggests photosensitivity. This can also be caused by SLE, porphyria, rosacea and drugs (amiodarone, thiazides, and phenothiazines).

4.16 Answer: D

Inflammation affects the dermis and subcutaneous layers (panniculitis), and is usually tender. The lesions vary in size and have the appearance of slightly raised bruises.

4.17   A 17-year-old woman is referred to the Dermatology Clinic for assessment of severe acne vulgaris affecting her face, shoulders and back. She is asking if isotretinoin could be given. Which of the following statements is most accurate with regard to retinoid treatment?

    A   Around 35% of patients respond to treatment

    B   Euphoria is a characteristic adverse effect

    C   It lessens the likelihood of conception

    D   It should normally only be prescribed by dermatology specialists

    E   Patients should avoid pregnancy until treatment is stopped

4.18   A 43-year-man presents with a rash between his first and second toes of the left foot, associated with erythema, discoloration and flaking of local skin. There is bright pink fluorescence under ultraviolet light. What is the most likely diagnosis?

    A   *Candida albicans* infection

    B   Erysipelas

    C   Erythrasma

    D   Psoriasis

    E   Tinea pedis

4.19   Which of the following is best recognised as a feature of Stevens–Johnson syndrome?

    A   Cutaneous target lesions

    B   Necrotic genital ulcers

    C   Preceding streptococcal infection in most patients

    D   Sparing of the mucous membranes

    E   Underlying tuberculosis in 30% of patients

4.17   Answer: D
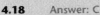

Retinoids are highly effective with a 90% response rate and two-thirds cure rate. They are teratogenic and patients should avoid conception during and up to 2 years after stopping acitretin treatment. They may impair liver biochemical tests and are associated with myalgia and depression.

4.18   Answer: C

The condition often mimics tinea infection, but the UV light findings are diagnostic. Caused by *Corynebacterium minutissimum* and treated with topical fusidic acid or oral erythromycin.

4.19   Answer: B

Often associated with mucosal involvement but, unlike erythema multiforme, there are few cutaneous target lesions. Most cases are drug-induced, eg sulphonamides, NSAIDs and the oral contraceptive pill.

4.20 You are reviewing a 55-year-old woman in the Outpatient Department when you notice that she has patchy areas of depigmentation overlying her hands and abdomen. You suspect that this appearance is due to vitiligo. Which one of these statements is most accurate regarding this condition?

- ☐ **A** It is post-inflammatory in most patients
- ☐ **B** Skin involvement is most noticeable in Caucasians
- ☐ **C** Repigmentation can occur spontaneously
- ☐ **D** Topical corticosteroids are effective in most patients
- ☐ **E** Usually associated with high anti-melatonin antibody titre

4.21 A 45-year-old woman is noted to have dry, erythematous skin overlying the volar surfaces of both wrists. A diagnosis of atopic dermatitis is suspected. Which of the following features is most consistent with this diagnosis?

- ☐ **A** Hepatomegaly
- ☐ **B** Intensive itch
- ☐ **C** Local lymphadenitis
- ☐ **D** Nodules overlying the distal interphalangeal joints
- ☐ **E** Small vesicles with clear fluid

4.22 Which one of the following statements regarding atopic dermatitis is most correct?

- ☐ **A** Affects 15–25% of adults
- ☐ **B** B-lymphocyte dysfunction is responsible
- ☐ **C** Inflammation is mediated by IgM
- ☐ **D** Normally associated with raised serum uric acid concentrations
- ☐ **E** Prevalence has increased 2-fold in past 20 years

4.23 Which of the following statements most correctly describes the role of tacrolimus in treating skin disease?

- ☐ **A** Inhibits eosinophil activity
- ☐ **B** Herpes simplex infection is a recognised complication of topical treatment
- ☐ **C** Is ineffective in acne rosacea
- ☐ **D** It is a preferred first-line agent for atopic dermatitis
- ☐ **E** Oral treatment is reserved for psoriasis with joint involvement

4.20   Answer: C

Effects are most pronounced in Afro-Caribbean patients and those with tanned skin. The margins often appear hyper-pigmented, but there is no evidence that this is the case. Patients should be advised to protect themselves against sunburn.

4.21   Answer: B

Affects 1–6% of adults. Distribution may be more atypical than in childhood, eg non-flexural sites, and family history of atopy less strong than in childhood atopic dermatitis.

4.22   Answer: E

Caused by excess T-helper cell (subtype 2) activity, mediated by IgE. Affects 1–6% of adults, many of whom have had childhood eczema.

4.23   Answer: B

Topical treatment is reserved for severe atopic dermatitis, and appears effective also for rosacea, psoriasis and other skin disorders. It inhibits T-cell activation and cytokine release, and systemic absorption can cause renal impairment.

4.24 A 41-year-old woman is reviewed in the Dermatology Outpatient Department with easy bruising. She has had longstanding rheumatoid arthritis, which is quiescent at present. Which of the following features is most likely a complication of repeated use of high-dose corticosteroid treatment?

- [ ] **A** Abdominal white striae
- [ ] **B** Acne
- [ ] **C** Gum hyperplasia
- [ ] **D** Hirsutism
- [ ] **E** Paper-thin skin

4.25 Which one of these aspects of lifestyle advice would be most effective in controlling the extent of psoriasis in a 42-year-old woman with extensive plaques over her buttocks and lower limbs?

- [ ] **A** Lose weight
- [ ] **B** Moderate alcohol intake
- [ ] **C** Reduce salt intake
- [ ] **D** Stop smoking cigarettes
- [ ] **E** Take more regular aerobic exercise

4.26 A 51-year-old man attends the Dermatology Outpatient Department for routine follow-up of his psoriasis. Which of the following features is the strongest indicator of a severe flare-up?

- [ ] **A** Flaking of dry skin layers
- [ ] **B** Involvement of 15% of body surface area
- [ ] **C** Serum uric acid is 468 μmol/l
- [ ] **D** Signs of arthritis on examination of the right knee
- [ ] **E** Temperature 37.4°C

4.27 Which one of the following skin disorders is most likely to be worsened by exposure to strong sunlight?

- [ ] **A** Acne vulgaris
- [ ] **B** Eczema
- [ ] **C** Pityriasis versicolor
- [ ] **D** Psoriasis
- [ ] **E** Rosacea

4.24   Answer: E

Although the others are recognised features, they are less specific. Of note, white striae are 'inactive', whilst purple-red striae are 'active'.

4.25   Answer: D

Cigarette smoking confers a 3-fold increased risk in women with psoriasis, and smoking cessation allows better recovery in both men and women.

4.26   Answer: B

Involvement of more than 10% BSA (5% in some cases) is sufficient to warrant systemic treatment.

4.27   Answer: E

Although this may be less important in most cases than was previously believed. Sunlight may worsen the other conditions, but is generally thought beneficial in eczema and psoriasis.

4.28 A 29-year-old woman presents to the Dermatology Clinic with a 2–4 week history of intermittent abdominal pain associated with transient blanching erythematous rash overlying face, neck and trunk. She has noted a number of distinct weals over her chest wall, but these have settled. What is the most likely diagnosis?

- [ ] **A** Acute intermittent porphyria
- [ ] **B** Angioedema
- [ ] **C** Atopic dermatitis
- [ ] **D** Atypical migraine
- [ ] **E** Recurrent anaphylaxis

4.29 A 56-year-old man presents with a 4-month history of rash overlying his trunk and upper and lower limbs. A skin biopsy is reported to show a leukocytoclastic vasculitis pattern. What is the most likely underlying cause?

- [ ] **A** Adverse drug reaction
- [ ] **B** Cryoglobulinaemia
- [ ] **C** Discoid lupus erythematosus
- [ ] **D** Polyarteritis nodosum
- [ ] **E** Wegener's granulomatosis

4.30 A 22-year-old woman is noted to have an urticarial rash overlying both forearms and hands, which is intensely itchy. Which of the following statements is correct regarding treatment in this condition?

- [ ] **A** Corticosteroids are highly effective
- [ ] **B** Histamine-2 (H₂) receptor antagonists are ineffective
- [ ] **C** Leukotriene antagonists have no role in treatment
- [ ] **D** Non-sedating antihistamines are less effective in controlling itch
- [ ] **E** Tricyclic antidepressants exaggerate skin response to histamine

4.28   Answer: B

Acute angioedema (< 6 weeks) is common, affecting up to one-third of adults at some point. Can be associated with skin, abdominal and respiratory symptoms.

4.29   Answer: A

Can occur as an adverse effect of any one of a large range of different drugs. Also a characteristic finding in urticarial vasculitis.

4.30   Answer: D

H_1-receptor antagonists are the mainstay of treatment, although addition of H_2-receptor or leukotriene antagonists may be of benefit. TCAs have some antihistamine properties. Immunomodulatory drugs, including corticosteroids, may be of limited value.

4.31 A 43-year-old man presented to the Dermatology Outpatient Department for assessment of multiple red–yellow papules which had developed over his lower limbs over the past 3 months. The appearance of the lesions is strongly suggestive of eruptive xanthomata. What underlying metabolic disturbance is most likely to be associated with these findings?

  A High LDL cholesterol

  B High serum triglycerides

  C High VLDL particle fraction

  D Low HDL cholesterol

  E Low lipoprotein-a concentrations

4.32 A 19-year-old woman develops a painful rash at the left angle of her mouth, associated with a cluster of small fluid-filled vesicles. The laboratory reports that a Tzanck test is positive. What is the most likely diagnosis?

  A Chicken pox

  B Dermatitis herpetiformis

  C Erysipelas

  D Herpes simplex

  E Measles

4.33 During pre-operative assessment before hip replacement surgery, a 79-year-old woman is noted to have thickening and disfiguration of a number of her toenails, and fungal infection is suspected. What is the most rapid means of confirming the diagnosis?

  A Fungal blood cultures

  B Fungal culture of toe scrapings

  C Plain X-ray of the foot and toes

  D Potassium hydroxide test

  E Wood's light

4.31   Answer: B

Sudden crops of red–yellow papules with erythematous halos, usually over buttocks or extensor surfaces of the limbs. Lesions contain lipids and lymphocytic infiltrate. Increased risk of pancreatitis.

4.32   Answer: D

The Tzanck test is a direct smear test for herpesvirus, but cannot distinguish VZV from HSV. Localisation of the lesions to one site, with perioral distribution, makes HSV more likely.

4.33   Answer: D

Nail sample is placed on a slide with potassium hydroxide and gently heated to dissolve the skin and nail cells, leaving the fungal cells, which may be visualised on light microscopy. Fungal culture may take 3–6 weeks.

4.34 A 36-year-old woman with longstanding diabetes presented with plaques over both shins. She was found to have a 12 cm, yellow, atrophic, centrally scarred plaque over each shin, associated with surrounding swelling. What is the most likely diagnosis?

- A Dermatomyositis
- B Diabetic lipoatrophy
- C Necrobiosis lipoidica
- D Polymyositis
- E Sarcoidosis

4.35 A 64-year-old woman is under investigation in the General Medical Outpatient Department for fatigue and lethargy. On examination, you find that all her fingernails appear concave and brittle. What is the most likely cause?

- A Calcium deficiency
- B Iron deficiency
- C Iron poisoning
- D Trauma
- E Vitamin B_{12} deficiency

4.36 Which of the following factors is most likely to diminish the severity of skin disease in a patient with longstanding psoriasis?

- A Alcohol excess
- B Corticosteroid withdrawal
- C Pregnancy
- D Streptococcal throat infection
- E Trauma

4.37 What is the most likely cause of angular chelitis in a 56-year-old woman who is also found to have a bright red tongue?

- A Folate deficiency
- B Iron deficiency
- C Rifampicin treatment
- D Streptococcal infection
- E Vitamin B_{12} deficiency

4.34   Answer: C

Occurs predominantly (but not exclusively) in patients with diabetes. Three-fold greater prevalence in women. Spontaneous remission occurs in one-quarter of patients, and scarring is common.

4.35   Answer: B

Other recognised causes of koilonychia include trauma (unlikely to affect all nails), lead poisoning, and it is associated with recurrent pleural effusions in yellow nail syndrome.

4.36   Answer: C

Although the disease can flare up during the immediate post-partum period. The other listed causes are generally associated with worsening of psoriasis skin disease, also use of β-blockers or lithium.

4.37   Answer: B

Classically, this leads to a cherry red tongue appearance. Of note, rifampicin is associated with pink discoloration of body fluids and secretions, rather than organ discoloration.

4.38   A 43-year-old man is noted to have a painless white plaque along the left lateral border of his tongue. It is firmly adherent to the tongue, with a fine overlying pattern of striation visible on close inspection. What is the likeliest diagnosis?

- [ ] A Candidiasis
- [ ] B Leukoplakia
- [ ] C Lichen planus
- [ ] D Phosphorus burn
- [ ] E Streptococcal stomatitis

4.39   A 42-year-old man has recently been discharged from hospital after presenting with features of alcohol withdrawal and abdominal pain. He had been commenced on a number of new medications. He now re-attends the Emergency Department with fever symptoms. On examination, there is a new diffuse erythematous rash over his trunk and limbs, and investigations show white cell count $9.7 \times 10^9/l$, and eosinophils $0.8 \times 10^9/l$. Which of the following drugs is most likely to have caused his rash?

- [ ] A Diazepam
- [ ] B Metronidazole
- [ ] C Phenytoin
- [ ] D Quinine
- [ ] E Thiamine

4.40   A 34-year-old man is referred to the General Medicine Outpatient Clinic for investigation of urticarial symptoms. He has had a number of attacks over the past 3 months, characterised by swelling of the lips and tongue associated with a non-specific generalised rash. During the episodes, he experiences severe colicky abdominal pain for around 6–8 hours. Which of the following investigations might be most helpful?

- [ ] A Antibody to house dust mite antigen
- [ ] B Eosinophil count
- [ ] C C1 esterase inhibitor
- [ ] D IgE
- [ ] E Urinary porphyrins

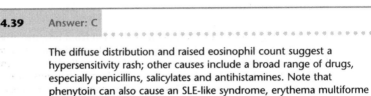

4.38   Answer: C

This is a common condition. It is usually painless (unlike stomatitis) and firmly adherent to the tongue (unlike candidiasis). Phosphorus burns are often painless but associated with ulceration and sloughing. Wickham's striae are pathognomonic for lichen planus. Leukoplakia is a diagnosis of exclusion.

4.39   Answer: C

The diffuse distribution and raised eosinophil count suggest a hypersensitivity rash; other causes include a broad range of drugs, especially penicillins, salicylates and antihistamines. Note that phenytoin can also cause an SLE-like syndrome, erythema multiforme and fixed drug eruptions.

4.40   Answer: C

C1 esterase inhibitor deficiency is a rare condition that predisposes to urticarial reactions with prominent respiratory and gastrointestinal features. As with chronic urticaria, trigger factors are varied including aspirin, NSAIDs, codeine, food additives, exercise and trauma.

5. ENDOCRINOLOGY

5.1 You are asked to interpret thyroid function test results from a 42-year-old woman who has been attending the Medical Outpatient Department with weight loss. These show thyroid stimulating hormone (TSH) undetectable and free T_4 18 pmol/l. What is the most likely underlying diagnosis?

- [ ] A Early primary hypothyroidism
- [ ] B Graves' disease
- [ ] C Primary hyperthyroidism
- [ ] D Subclinical hyperthyroidism
- [ ] E T3 thyrotoxicosis

5.2 A previously healthy 42-year-old man is referred to the Medical Outpatient Department with a 3-month history of weight loss and persistent sinus tachycardia. Thyroid function tests show TSH 2.4 mIU/l, free T_4 25 pmol/l and free T_3 6.2 pmol/l. What is the most likely underlying diagnosis?

- [ ] A Primary hyperthyroidism
- [ ] B Secondary hyperthyroidism
- [ ] C Sick euthyroidism
- [ ] D Subclinical hypothyroidism
- [ ] E Viral thyroiditis

5.3 A 51-year-old woman is being investigated for obesity and hypertension in the Medical Outpatient Department. Investigations indicate hypothyroidism, and antibody tests are positive for anti-thyroid peroxidase (anti-TPO), positive for anti-thyroglobulin and negative for anti-TSH receptor. What is the most likely underlying diagnosis?

- [ ] A Autoimmune hypothyroidism
- [ ] B Graves' disease
- [ ] C Hashimoto's thyroiditis
- [ ] D Pituitary failure
- [ ] E SLE

5.1 Answer: E

5% of hyperthyroidism. T_4 is often normal, whereas free T_3 concentrations are abnormally high. Complete suppression of TSH can, less commonly, be associated with primary hyperthyroidism where free T_4 is in the upper part of the normal reference range.

5.2 Answer: B

In the setting of primary hyperthyroidism, TSH would be completely suppressed. Detectable levels strongly suggest secondary hyperthyroidism (excess pituitary TSH secretion) or, in rare cases, tertiary hyperthyroidism (excess hypothalamic TRF secretion).

5.3 Answer: A

Not definitive, but anti-TSH receptor antibodies are more usually positive in Grave's disease, whereas the others are less commonly so.

5.4 A 41-year-old woman is referred for radionuclide thyroid scanning, and the report shows enlarged thyroid gland size, with homogeneously increased radionuclide uptake. What is the most likely diagnosis?

☐ **A** de Quervain's thyroiditis

☐ **B** Graves' hyperthyroidism

☐ **C** Primary hypothyroidism

☐ **D** Thyroid carcinoma

☐ **E** Toxic nodule

5.5 A 47-year-old woman is noted to have a non-tender thyroid nodule during a routine physical examination. Which of the following statements best describes the role of fine needle aspiration cytology (FNAC)?

☐ **A** Around 20–30% specificity

☐ **B** Infection occurs after the procedure in 5–10% of patients

☐ **C** Outdated modality now being replaced by MRI scanning

☐ **D** Overall diagnostic accuracy more than 90%

☐ **E** Virtually 100% sensitivity

5.6 You review a 30-year-old man in the Endocrinology Outpatient Department, who has recently been diagnosed with Graves' ophthalmopathy. Which of these statements is correct regarding this condition?

☐ **A** Corneal ulceration is a recognised complication

☐ **B** Most patients have biochemical hyperthyroidism

☐ **C** Only 5–10% ever develope extra-ocular features of Graves' disease

☐ **D** Targeted radiotherapy is useful in most patients

☐ **E** Smoking cessation can worsen progression

5.7 Which of the following is most commonly found in patients with Hashimoto's thyroiditis?

☐ **A** Anti-TSH receptor antibodies inhibit thyroid release

☐ **B** Extensive thyroid gland infiltration by plasma cells

☐ **C** Early fibrosis and scarring of the thyroid gland

☐ **D** Pretibial swelling and skin thickening

☐ **E** Proptosis

5.4   Answer: B

Thyroiditis and hypothyroidism are associated with attenuated radionuclide uptake.

5.5   Answer: D

Values vary between centres and operators, but sensitivity and specificity are both around 90% too, and false negative rate is around 5%.

5.6   Answer: A

Due to non-closure of the eyelid and corneal dryness. Specific treatment is usually not required for Graves' ophthalmopathy in most cases, other than to ensure corneal lubrication. Corticosteroids and radiotherapy may be effective in severe cases complicated by optic nerve compression.

5.7   Answer: B

Typically associated also with anti-TPO and anti-thyroglobulin antibodies and, less commonly, anti-TSH receptor antibodies (unlike those in Graves' disease, these tend to be stimulatory).

5.8 A 34-year-old man is referred from the Endocrinology Outpatient Department to the local surgical unit for excision of a solitary thyroid nodule. What histological type is associated with the best outcome?

- [ ] A Adenocarcinoma
- [ ] B Anaplastic
- [ ] C Follicular
- [ ] D Papillary
- [ ] E Squamous cell

5.9 Which of the following treatments is most likely to be useful in the management of non-toxic multinodular goitre?

- [ ] A Carbimazole
- [ ] B Non-selective β-blockers
- [ ] C Radioiodine may reduce goitre
- [ ] D Surgery is not indicated because the patient is not hyperthyroid
- [ ] E Thyroxine should be avoided

5.10 A 51-year-old woman is found to have bitemporal hemianopsia and is being investigated for a suspected pituitary tumour. Which of the following investigations provides optimal views to determine whether the pituitary gland is enlarged?

- [ ] A Contrast-enhanced CT brain
- [ ] B Functional PET scan
- [ ] C Plain skull X-ray
- [ ] D T1-weighted MRI scan
- [ ] E Transcranial Doppler ultrasound

5.11 Which of the following tests would most reliably detect a deficiency of the growth hormone axis in a 19-year-old man?

- [ ] A ACTH stimulation test
- [ ] B Arginine test
- [ ] C Glucagon test
- [ ] D Insulin tolerance test
- [ ] E Thyroid releasing hormone (TRH) administration test

5.8   Answer: D

Metastases are found in only 1% of patients, and treatment involves near-total thyroid resection and post-operative thyroid hormone replacement (additional ablative I^{131} treatment is considered in high risk patients).

5.9   Answer: C

Useful in shrinking the goitre in most patients. Surgery is often indicated for cosmetic reasons or to reduce underlying tissue compression, and thyroid hormone can suppress TSH and reduce goitre in certain cases.

5.10   Answer: D

T1-weighted MRI shows brain tissue as white, and pituitary adenomata typically are of lower signal intensity than surrounding tissue. Contrast-enhancement may help distinguish the nature of larger tumours.

5.11   Answer: D

Insulin is administered to provoke a stress response, with subsequent release of growth hormone and ACTH. Glucagon also stimulates growth hormone release, but less directly. Arginine stimulates growth hormone secretion, and may be used as a second-line test.

5.12   You see a patient in the Outpatient Department with blood pressure 102/64 mmHg who is found to have Na$^+$ 132 mmol/l and K$^+$ 5.1 mmol/l. You suspect a diagnosis of hypopituitarism. Which of the following would be the most appropriate next step in the patient's management?

- [ ] **A** CT brain
- [ ] **B** Glucagon test
- [ ] **C** Insulin tolerance test
- [ ] **D** MRI brain scan
- [ ] **E** Short synacthen test

5.13   A 52-year-old man attends the Endocrinology Outpatient Department for review of his hypopituitarism. He is currently taking prednisolone 4 mg in mornings and 2 mg in evenings. What is the most reliable test to ensure that his glucocorticoid treatment is not excessive?

- [ ] **A** ACTH concentrations in serum
- [ ] **B** Blood pressure
- [ ] **C** Dipstick urinalysis for glucose
- [ ] **D** Random plasma glucose
- [ ] **E** Urinary free cortisol measurements

5.14   A 16-year-old boy attends the Endocrinology Clinic for the first time, having previously attended a specialist paediatric unit for review of his growth hormone deficiency. Which of the following statements most accurately describes the effect of growth hormone treatment in this condition?

- [ ] **A** Hypercholesterolaemia is a recognised feature
- [ ] **B** May become unnecessary in around 50% of patients in whom deficiency resolves
- [ ] **C** Impaired quality of life is a recognised adverse effect of treatment
- [ ] **D** Tends to cause obesity in most patients
- [ ] **E** Treatment is generally unnecessary in adults

5.12   Answer: C

Hypoglycaemia stimulates ACTH and GH release. Glucagon gives a similar, although less potent, stimulus. Short synacthen test provides information about the glucocorticoid axis only, and not the growth hormone axis.

5.13   Answer: E

Aiming to keep these within the normal daily limits, so as to avoid development of diabetes, hypertension and reduced bone mineral density.

5.14   Answer: B

Therefore, retesting should be considered. Associated with improved quality of life, exercise capacity, increased lean body mass and reduced fat mass and serum cholesterol.

5.15 Which of the following factors is most likely to cause hyperprolactinaemia?

- [ ] A Breast stimulation
- [ ] B Cranial irradiation
- [ ] C Hyperthyroidism
- [ ] D Levodopa
- [ ] E Obstructive jaundice

5.16 Which of the following is most likely to be a feature associated with acromegaly?

- [ ] A Three-fold increased prevalence in women
- [ ] B Histology shows adenocarcinoma in 15–20%
- [ ] C Local invasion is common
- [ ] D Most cases are diagnosed at 18–30 years age
- [ ] E Pituitary adenoma is found in fewer than 30% of cases

5.17 A 43-year-old woman has suffered deterioration of her vision over the past 6 months, and investigations have established a diagnosis of acromegaly secondary to a functional pituitary adenoma. What initial treatment is most appropriate?

- [ ] A High-dose corticosteroids
- [ ] B Radiolabelled growth hormone
- [ ] C Somatotropin
- [ ] D Targeted radiotherapy
- [ ] E Trans-sphenoidal resection

5.18 A 46-year-old man is referred to the Medical Outpatient Department for advice on the management of his hypertension and diabetes. On examination, he is noted to have a plethoric face, hirsutism, thin skin, multiple bruises and active striae across the abdominal wall. What is the most likely underlying cause?

- [ ] A ACTH-dependent pituitary adenoma
- [ ] B Adrenal carcinoma
- [ ] C Alcoholism
- [ ] D Depression
- [ ] E Ectopic ACTH syndrome

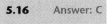

5.15   Answer: A

Other causes include dopamine antagonists (antipsychotics and antiemetics), opiates, primary hypothyroidism (TSH stimulates prolactin release), and renal failure (accumulation).

5.16   Answer: C

Most cases are diagnosed aged 40–60 years. Carcinoma is rare, and pituitary adenoma is found in >99% of cases. Equal gender prevalence.

5.17   Answer: E

Radiotherapy is appropriate for patients in whom surgery is unsuccessful or inappropriate. Pre-operative octreotide is thought to improve outcome.

5.18   Answer: A

Alcoholism and severe depression account for around 1% of all cases of Cushing's syndrome, whereas ACTH-dependent pituitary adenoma is found in around two-thirds of patients.

5.19 A 44-year-old woman is undergoing investigations for an underlying cause of obesity. Thyroid function tests and 24-h urinary free cortisol and overnight dexamethasone tests are all normal. Which one of these statements is correct?

- [ ] A 24-h urinary free cortisol test has 5–10% false negative rate
- [ ] B Cushing's syndrome has been excluded
- [ ] C Low-dose dexamethasone suppression test may provide additional information
- [ ] D Midnight cortisol measurement has low sensitivity but is highly specific
- [ ] E Overnight dexamethasone suppression test is more sensitive in obese patients

5.20 Which one of the following drugs is most likely to stimulate prolactin release?

- [ ] A Bromocriptine
- [ ] B Cabergoline
- [ ] C Levodopa
- [ ] D Metoclopramide
- [ ] E Ropinirole

5.21 A 30-year-old woman is referred to the Medical Outpatient Department for investigation of excessive thirst and polydipsia. A fluid deprivation test is performed and shows urine osmolality 280 mOsm/kg. After administration of desmopressin, urine osmolality is 920 mOsm/kg. What is the most likely underlying diagnosis?

- [ ] A Cranial diabetes insipidus
- [ ] B Nephrogenic diabetes insipidus
- [ ] C Psychogenic polydipsia
- [ ] D Syndrome of inappropriate ADH
- [ ] E Sample contamination giving an erroneous result

5.19   Answer: C

Overnight suppression test has false negative rate of 2% (similar rate to low-dose dexamethasone suppression test) but this is higher in obese patients. Midnight cortisol has virtually 0% false negative rate, ie highly sensitive.

5.20   Answer: D

Dopamine antagonist. The others have dopamine agonist effects, which suppress prolactin release.

5.21   Answer: A

Low urine osmolality due to lack of ADH effect, indicative of diabetes insipidus; restoration by ADH indicates cranial cause, lack of response to ADH would indicate nephrogenic DI (insensitivity to ADH). After fluid deprivation, osmolality is high in psychogenic water drinking.

5.22 A 68-year-old man is admitted with acute confusional state, and found to have serum sodium 128 mmol/l. He has been taking no regular medications. Urine sodium concentration is 2 mmol/l. What is the most likely cause?

- [ ] A Cirrhosis
- [ ] B Dehydration
- [ ] C Nephrotic syndrome
- [ ] D Salt-losing nephropathy
- [ ] E Syndrome of inappropriate ADH secretion

5.23 Which of the following features is most strongly suggestive of the syndrome of inappropriate ADH secretion?

- [ ] A Headache
- [ ] B Hyponatraemia with raised plasma osmolality
- [ ] C Hypovolaemia
- [ ] D Impaired renal function
- [ ] E Normal urine osmolality despite abnormally low serum osmolality

5.24 A 72-year-old man with known diabetic nephropathy presents to hospital with a history of diarrhoea and vomiting over the last 3 days. He reports he is not passing much urine. His temperature is 38.7°C, and laboratory investigations show glucose 26 mmol/l, Na^+ 137 mmol/l, K^+ 7.0 mmol/l, urea 18.2 mmol/l, creatinine 320 μmol/l and CRP 150 IU/l. What is the most appropriate immediate treatment?

- [ ] A Calcium gluconate
- [ ] B Co-amoxiclav
- [ ] C Insulin and dextrose infusion
- [ ] D Intravenous hydration
- [ ] E Urethral catheter insertion and monitoring of urine output

5.22   Answer: B

Low urinary sodium is a feature of excess aldosterone activity, which is an appropriate compensatory response to volume depletion.

5.23   Answer: E

Normal osmolality is inappropriate, and would be expected to be low.

5.24   Answer: A

The immediate risk is arrhythmia secondary to hyperkalaemia. Thereafter, dextrose infusion and insulin should be used to shift potassium into tissues to reduce circulating potassium concentrations, in addition to controlling circulating glucose concentrations.

5.25 A 64 year old with type 2 diabetes attends the Outpatient Department for review. He is taking twice daily NovoMix 30 and metformin 500 mg tds, and reports high fasting blood glucose readings in the morning and regularly feeling sweaty and unwell overnight. What is the most appropriate step in his management?

- A Increase evening insulin dose
- B Increase morning insulin dose
- C Omit night time snack
- D Reduce evening insulin dose
- E Stop metformin

5.26 An obese 55-year-old man presents with a 6-week history of thirst and polyuria. His fasting glucose is 7.6. Which of the following is the best initial treatment?

- A Advise that results are satisfactory and offer reassurance
- B Institute lifestyle modification to lose weight and increase fitness
- C Start glipizide
- D Start metformin
- E Start rosiglitazone

5.27 A 24-year-old woman is referred to the Diabetic Clinic by her GP, who has diagnosed diabetes on the basis of glycosuria, and a 6-month history of polyuria and polydipsia. Her weight has been stable for the past year. There is a strong family history of diabetes. A glucose tolerance test is positive, with a post-prandial glucose of 12.6. Which of the following diagnoses is most likely?

- A Type 1 diabetes
- B Type 2 diabetes
- C Monogenic diabetes (MODY)
- D Latent auto-immune diabetes of adulthood (LADA)
- E Secondary diabetes

5.25   Answer: D

Scenario suggests nocturnal hypoglycaemia and reflex morning hyperglycaemia. A reduction in the evening insulin dose should prevent this. Metformin may be helpful in reducing insulin resistance and preventing rebound hyperglycaemia.

5.26   Answer: B

A fasting glucose > 7 mmol/l confirms diabetes mellitus. Advice regarding diet, weight loss and exercise is appropriate first-line treatment and, if this is insufficient, then oral hypoglycaemics could be introduced.

5.27   Answer: C

The lack of weight loss despite prolonged osmotic symptoms makes type 1 DM less likely. Normal BMI without hypertension or hyperlipidaemia makes type 2 less likely. Family history makes MODY more likely than LADA.

5.28 An 18-year-old male with known type I diabetes presents to the Emergency Department with general malaise. Dipstick urinalysis is strongly positive for ketones, and an arterial blood gas confirms a metabolic acidosis. You suspect diabetic ketoacidosis. Which one of the following findings would be LEAST likely to occur, and might suggest an alternative diagnosis?

- [ ] A CRP 50
- [ ] B Leukocyte count $16.2 \times 10^9/l$
- [ ] C Serum glucose 36 mmol/l
- [ ] D Serum sodium 162 mmol/l
- [ ] E Urea 13.8 mmol/l

5.29 A 46-year-old obese patient with type 2 diabetes is referred to the New Patient Diabetic Clinic. His BMI is 36, he drinks 30 units of alcohol per week and he smokes 20 cigarettes per day. His blood pressure has been around 170/90 on at least three occasions in the last 6 months. His HbA1c at clinic is 9.6% and fasting cholesterol is 7.0 mmol/l. Which measure would most reduce his future risk of stroke?

- [ ] A Blood pressure control
- [ ] B Metformin
- [ ] C Moderating alcohol intake
- [ ] D Simvastatin
- [ ] E Smoking cessation

5.30 A 34-year-old man is referred to the Endocrinology Clinic for investigation of gynaecomastia. Which of the following investigations would be most appropriate in his initial management?

- [ ] A 24-h urinary cortisol
- [ ] B Chest X-ray
- [ ] C Mammography
- [ ] D Serum testosterone
- [ ] E Testicular ultrasound

5.28   Answer: D

It is unusual to see hypernatraemia in DKA, which is normally more suggestive of hyperosmotic, non-ketotic syndrome (HONK).

5.29   Answer: A

Treatment to target blood pressure of < 135 mmHg for systolic BP and < 85 mmHg would reduce future stroke risk by more than 35%. All of the above measures are important in reducing global cardiovascular risk.

5.30   Answer: D

Other tests include liver biochemistry, serum oestradiol, luteinising hormone (LH) and follicle stimulating hormone (FSH), prolactin, human chorionic gonadotrophin (HCG) and sex hormone binding globulin (SHBG).

5.31 A 65-year-old man is found to have serum calcium of 2.72 mmol/l and albumin 34 g/l. Further investigation shows chest X-ray is normal and serum parathyroid hormone is 0.7 IU/l. What is the most likely diagnosis?

- A Primary hyperparathyroidism
- B Medullary thyroid carcinoma
- C Small cell lung carcinoma
- D Squamous cell lung carcinoma
- E Dietary vitamin D excess

5.32 A 34-year-old woman is found to have serum calcium 2.64 mmol/l and phosphate 0.3 mmol/l. Which of the following statements regarding the aetiology of hypercalcaemia is correct?

- A Hyperthyroidism is the commonest cause in young adults
- B Is less common in patients taking calcium channel blockers
- C It is a recognised feature of vitamin A toxicity
- D Milk–alkali syndrome has become increasingly common recently
- E Sarcoidosis is a recognised cause due to delayed calcium excretion

5.33 Which of the following is a recognised adverse effect of chronic hypercalcaemia?

- A Asthma
- B Fatty liver infiltration
- C Osteoarthritis
- D Peptic ulcer disease
- E Varicose veins

5.34 A 29-year-old woman is being investigated for muscle cramps and fatigue in the General Medical Outpatient Clinic. Investigations show modest elevation of PTH and calcium concentrations, and normal creatinine phosphokinase. What is the most likely underlying diagnosis?

- A Diffuse parathyroid hyperplasia
- B Functional parathyroid adenoma
- C Hyperthyroidism
- D Multiple myeloma
- E Multiple parathyroid adenomata

5.31 Answer: A

Hypercalcaemia suppresses parathyroid hormone (PTH) release, which should be undetectable. Hypercalcaemia is often seen in squamous cell carcinoma, breast and renal carcinoma and is thought due to PTH-related peptide.

5.32 Answer: C

Hypercalcaemia in sarcoidosis is thought due to production of active 1,25-D3 by granulomata. Common causes include hyperparathyroidism and malignancy. Rarer causes include hyperthyroidism, phaeochromocytoma, Addison's disease and thiazide use.

5.33 Answer: D

Due to excess gastrin production. Other features include myopathy, constipation, nephrolithiasis and nephrogenic diabetes insipidus.

5.34 Answer: B

The absence of PTH suppression in the presence of raised serum calcium is strongly suggestive of primary hyperparathyroidism. The vast majority of cases arise from a solitary functional nodule, and less commonly due to multiple adenomata or diffuse hyperplasia.

5.35 Which of the following is most likely to cause raised circulating serum calcium concentrations?

☐ **A** Chronic renal failure

☐ **B** Malabsorption

☐ **C** Rhabdomyolysis

☐ **D** Tertiary hyperparathyroidism

☐ **E** Tumour lysis syndrome

5.36 A 61-year-old man is investigated for unexplained leg weakness and muscle cramps. Investigations show ALP 234 IU/l, ALT 39 IU/l, albumin 41 g/l, and serum calcium 1.98 mmol/l. What is the most likely cause for these findings?

☐ **A** Alcoholic liver disease

☐ **B** Osteomalacia

☐ **C** Osteoporosis

☐ **D** Paget's disease

☐ **E** Primary biliary cirrhosis

5.37 A 71-year-old woman has recently sustained a fractured left femoral head after a minor fall. Dual enery X-ray absorptiometry scanning shows femoral neck bone density T-score of –2.8. What does this mean?

☐ **A** 2.8% of the population have lower bone density

☐ **B** Bisphosphonates should be considered

☐ **C** Less than normal but treatment not required

☐ **D** Lifestyle modification is ineffective beyond 60 years of age

☐ **E** Ten-year fracture risk is 2.8%

5.38 Which of the following conditions is most likely to account for a serum magnesium concentration of 1.7 mmol/l?

☐ **A** Acute pancreatitis

☐ **B** Bartter's syndrome

☐ **C** Chronic renal impairment

☐ **D** Diarrhoea

☐ **E** Thiazide diuretics

5.35 Answer: D

A feature of primary and tertiary hyperparathyroidism (autonomous PTH production regardless of serum calcium), whereas calcium is often slightly low or normal in secondary hyperparathyroidism. The other listed options are all recognised causes of hypocalcaemia.

5.36 Answer: B

Commonly associated with high ALP (bone turnover) and low serum calcium. Calcium and phosphate are usually normal in osteoporosis and Paget's disease, in the absence of fractures.

5.37 Answer: B

2.8 standard deviations lower than gender-matched population mean. Bisphosphonate therapy can reduce the risk of subsequent fracture by up to 50%.

5.38 Answer: C

Uncommon, but usually associated with excess iv administration. The other listed causes are recognised causes of hypomagnesaemia.

5.39 A 56-year-old patient presents to the Emergency Department with profound malaise and confusion. Initial investigations show Na$^+$ 144 mmol/l, K$^+$ 4.3 mmol/l, Cl$^-$ 97 mmol/l and HCO$_3^-$ 10 mmol/l. What is the most likely explanation for these findings?

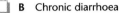

- ☐ **A** Acute pneumonia
- ☐ **B** Chronic diarrhoea
- ☐ **C** Lactic acidosis
- ☐ **D** Pulmonary embolus
- ☐ **E** Renal tubular acidosis

5.40 A 24-year-old man attends the Endocrinology Outpatient Department for a routine follow-up appointment for alkaptonuria. Which of these is the most common feature of the condition?

- ☐ **A** Gastrointestinal obstruction
- ☐ **B** Haematuria
- ☐ **C** Liver disease
- ☐ **D** Nephrolithiasis
- ☐ **E** Psoriatic arthropathy

5.41 A 20-year-old man is admitted to hospital with colicky abdominal and flank pain, and a CT scan shows calculus partially obstructing the distal left ureters. He has had two previous hospital admissions for ureteric calculi. Which of the following conditions is most likely to predispose to nephrolithiasis?

- ☐ **A** Diabetes insipidus
- ☐ **B** Ketoacidosis
- ☐ **C** Homocysteinuria
- ☐ **D** Lactic acidosis
- ☐ **E** Oxalosis

5.39 Answer: C

The findings are consistent with a severe metabolic acidosis and increased anion gap $[(Na + K) - (Cl + HCO_3)]$. Other causes include ketoacidosis, renal failure and ingestion of methanol, ethanol and aspirin.

5.40 Answer: D

Rare disorder with autosomal recessive inheritance, deficiency of enzyme homogentisic acid oxidase. Homogentisate polymers, alkapton, accumulate in urine (darkens on standing) and cartilage (osteoarthritis). Rarer features include ocular involvement and aortic valve incompetence.

5.41 Answer: E

Metabolic abnormality causing overproduction of oxalate. Features include bone disease, recurrent nephrolithiasis and premature cardiovascular disease.

5.42 A 53-year-old woman presents with sudden onset of pain in the first metatarsophalangeal joint in her left foot. The pain is severe and she is unable to weight-bear. On examination, the joint is swollen and red with limited mobility, and temperature is 37.1°C. Serum calcium is 2.26 mmol/l, albumin 42 g/l and urate 0.26 mmol/l. What is the most likely diagnosis?

☐ **A** Acute gout
☐ **B** Atheroembolism
☐ **C** Osteoarthritis
☐ **D** Septic arthritis
☐ **E** Subluxation

5.43 A 56-year-old woman is referred to the General Medical Outpatient Department because of a recent episode of acute gout diagnosed by her GP. Pain and swelling of the affected joint have now subsided, and examination appears normal. Serum urate is 0.36 mmol/l. What is the most appropriate step in her initial management?

☐ **A** Allopurinol
☐ **B** Ibuprofen
☐ **C** Myeloma screen
☐ **D** Offer lifestyle advice
☐ **E** Urate oxidase

5.44 An 18-year-old man is being investigated in the Medical Outpatient Department for abnormal liver function tests. Which of the following most strongly suggests an underlying diagnosis of Wilson's disease?

☐ **A** Decreased urinary copper excretion
☐ **B** Dilatation of the biliary tree on ultrasound scan
☐ **C** Hypoparathyroidism
☐ **D** Increased serum caeruloplasmin
☐ **E** Scattered corneal microdeposits

5.42 Answer: A

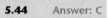

The site and characteristics are strongly suggestive. There is no correlation between serum urate and risk of gout; risk is dependent on total body urate, which varies from 0.5–1.0 g in healthy individuals to 10–30 g in patients with hypertension or heart failure.

5.43 Answer: D

Avoidance of excess alcohol, weight loss and a low purine diet are appropriate, and consideration should be given to withdrawal of drugs that predispose (eg thiazides). Allopurinol is generally only used if more than one episode. Urate oxidase given intravenously to prevent tumour lysis syndrome.

5.44 Answer: C

Other features include cirrhosis and chronic hepatitis, haemolysis, tremor, chorea, seizures, arthropathy and Kayser–Fleischer corneal rings. Diagnosis is usually based on decreased serum caeruloplasmin and increased urinary copper excretion, and copper deposition can be demonstrated on liver biopsy.

5.45 A 46-year-old man is referred to the Medical Outpatient Clinic for investigation of hepatomegaly. You note that he appears to have excessive skin pigmentation. Which of these most strongly suggests haemochromatosis?

A   ESR 38 mm/h

B   Haematocrit 0.58

C   Hb 161 g/l

D   Serum ferritin 560 µg/l

E   Transferrin saturation 76%

5.46 Which of the following statements most correctly describes the pathophysiology of primary haemochromatosis?

A   Hepatocellular carcinoma is a rare complication

B   *HFE* gene on chromosome 6 is responsible

C   Inherited in autosomal dominant pattern

D   Presents in late teens and early 20s

E   Women have a 2-fold risk compared to men

5.47 A 55-year-old woman is found to have serum transferrin 66% and serum ferritin 620 µg/l. You suspect a possible diagnosis of haemochromatosis. Which of the following is most likely to be responsible?

A   Alcohol excess

B   Chronic obstructive airways disease

C   Excessive iron intake

D   Living at high altitude

E   Longstanding smoking

5.48 A 45-year-old woman is admitted to hospital with generalised abdominal pain. Physical examination is normal. Her urine is found to turn dark red on standing. What is the most likely explanation for these features?

A   Acute intermittent porphyria

B   Acute interstitial nephritis

C   Alkaptonuria

D   Porphyria cutanea tarda

E   Rifampicin overdose

5.45 Answer: E

Features also include raised ferritin (this is less specific) and liver iron concentrations > 180 μmol/g on biopsy specimens. There is increased prevalence of diabetes mellitus, hypogonadism and cardiomyopathy.

5.46 Answer: B

Autosomal recessive. Gene frequency is around 5%, and disease frequency 1 in 220. Around 30% of patients with cirrhosis will develop hepatocellular carcinoma.

5.47 Answer: A

Other causes of secondary haemochromatosis include liver disease, parenteral iron overload (eg in patients with chronic renal disease), and ineffective erythropoiesis (eg β-thalassaemia).

5.48 Answer: A

Unlike porphyria cutanea tarda, there is no skin involvement or photosensitivity. Rifampicin causes pink-red discoloration of body fluids and urine, whereas urine in alkaptonuria turns black on standing.

5.49 A 61-year-old woman attending the Cardiovascular Risk Clinic is found to have fasting total cholesterol 6.2 mmol/l, HDL cholesterol 1.3 mmol/l and triglycerides 6.6 mmol/l. Which of the following statements is correct?

A Addition of a fibrate reduces the risk of statin-induced myositis

B Fibrate therapy lowers triglycerides but increases cholesterol

C Raised triglycerides alone do not merit treatment

D Statins lower total cholesterol but have equivocal effects on outcome

E Total : HDL cholesterol ratio correlates well with cardiovascular risk

5.50 A 56-year-old man is given radio-labelled iodine treatment for hyperthyroidism associated with a diffuse multinodular goitre. Which of these is most frequently recognised as a feature of this treatment?

A Doses up to 800 MBq do not cause extracorporeal radiation emission

B Most patients require repeated administration

C Risk of cancer is increased by around 1% per year

D Should be avoided in pregnant women

E There is predominantly α-particle emission

5.51 A 54-year-old woman is referred to the Hypertension Clinic because she has failed to respond to combination of three anti-hypertensive agents. Blood pressure is 168/98 mmHg in her right arm, and initial investigations show Na⁺ 146 mmol/l, K⁺ 3.0 mmol/l and bicarbonate 32 mmol/l. What is the most likely diagnosis?

A Addison's disease

B Conn's syndrome

C Cushing's disease

D Phaeochromocytoma

E Renal artery stenosis

5.49   Answer: E

Hypertriglyceridaemia is associated with increased cardiovascular risk (possibly not a causal association) and predisposes to pancreatitis. Statins and fibrates independently increase the risk of myositis, and the combination is potentially hazardous.

5.50   Answer: D

Causes emission of α-particles predominantly (poor penetration and range) and, to a lesser extent, gamma rays (higher penetration). 10–15% require further radio-iodine. Women of childbearing age should avoid pregnancy for at least 4 months.

5.51   Answer: B

Typically, patients have hypertension resistant to conventional therapy and thought present in 2–10% of all hypertensive patients. Good blood pressure and electrolyte response to spironolactone. Cushing's could cause the same abnormalities, but would be expected to manifest other clinical features.

5.52 A 60-year-old man is found to have resistant hypertension, and investigations show hypokalaemic alkalosis. Two weeks after commencing spironolactone therapy his blood pressure is found to have decreased from 182/95 mmHg to 156/82 mmHg and his metabolic disturbance has resolved. What is the most likely underlying cause of his hypertension?

A Adrenal carcinoma

B Benign adenoma in adrenal cortex

C Diffuse hyperplasia of the adrenal medulla

D Phaeochromocytoma

E Severe essential hypertension

5.53 A 24-year-old man is referred to the Medical Outpatient Department for assessment of anorexia and weight loss over the past 6 months. On examination, he is found to have 22 mmHg difference between seated and standing systolic blood pressure readings. Investigations show Na⁺ 132 mmol/l, K⁺ 4.7 mmol/l and ESR 28 mm/h. What is the most likely diagnosis?

A Addison's disease

B Conn's syndrome

C Diabetes insipidus

D Diabetes mellitus

E Tuberculosis

5.54 A 34-year-old man is found to have adrenal insufficiency. He is taking no regular treatments, and has never taken corticosteroid therapy. Which of these is the most likely underlying cause?

A Adrenal infarction secondary to hyperviscosity syndrome

B Adrenal metastases from prostatic carcinoma

C Anti-aldosterone antibody production in SLE

D Autoimmune polyglandular syndrome type 1

E Haemorrhagic adrenal infarction secondary to sepsis

5.52   Answer: B

Scenario strongly suggestive of hyperaldosteronism. Single functional adrenocortical adenoma (Conn's syndrome) accounts for 75% of cases.

5.53   Answer: A

Other features include pigmentation (generalised or in creases), arthralgia, symptoms resembling hypoglycaemia, and investigations also show modestly elevated urea and calcium, and eosinophilia.

5.54   Answer: D

70% cases of primary hypoaldosteronism are autoimmune, which can be part of APS type 1 or 2. Adrenal metastases can occur from lung, renal or breast carcinoma or lymphoma, but this is uncommon in young patients.

5.55   A 43-year-old woman is found to have adrenal insufficiency in the context of a number of other autoimmune disorders. Which of the following features most strongly suggests autoimmune polyglandular syndrome type 1?

☐ **A**   Autosomal dominant familial pattern

☐ **B**   Diabetes insipidus

☐ **C**   Hypoparathyroidism

☐ **D**   Primary gonadal failure

☐ **E**   Vitiligo

5.56   A 32-year-old woman is referred to the local Hypertension Clinic for investigation of high blood pressure. Recordings have been highly variable ranging from 148/86 to 182/106 mmHg with no obvious diurnal pattern. Which of the following is the most appropriate initial test in screening for underlying phaeochromocytoma?

☐ **A**   24-h urinary free catecholamine measurement

☐ **B**   24-h urinary metanephrine measurement

☐ **C**   Clonidine suppression test

☐ **D** ^{123}I-labelled MIBG scan

☐ **E**   Plasma catecholamines

5.57   A 46-year-old man presents with a 1-year history of intermittent headaches and dizziness. Blood pressure is found to be 144/92 mmHg seated, and 126/84 mmHg standing. 24-h cardiac monitoring shows pulse rate varying between 92 and 132 per min in sinus rhythm. What is the most likely underlying diagnosis?

☐ **A**   Addison's disease

☐ **B**   Adrenal carcinoma

☐ **C**   Generalised anxiety disorder

☐ **D**   Hyperthyroidism

☐ **E**   Phaeochromocytoma

5.55 Answer: C

Not seen in APS-2. The features of APS-1 are chronic candidiasis, adrenal insufficiency, hypoparathyroidism, primary hypogonadism and hypothyroidism, and (rarely) hypopituitarism and diabetes insipidus.

5.56 Answer: A

Should be performed at least twice because of variability in readings. Free catecholamine assay is more sensitive than metabolites (metanephrine and vanillyl mandelic acid (VMA)). Suppression tests are reserved for cases were diagnosis is questionable, and MIBG scans are used for localisation rather than diagnosis.

5.57 Answer: E

Hypertension and postural hypotension are characteristic features, the latter due to functional stiffening of the blood vessels. Diagnosis should be confirmed by at least 2×24-h urinary catecholamine assays.

5.58 A 36-year-old woman attends the Obesity Clinic for assessment. She has had amenorrhoea for 5 months. On examination, she weighs 92 kg, blood pressure is 156/86 mmHg and she has marked hirsutism. What is the most likely cause?

A Androgen-secreting ovarian tumour

B Congenital adrenal hyperplasia

C Cushing's syndrome

D Polycystic ovary disease

E Pregnancy

5.59 A 23-year-old woman is referred to the Endocrinology Department for assessment of amenorrhoea for the past 4 months. Her weight has decreased from 72 kg to 58 kg over the past 6 months. What is the most likely cause of her amenorrhoea?

A Excessive exercise

B Gastric carcinoma

C Pregnancy

D Premature ovarian failure

E Turner's syndrome

5.60 You are asked for advice regarding hormone replacement therapy (HRT) in a 61-year-old woman with symptoms of hot flushes. Which statement most correctly describes the role of HRT?

A Can lower systemic blood pressure

B Improves overall survival

C Increases overall cardiovascular risk

D Reduces symptoms of vaginal dryness

E Should be considered in all women aged 45 years or more

5.58 Answer: D

If virilisation features are prominent, then an androgen-secreting tumour may need to be sought (eg adrenal or ovarian). Amenorrhoea is not a characteristic feature of Cushing's syndrome.

5.59 Answer: A

Although weight loss alone would be sufficient; may suggest anorexia. Pregnancy should be excluded; however, weight loss makes this less likely. Turner's syndrome and Kallman's syndrome cause primary amenorrhoea.

5.60 Answer: D

HRT offers effective symptomatic relief for hot flushes and other post-menopausal symptoms. There is a reduction in cardiovascular disease risk and improvement in bone mineral density, offset by an increased risk of hepatobiliary disease and thromboembolism.

5.61 A 23-year-old man is undergoing investigation of hypogonadism in the Medical Outpatient Department. He is taking no prescribed medications, and there is no family history of note. He has noted altered taste sensation over the past few months. On examination, he is found to have a cleft palate and mild impairment of coordination in upper and lower limbs. What is the most likely diagnosis?

- [ ] A Anabolic steroid misuse
- [ ] B Haemochromatosis
- [ ] C Kallman's syndrome
- [ ] D Prader–Willi syndrome
- [ ] E Recreational drug use

5.62 A 61-year-old man attends the Diabetic Outpatient Department for routine follow-up. He mentions that he has been impotent for some time, and is interested in possible treatment. Which of these statements best characterises the role of sildenafil in this situation?

- [ ] A Ineffective in patients with type 2 diabetes
- [ ] B Normally taken orally 12 h before intercourse attempted
- [ ] C Sudden cardiac death is a recognised adverse effect
- [ ] D Therapeutic effects enhanced by nitrate co-administration
- [ ] E Therapeutic effects mediated by enhanced cyclic AMP

5.63 Which of the following factors most strongly indicates the need for surgical intervention in primary hyperparathyroidism?

- [ ] A Chronic renal impairment
- [ ] B Impaired liver function
- [ ] C Patient < 50 years age
- [ ] D Serum calcium 2.60 mmol/l or above
- [ ] E Single episode of ureteric colic

5.61   Answer: C

Genetic defect resulting in anosmia (manifests as loss of smell and taste), cleft lip and palate, sensorineural deafness and cerebellar ataxia. Recreational drug use and haemochromatosis are recognised causes of hypogonadism, but do not account for the other features.

5.62   Answer: C

Mostly in patients with pre-existing heart disease. Potentially hazardous interaction with nitrate therapy causing hypotension. Treatment is given as a single 50–100 mg dose 1 h before intercourse.

5.63   Answer: A

Other criteria are serum calcium > 3.00 mmol/l, urinary calcium excretion of > 10 mmol/day, nephrocalcinosis, recurrent ureteric calculi and evidence of bone disease. Less strict criteria are young age, patient preference and single episode of calculus disease.

5.64 A 43-year-old woman is referred to the Endocrinology Outpatient Department for assessment of a number of metabolic abnormalities. Ca^{2+} is 2.45 mmol/l, phosphate is 0.2 mmol/l, bicarbonate 12 mmol/l and dipstick urinalysis shows ketones + and glucose +++. What is the most likely underlying diagnosis?

- [ ] **A** Bartter's syndrome
- [ ] **B** Diabetic ketoacidosis
- [ ] **C** Fanconi's syndrome
- [ ] **D** Felty's syndrome
- [ ] **E** Lactic acidosis

5.65 You are reviewing a 56-year-old woman in the Outpatient Department following a recent fall and fractured left hip. You suspect probably underlying osteoporosis. Which lifestyle modification is most likely to be effective in delaying further bone loss in this condition?

- [ ] **A** Daily calcium 10 mg supplementation
- [ ] **B** High-protein diet
- [ ] **C** Increased fresh fruit in the diet
- [ ] **D** Non-weight-bearing exercise
- [ ] **E** Smoking cessation

5.66 A 51-year-old man with longstanding diabetes is referred to the Medical Outpatient Department for investigation of his right foot. He had fallen 4 weeks earlier, and X-rays of the foot and ankle at that time showed no fractures. On examination, the left foot feels warmer than the right, and peripheral pulses are intact. A repeat X-ray is normal, and bone scintigraphy shows increased uptake overlying the left foot. What is the most likely diagnosis?

- [ ] **A** Avascular necrosis
- [ ] **B** Charcot neuroarthropathy
- [ ] **C** Osteomyelitis
- [ ] **D** Reflex sympathetic dystrophy
- [ ] **E** Stress fracture

5.64 Answer: C

Characteristic renal wasting of glucose, bicarbonate, phosphate and amino acids due to tubular defect, often leading to osteomalacia.

5.65 Answer: E

Other measures that can be effective include moderation of alcohol intake, weight-bearing and high-impact exercise (eg skipping, jogging) and calcium-rich diet: calcium 1 g daily reduces fracture risk in older patients.

5.66 Answer: B

Diabetes is the commonest cause of this disorder. Peripheral pulses are often intact, whereas there is usually evidence of a sensory neuropathy. It may be precipitated by minor trauma.

5.67 A 43-year-old man presents to the Emergency Department with a 12-h history of loin and back pain, fever and rigors. Examination shows temperature 39.4°C. Investigations show Na⁺ 134 mmol/l, K⁺ 5.4 mmol/l, urea 25 mmol/l, creatinine 164 µmol/l, bicarbonate 12 mmol/l, serum osmolality 332 mOsm/kg. What is the most likely diagnosis?

- A   Alcoholic hepatitis
- B   Diabetic ketoacidosis
- C   Lactic acidosis
- D   Methanol ingestion
- E   Pancreatitis

5.68 A 45-year-old man has had well-controlled diabetes, since age 18 years of age. What finding would be most likely on physical examination?

- A   Background diabetic retinopathy
- B   Hepatomegaly
- C   Hypertension
- D   Lipoatrophy
- E   Peripheral sensorimotor neuropathy

5.69 A 28-year-old man is admitted to the High Dependency Unit via the Emergency Department with diabetic ketoacidosis. Which one of these statements is most accurate with respect to his initial management?

- A   Hydration should provide 1.5 l in the first 24 h
- B   Hyponatraemia should be corrected rapidly
- C   Potassium supplements should be withheld in the first hour
- D   Resuscitation should be with saline only
- E   Urine output should be monitored at least hourly in the first 24 h

5.67   Answer: B

Osmolality is very high. Estimated by [(Na + K) × 2 + urea + glucose], therefore glucose is probably 27 mmol/l.

5.68   Answer: A

Background (non-proliferative) retinopathy is dependent on the duration of diabetes, and is present in around 80% of patients who have had diabetes for 20 years or more.

5.69   Answer: E

The mainstay of treatment is fluid replacement, insulin administration and careful monitoring of fluid balance and electrolyte status.

5.70 A 34-year-old man is admitted via the Emergency Department following a collapse and reduced conscious level. He has had longstanding diabetes, which has been well controlled with insulin. On arrival in the Emergency Department, a BM glucose reading was 1.0 mmol/l and his conscious level responded rapidly to administration of intravenous glucose. What test will be most helpful in establishing the underlying cause of his hypoglycaemia?

   A HbA1c

   B Post-prandial glucose

   C Serum insulin concentration

   D Short synacthen test

   E Urinary C-peptide excretion

5.71 A 30-year-old woman is referred to the Endocrinology Department for investigation of weight loss despite a healthy appetite. Thyroid function tests show free T_4 = 36 pmol/l and TSH is undetectable. Which of the following signs is most likely to be present on examination?

   A Atrial fibrillation

   B Bitemporal hemianopia

   C Exophthalmos

   D Lid lag

   E Pretibial myxoedema

5.72 A 55-year-old woman attending the Hypertension Clinic is found to have elevated 24-h urinary catecholamine excretion on two successive tests, suggesting a diagnosis of phaeochromocytoma. Which of the following statements is most accurate regarding this condition?

   A Around one-third are malignant

   B Family history is common

   C More than 85% are solitary adrenal medullary tumours

   D Radiolabelled iodine is a recognised treatment

   E Surgical resection normalises blood pressure in > 95% of patients

5.70   Answer: A

The most common explanation for hypoglycaemia is overly-aggressive insulin therapy, which will be reflected by a low HbA1c concentration. In some cases, Addison's disease should be considered an alternative diagnosis.

5.71   Answer: D

This is a feature of hyperthyroid states, as is tachycardia. Atrial fibrillation is a less consistent complication, and exophthalmos and pretibial skin changes are features of Graves' disease regardless of thyroid state.

5.72   Answer: C

Around 10–15% are diffuse, bilateral or extramedullary. Between 8 and 12% are malignant. Radioiodine-labelled metaiodobenzylguanidine MIBG can help localise functionally active tumour. Surgical correction alleviates symptoms and can make hypertension easier to control with conventional therapy; in only a small proportion of patients can treatment be completely withdrawn.

5.73 A 56-year-old man with diabetes since childhood is referred to the General Medical Outpatient Department for assessment. Over the past 6 weeks, he has been complaining of increased sweating and abdominal bloating. He also describes blurred vision on rising from bed in the mornings associated with dizziness. What is the best explanation for his symptoms?

- [ ] A Addison's disease
- [ ] B Autonomic neuropathy
- [ ] C Nocturnal hypoglycaemia
- [ ] D Postural hypotension
- [ ] E Thyrotoxicosis

5.74 A 34-year-old woman is 24 weeks pregnant. She is referred for further assessment because her weight gain has been much greater than anticipated. In addition, her husband is concerned that she has become harder to rouse from sleep in the mornings and has been rather confused after waking. What is the most likely diagnosis?

- [ ] A Alcoholism
- [ ] B Gestational diabetes
- [ ] C Glucagonoma
- [ ] D Hepatic failure
- [ ] E Insulinoma

5.75 Which of the following is most likely to be associated with increased insulin sensitivity?

- [ ] A Acromegaly
- [ ] B Smoking cessation
- [ ] C Phaechromocytoma
- [ ] D Polycystic ovary disease
- [ ] E Weight loss

5.73   Answer: B

Blurred vision and dizziness are suggestive of postural hypotension; additional features of excessive sweating and abdominal bloating suggest a more generalised autonomic impairment. Other features include gustatory sweating, gastroparesis, vomiting and diarrhoea.

5.74   Answer: E

Uncommon cause of hypoglycaemia, typically associated with weight gain. Can be demonstrated by prolonged fasting, up to 72 h. Other causes of hypoglycaemia include soft tissue sarcomata that secrete insulin-like growth factor, liver disease and alcoholism.

5.75   Answer: E

This has been shown to completely normalise insulin sensitivity in obese patients with impaired glucose tolerance. Smoking cessation would be expected to increase sensitivity, but this has not been demonstrated so convincingly. The other listed condtions are associated with increased insulin resistance.

6. GASTROENTEROLOGY

6.1 You see a 65-year-old woman in the Medical Outpatient Department who has been referred for investigation of weight loss, anorexia and iron deficiency anaemia. Which of these initial investigations would be most helpful?

- [ ] **A** Abdominal ultrasound scan
- [ ] **B** Barium enema
- [ ] **C** Faecal fat measurement
- [ ] **D** Mesenteric angiography
- [ ] **E** Sigmoidoscopy

6.2 A 34-year-old woman attends the Gastroenterology Clinic for investigation of intermittent crampy abdominal pain. On examination, you note that she has oral ulceration, glossitis and angular stomatitis. Which of the following diagnoses is most likely to cause these physical findings?

- [ ] **A** Coeliac disease
- [ ] **B** Erythema multiforme
- [ ] **C** Peutz–Jeghers syndrome
- [ ] **D** Porphyria
- [ ] **E** Ulcerative colitis

6.3 A 65-year-old man attends his GP complaining of 'food sticking in his throat'. Which of the following is correct regarding oesophageal dysphagia?

- [ ] **A** Bolus transit time is usually not affected
- [ ] **B** Characteristically there is difficulty initiating swallowing
- [ ] **C** Dysphagia for solids is usually due to altered oesophageal motility
- [ ] **D** Functional dysphagia can be intermittent and non-progressive
- [ ] **E** Stricture (benign or malignant) is an uncommon cause

6.1   Answer: B

Need to exclude caecal carcinoma; colonoscopy is an alternative. Angiography technically difficult, false positives.

6.2   Answer: A

Coeliac disease also associated with dermatitis herpetiformis. Erythema multiforme gives target-like rash with mucosal blistering and ulceration. Peutz–Jeghers syndrome involves mucosal freckling and intestinal polyposis. Oral ulceration can be a feature of Crohn's disease, but not ulcerative colitis.

6.3   Answer: D

Bolus transit time is reduced, or completely impeded. Dysphagia for solids is most commonly due to structural lesion, most commonly a stricture. Oropharyngeal dysphagia more typically causes difficulty initiating swallowing, and may be associated with nasopharyngeal regurgitation.

6.4   A 37-year-old woman attends the Emergency Department after sudden onset of moderately severe central chest pain associated with nausea and sweating. Physical examination is normal, and serial ECGs show sinus rhythm and normal morphology. Oesophageal spasm is thought the most likely explanation for her symptoms. Which of the following statements related to oesophageal spasm is correct?

◻ A   10% of patients with recurrent non-cardiac chest pain have oesophageal dysfunction

◻ B   Can be provoked by food ingestion

◻ C   It is a recognised cause of globus

◻ D   Pain can be relieved by sublingual GTN

◻ E   Rarely associated with gastro-oesophageal reflux

6.5   A 32-year-old nurse on your ward has been self-administering omeprazole, bought as an over-the-counter preparation for intermittent dyspepsia. She has experienced good relief from her symptoms and asks you for some advice. To what extent are proton pump inhibitors capable of reducing gastric acid secretion?

◻ A   25–30%

◻ B   55–60%

◻ C   75–80%

◻ D   90–95%

◻ E   > 99%

6.6   You review a 56-year-old woman in the Medical Outpatient Department following recent inpatient investigation of dyspepsia. At that time she had been commenced on regular therapy with omeprazole 20 mg bd. Which of the following is a characteristic adverse effect of proton pump inhibitor therapy?

◻ A   Constipation

◻ B   Headache

◻ C   Salmonellosis

◻ D   Viral gastroenteritis

◻ E   Visual disturbance

6.4   Answer: B

Can be provoked by food ingestion or reflux, but no obvious precipitant in most cases. Up to 50% of patients with recurrent non-cardiac chest pain have oesophageal dysfunction. Globus (lump in throat sensation) occurs at laryngeal level.

6.5   Answer: E

pH would increase by 3 following a 1000-fold reduction in H^+ secretion, and rise by 4 after a 10,000-fold reduction.

6.6   Answer: C

Reduced stomach acid defences predispose to gastroenteritis, particularly that caused by salmonella and other bacteria. Diarrhoea is a characteristic adverse effect, particularly in patients treated with lansoprazole. Administration of lansoprazole 30 mg daily suppresses gastric acid production by 50–75% overall, whereas administration of omeprazole 40 mg daily suppresses acid production by 75–100%.

6.7 You see a 56-year-old woman in the General Medical Clinic, who presents with a 9-month history of dyspepsia, aggravated by spicy food. You diagnose reflux oesophagitis and treat her with regular oral omeprazole, which gives good relief of her symptoms. Which of the following statements best describes the role of long-term proton pump inhibitor treatment of reflux?

- A   Causes complete regression of Barrett's metaplasia
- B   Increases the risk of gastric cancer
- C   Offers symptomatic relief in most cases
- D   Reduces the need for endoscopy examination
- E   This is the optimal treatment for reflux

6.8 A 56-year-old woman is investigated for symptoms of progressive dysphagia, and is diagnosed with benign oesophageal stricture. Which of the following conditions is most likely to have caused this disorder?

- A   Accidental ingestion of bleach 6 years before
- B   Achalasia
- C   Barrett's oesophagus
- D   Longstanding gastro-oesophageal reflux
- E   Prolonged nasogastric tube insertion 1 year earlier

6.9 A 32-year-old woman attends the Gastroenterology Outpatient Department for investigation of retrosternal pain after swallowing, which is worst after solid foods. Which of the following conditions is most likely to account for her symptoms?

- A   Achalasia
- B   Herpes simplex oesophagitis
- C   Mallory–Weiss syndrome
- D   Oesophageal pouch
- E   Plummer–Vinson syndrome

6.7 Answer: C

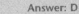

Around 25% of patients respond to simple antacids and addressing lifestyle factors. There is no clear evidence that treatment reduces Barrett's metaplasia, and endoscopy surveillance is still required. Long-term omeprazole does not appear to increase gastric cancer risk in humans.

6.8 Answer: D

So-called peptic stricture is the most common cause. Other recognised causes include corrosive ingestion, prolonged nasogastric tube insertion and radiotherapy.

6.9 Answer: B

Oesophagitis can cause severe pain on swallowing, whereas the other conditions listed are typically painless.

6.10 You are asked to review a 38-year-old man, who has regularly been attending the Infectious Diseases Unit for the past 4 years. He has been complaining of progressively worsening odynophagia over the past 5 weeks. Which of the following conditions is most likely to account for his symptoms?

- [ ] **A** Benign oesophageal stricture
- [ ] **B** Gastro-oesophageal reflux
- [ ] **C** Herpes simplex oesophagitis
- [ ] **D** Oesophageal lymphoma
- [ ] **E** Oesophageal perforation

6.11 You are asked to review a 62-year-old man in the Medical Outpatient Department. For the past 7 weeks, he has complained of progressive difficulty swallowing. He has lost around 15 kg weight in the past year. Which of the following factors is most strongly associated with underlying oesophageal carcinoma?

- [ ] **A** Abstinent from alcohol
- [ ] **B** Achalasia
- [ ] **C** High dietary intake of root vegetables
- [ ] **D** History of intermittent febrile illness
- [ ] **E** Hypertension

6.12 You are asked to review a male patient in your Gastroenterology Outpatient Clinic for consideration of an upper GI endoscopy. He has been complaining of progressive dysphagia for 4 months, associated with intermittent dyspepsia. Which of the following factors is most likely to increase the risk of underlying oesophageal carcinoma?

- [ ] **A** 5 kg weight loss in past 4 months
- [ ] **B** Age 60–70 years
- [ ] **C** History of intermittent dysphagia
- [ ] **D** Strong family history of oesophageal carcinoma
- [ ] **E** Dysphagia for liquids only

6.10 Answer: C

Oesophagitis is particularly common in immunocompromised patients, eg HIV positive, corticosteroid users, and can be due to candida, HSV, CMV.

6.11 Answer: B

Other risk factors are tobacco use, heavy alcohol intake, Plummer–Vinson syndrome, coeliac disease and long-standing gastro-oesophageal reflux. Diets high in cereal and N-nitroso compounds appear to increase risk.

6.12 Answer: B

Weight loss is common in dysphagia, typically associated with increased appetite with benign strictures, and anorexia with carcinoma.

6.13 An elderly female patient is referred to the Medical Outpatient Department for investigation of progressive weight loss and dysphagia over the past 6 months. Which of the following investigations is most appropriate for initial investigation of her symptoms?

  A   Abdominal ultrasound scan

  B   Barium swallow

  C   Cervical lymph node biopsy

  D   CT scan thorax

  E   Plain chest X-ray

6.14 You refer a 32-year-old man for upper GI endoscopy for investigation of dyspepsia. A report indicates that he is positive for *Helicobacter pylori*, and you wish to explain the significance of this finding to him at a subsequent review. Which of the following statements is most accurate with respect to *H. pylori*?

  A   Faeco–oral transmission is thought to be common

  B   Infection confers a 3- to 4-fold increased risk of gastric carcinoma

  C   Nasal droplet spread is believed to be the main route of transmission

  D   Prevalence is around 10–15% in Western societies

  E   Prevalence is highest in young people, aged < 35 years

6.15 One of the nursing staff on your ward has been experiencing intermittent dyspepsia. She has read some information on the internet about *H. pylori* infection, and wondered how to test for this. Which of the following is the most sensitive test for detecting gastrointestinal infection with *H. pylori*?

  A   Blood culture and sensitivities

  B ^{13}C-urea breath test

  C   IgG antibody titres

  D   IgM antibody titres

  E   Stool culture

6.13   Answer: B

Alternatively, endoscopy is a useful first investigation that allows biopsy, but intraluminal tumour (eg lymphoma) can be overlooked. CT or endoscopic ultrasound is useful for assessing the extent of spread and lymph node involvement.

6.14   Answer: A

Route of transmission not entirely clear, but thought most likely due to ingestion of fomites, oral–oral or faeco–oral routes. Prevalence is 40–70% in developed nations, 80–90% in developing nations. Prevalence is much higher in older patient groups.

6.15   Answer: B

Sensitivity 98%, specificity 95%. Stool cultures have 90% sensitivity and 95% specificity, and IgG titres have 85% sensitivity. Breath testing can be used to confirm eradication after treatment.

6.16   A 64-year-old lifelong smoker presents with a 3-month history of weight loss and progressive dysphagia. He is found to weigh 46 kg and an irregular, hard liver edge is palpable. Which of the following is the most likely explanation for his symptoms?

☐ A   Adenocarcinoma of the upper oesophagus

☐ B   Adenocarcinoma of the lower third of the oesophagus

☐ C   Metastatic thyroid carcinoma

☐ D   Oesophageal lymphoma

☐ E   Squamous carcinoma of the lower third of the oesophagus

6.17   A 51-year-old man presents with a 2-month history of 14 kg weight loss and fatigue. Upper GI endoscopy is reported as normal. He is seen in Clinic and reports progressive dysphagia for solids over the past 4 weeks. Which of the following investigations would be most helpful next?

☐ A   Barium swallow

☐ B   Coeliac antibody screening

☐ C   CT scan of thorax

☐ D   Iron studies

☐ E   Plain chest X-ray

6.18   A 34-year-old patient presents with epigastric pain radiating to the back, associated with haematemesis. Endoscopy reveals a 2 × 2 cm peptic ulcer and he is commenced on omeprazole 40 mg daily. Which of the following statements regarding its mechanism of action is correct?

☐ A   Blocks H^+ release from G-cells

☐ B   Enhances HCO_3^- release from G-cells

☐ C   Increases chief cell secretions

☐ D   Inhibits H^+ release from parietal cells

☐ E   Potentiates the effects of gastrin

6.16   Answer: B
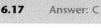

These account for around 45% of all oesophageal malignancies. Squamous carcinoma of the middle part of the oesophagus accounts for around 40%. Lymphoma is less common and can be more diffuse and submucosal.

6.17   Answer: C

Endoscopy can miss important diagnoses: extrinsic compressive tumours, and submucosal intrinsic oesophageal lesions (eg lymphoma). Obstruction can be demonstrated in some cases by barium swallow, but CT is more detailed and the investigation of choice, or endoscopic ultrasound.

6.18   Answer: D

Parietal cells are responsible for H^+ and intrinsic factor secretion, chief cells secrete pepsinogen, whilst G-cells secrete gastrin (which stimulates parietal cell H^+ secretion).

6.19 A 52-year-old man is admitted to hospital after suspected haematemesis. Which of the following statements most accurately describes this condition?

☐ A 20–30% of patients require surgery to stop blood loss

☐ B 75% of patients have had a similar admission in the past 12 months

☐ C Bleeding resolves spontaneously in 30–40% within 48 h

☐ D Early endoscopy is recommended for all patients

☐ E Shock suggests a significant volume blood loss

6.20 A 26-year-old man is admitted at the weekend with a short history of vomiting and haematemesis. At 24 h after admission, his vomiting has settled and you are asked to decide if he can be discharged. Which of the following factors most strongly suggests the patient is medically fit for discharge?

☐ A Abdominal examination normal

☐ B Blood pressure normal

☐ C Endoscopy finds no evidence of recent bleeding

☐ D Family history of peptic ulcer disease

☐ E Repeat haemoglobin is 12.2 g/dl

6.21 A GP telephones you for advice. One of his patients has been found to have a positive 'faecal occult blood (FOB)' stool test during a general health-check. The patient is a 42-year-old banker who does not report any specific abdominal symptoms. Which of the following represents the best course of initial action?

☐ A Admit for urgent inpatient investigation

☐ B Arrange outpatient barium enema

☐ C Arrange outpatient colonoscopy

☐ D Repeat further stool FOB test

☐ E Request mesenteric angiography

6.22 Which of the following statements is correct with regard to gastrin?

☐ A Causes gastric pH to increase

☐ B Concentrations fall significantly during proton pump inhibitor (PPI) treatment

☐ C Inhibits parietal cell secretion

☐ D Mainly located in the gastric cardia

☐ E Stimulates gastric mucosa growth

6.19   Answer: E

Bleeding resolves spontaneously in around 90% within 48 h, and the use of urgent endoscopy is best directed towards those requiring endoscopic treatment, or where the diagnosis will alter immediate patient management. Shocked patients should receive blood transfusion early.

6.20   Answer: C

Patients can normally be discharged safely at 24 h if they are haemodynamically stable (best assessed by heart rate in young person than BP alone) and the endoscopy suggest no ongoing blood loss.

6.21   Answer: D

FOB tests are generally only of value if there is suspected gastrointestinal blood loss or unexplained anaemia. There is a high false positive rate and, in the absence of symptoms or signs, investigations will have a very low yield.

6.22   Answer: E

Gastrin located mainly in the fundus, stimulates acid secretion by parietal cells, hence pH falls. Gastrin concentrations not altered directly by PPI treatment.

6.23 Which of the following statements best describes the role of motilin?

☐ A Causes smooth muscle relaxation

☐ B Circulating levels increase during erythromycin treatment

☐ C Decreases the rate of gastric emptying

☐ D Relaxes the lower oesophageal sphincter

☐ E Secreted only by pancreatic β cells

6.24 A number of peptides are involved in regulation of gut motility. Which of the following statements best describes their role in normal gastrointestinal physiology?

☐ A Cholecystokinin inhibits gut motility

☐ B Ghrelin enhances gastric emptying and appetite

☐ C Glucagon-like peptide 1 (GLP-1) inhibits insulin secretion

☐ D Motilin stimulates colonic propulsion

☐ E Vasoactive intestinal polypeptide (VIP) inhibits small bowel secretion

6.25 A 35-year-old woman is referred to the Gastroenterology Outpatient Department for investigation of intermittent abdominal pain and bloating over the past 6 months. On direct questioning, she reveals that her stools have been pale and more difficult to flush away than usual. Which of the following is the most likely explanation?

☐ A Achalasia of the oesophagus

☐ B Coeliac disease

☐ C Crohn's disease

☐ D Meckle's diverticulum

☐ E Ulcerative colitis

6.26 A 44-year-old woman has longstanding coeliac disease, and is referred to the General Medical Outpatient Department for investigation of anaemia. Her results show Hb 9.8 g/dl and MCV 97 fl. Which of the following initial investigations would be most helpful in determining her subsequent management?

☐ A Blood film microscopy

☐ B Dipstick urinalysis

☐ C Serum urea and electrolytes

☐ D Faecal occult blood test

☐ E ESR and serum calcium

6.23   Answer: B

Motilin stimulates gastric emptying and small bowel propulsion. It is secreted from the whole GI tract and metabolised by the liver. Erythromycin is an enzyme inhibitor that increases motilin levels (GI adverse effect of drug).

6.24   Answer: B

Ghrelin antagonists are being examined as potential adjuncts to aid weight loss. Cholecystokinin stimulates colonic motility, GLP-1 stimulates insulin release and VIP increases intestinal secretion.

6.25   Answer: B

The history of steatorrhoea strongly suggests small bowel malabsorption. This can be a feature of Crohn's disease, but is less likely in the absence of any other constitutional features.

6.26   Answer: A

This will help distinguish a normocytic anaemia from a diamorphic anaemia caused by mixed folate and iron deficiency.

6.27 A 52-year-old woman presents to the Outpatient Department with a 5-month history of passing pale stools that smell offensive and are difficult to flush away. Which of the following statements best describes confirmation of fat malabsorption?

A Breath $^{14}CO_2$ after labelled-fat administration can be used to indicate the extent of fat malabsorption

B Faecal fat > 8 g per day is diagnostic

C Impaired triglyceride absorption indicates pancreatic dysfunction

D Stool densiometry is a valuable diagnostic test

E Vitamin B_{12} deficiency often co-exists with fat malabsorption

6.28 A 59-year-old man is referred to the General Medical Outpatient Department for investigation of intermittent crampy abdominal pain and bloating over the past 9 months. Which one of the following is most appropriate regarding the possible diagnosis of coeliac disease?

A 1–2% of first-degree relatives will have the disease

B 90% of patients have HLA DQ2

C B cell lymphocytes play a central role in aetiology

D Oats typically cause small bowel mucosal atrophy

E Prevalence in Ireland is around 1 in 1500

6.29 You are reviewing a middle-aged woman in the Medical Outpatient Department, who is undergoing investigation of iron deficiency anaemia. Gastroscopy and colonoscopy investigations are normal. Which of the following factors would most strongly suggest a diagnosis of coeliac disease?

A Co-existent folate deficiency

B IgA endomysial antibodies

C Poor haemoglobin response to iron therapy

D Positive anti-reticulin antibody

E Thickened small bowel mucosal folds on barium follow-through

6.27   Answer: A

Diagnosis can be confirmed by faecal fat > 6 g/day during standard 100 g/day diet. Impaired triglyceride absorption is a feature of pancreatic and small bowel pathology. Often associated with malabsorption of fat-soluble vitamins (A, D, E and K).

6.28   Answer: B

This haplotype is found in only 25% of the normal population. 10–20% of first-degree relatives are affected, and the prevalence is around 1 in 250 in the UK and 1 in 150 in Ireland, although often clinically silent. Oats are not harmful; gluten is contained in cereals.

6.29   Answer: B

The other stems are recognised features, but only this test is sensitive and specific for coeliac disease. Up to 20% of patients are IgA deficient; this should be measured simultaneously to avoid false negative tests.

6.30   A 48-year-old woman has recently been attending the
Gastroenterology Department and is diagnosed with coeliac disease.
During a further attendance she asks for your opinion on a
blistering rash that has erupted around both elbows and her left
forearm. Which of the following is the most likely diagnosis?

☐ **A** Acne rosacea

☐ **B** Dermatitis herpetiformis

☐ **C** Erythema ab igne

☐ **D** Fixed drug eruption

☐ **E** Herpes simplex dermatitis

6.31   A 50-year-old man is admitted to the General Medical Ward for
investigations for weight loss and malabsorption. You note an
erythematous rash with multiple small vesicles, and suspect
dermatitis herpetiformis. Which of the following represents the best
immediate management of this patient?

☐ **A** Calorie controlled diet

☐ **B** Dapsone therapy

☐ **C** Gluten free diet

☐ **D** Oral co-amoxiclav

☐ **E** Topical hydrocortisone

6.32   You see a 42-year-old woman in the Medical Outpatient
Department. Her GP performed a full blood count and found Hb
9.2 g/dl and MCV 126 fl. Which of the following is the most likely
explanation for these findings?

☐ **A** Excess alcohol intake

☐ **B** Hepatic steatosis

☐ **C** Hypothyroidism

☐ **D** Intestinal bacterial overgrowth

☐ **E** Ulcerative colitis

6.30   Answer: B

This is an unusual non-infective condition, associated with similar jejunal morphology to coeliac disease and malabsorption, although typically less severe.

6.31   Answer: C

Both malabsorption and rash in dermatitis herpetiformis will improve. Dapsone is at least partly effective against the skin rash, but will not improve absorption.

6.32   Answer: D

The findings suggest folate or vitamin B_{12} deficiency, rather than a simple macrocytosis. Vitamin B_{12} is normally absorbed in the terminal ileum. Reduced absorption due to overgrowth can be established by performing a Schilling test before and after antibiotic treatment.

6.33 Which of the following diagnostic tests is the most useful for establishing a diagnosis of intestinal bacterial overgrowth?

☐ A ^{14}C-glycocholate breath test

☐ B Blood cultures

☐ C Hydrogen breath test

☐ D Intubation and aspiration of intestinal fluid

☐ E Stool culture

6.34 A 37-year-old man is admitted to the Acute Medical Assessment Unit complaining of abdominal pain and vomiting for 12 h. He has a past history of extensive Crohn's disease, and underwent small bowel resection 8 months earlier. Which of the following offers the most likely explanation for his current presenting symptoms?

☐ A Addisonian crisis

☐ B Bacterial peritonitis

☐ C Bowel obstruction

☐ D Sulfasalazine toxicity

☐ E Viral gastroenteritis

6.35 A 40-year-old woman has recently undergone massive intestinal resection for extensive Crohn's disease, resulting in ileostomy formation. Her Crohn's disease is now quiescent, and you are preparing to discharge her home. Which of the following is a frequently recognised long-term complication?

☐ A Constipation

☐ B Hypercalcaemia

☐ C Osteoporosis

☐ D Peptic ulcer disease

☐ E Urinary calculi

6.33   Answer: C

This has largely replaced the ^{14}C-glycocholate breath test and gut aspiration, and depends on liberation of hydrogen from lactulose by intestinal bacteria.

6.34   Answer: C

Post-operative risk of adhesions and bowel obstruction higher in Crohn's disease.

6.35   Answer: E

Reduced bile salt absorption stimulates increased bile turnover and more frequent gallstone formation. Reduced fat and vitamin absorption is important. Bile salts entering the colon stimulate oxalate absorption, increasing the risk of urinary calculi.

6.36 A 58-year-old man is undergoing radiotherapy for metastatic bowel cancer. Shortly after his irradiation course, he develops nausea, abdominal pain and diarrhoea. Which of the following statements is correct in relation to radiation enteritis?

- [ ] A   Bleeding risk increases due to peptic ulcer disease
- [ ] B   Corticosteroids should be avoided
- [ ] C   Early surgery is indicated in most patients
- [ ] D   Malabsorption can occur due to bacterial overgrowth
- [ ] E   Risk is unrelated to dose of radiation

6.37 A 56-year-old man is admitted with a 4-week history of progressive ankle oedema and breathlessness. Investigations show serum albumin 17 g/l and creatinine 69 μmol/l, and dipstick urinalysis is normal. Four months ago, his serum albumin was normal. Which of the following diagnoses is the most likely explanation for his current findings?

- [ ] A   Congestive heart failure
- [ ] B   Glomerulosclerosis
- [ ] C   Malnutrition
- [ ] D   Membranous glomerulonephritis
- [ ] E   Protein-losing enteropathy

6.38 A 22-year-old medical student has recently returned from her 'elective', and is complaining of persistent diarrhoea and steatorrhoea, abdominal bloating and weight loss. Which of the following diagnoses is the most likely cause of her symptoms?

- [ ] A   Coeliac disease
- [ ] B   Crohn's colitis
- [ ] C   Giardiasis
- [ ] D   Hyperthyroidism
- [ ] E   Tropical sprue

6.36   Answer: D

Enteritis is associated with ulceration and ischaemia, which heal by scarring and formation of telangiectasia (which increase bleeding risk). Partial obstruction is common, and surgery should be reserved for only cases of suspected perforation or complete obstruction.

6.37   Answer: E

Absence of significant proteinuria should be checked in a formal biochemical measurement. Causes of protein-losing enteropathy include coeliac disease, Crohn's disease, Ménétrier's disease and lymphangiectasis. Hypoalbuminaemia occurs when liver synthetic function cannot match protein loss.

6.38   Answer: C

Infection with *Giardia intestinalis* is the commonest parasitic infection in travellers returning to the UK. Tropical sprue presents with a similar malabsorptive syndrome, usually after viral gastroenteritis.

Gastroenterology answers

6.39 A 58-year-old woman presents to hospital with sudden onset of central abdominal pain and vomiting. Her pulse is irregular, blood pressure 102/68 mmHg and abdomen tender with absent bowel sounds. Which of the following diagnoses requires most urgent consideration?

A Aortic aneurysm rupture

B Intestinal ischaemia

C Myocardial infarction

D Perforated duodenal ulcer

E Severe gastroenteritis

6.40 A 52-year-old woman is referred to the Gastroenterology Outpatient Clinic for investigation of abdominal pain and recurrent episodes of profuse watery diarrhoea. On examination she is found to have facial telangiectasis. Which of the following diagnoses is most likely to account for her symptoms?

A Churg–Strauss syndrome

B Crohn's disease

C Functional enterochromaffin cell malignancy

D Hereditary haemorrhagic telangiectasia

E Scleroderma

6.41 A 33-year-old man is admitted via the Emergency Department with sudden onset of abdominal pain and bloating, associated with severe nausea and vomiting. A plain abdominal X-ray suggests dilated loops of small intestine. Which of the following underlying diagnoses is most likely to explain these findings?

A Coeliac disease

B Peri-appendix abscess

C Peutz–Jeghers syndrome

D Plummer–Vincent syndrome

E Ulcerative colitis

6.39 Answer: B

Acute small bowel ischaemia is most commonly caused by thromboembolic occlusion of the superior mesenteric artery, eg in atrial fibrillation. Mortality is high, and early surgical resection of ischaemic bowel is indicated.

6.40 Answer: C

The features are consistent with carcinoid syndrome, which occurs in 5% of patients with carcinoid tumour, usually when there are liver metastases. Other features include tricuspid incompetence and pulmonary stenosis.

6.41 Answer: C

The associated polyps are usually hamartomas, most commonly found in the small intestine, which predispose to intussusception and obstruction. Other features typically include mucocutaneous pigmentation.

6.42 A 29-year-old man attends the Gastroenterology Outpatient Clinic for follow-up. There is a strong family history of intestinal polyposis thought due to Peutz–Jeghers syndrome. Which of these statements is correct regarding this condition?

- A Endoscopy and X-ray follow-up should be undertaken every 5 years
- B Extensive polyposis is best treated by small bowel resection
- C Genetic testing is not yet available
- D It is inherited in an X-linked recessive manner
- E Malignant transformation of polyps is a recognised complication

6.43 A 40-year-old woman is under regular review in the Gastroenterology Outpatient Clinic for ulcerative colitis. Which of the following best describes the familial basis of inflammatory bowel disease?

- A 3-fold increased prevalence amongst women versus men
- B 10-fold increased risk in first-degree relatives
- C Heritability is greater in ulcerative colitis than Crohn's disease
- D Incidence is falling due to effective patient counselling
- E Inherited in autosomal dominant manner with incomplete expression

6.44 A 42-year-old male smoker attends the Gastroenterology Outpatient Clinic for review of his ulcerative colitis. His clinical condition is stable, and you discuss the potential health benefits of smoking cessation. Which of the following statements is correct?

- A Continued smoking will not have any adverse gastrointestinal effects
- B Nicotine patches increase the frequency of colitis flare-ups
- C Regular smokers are slightly less likely to develop Crohn's disease
- D Smoking cessation might cause exacerbation of his colitis
- E Inflammatory bowel disease protects against cardiovascular disease

6.45 Which of the following is *not* recognised as an effective treatment for patients with inflammatory bowel disease?

- A 6-Mercaptopurine
- B Balsalazide
- C Hydrocortisone
- D *Lactobacillus* spp.
- E Rofecoxib

6.42   Answer: E

The Peutz–Jeghers (gene LKB1) is inherited in an autosomal dominant manner. Follow-up should be at least every 2 years in view of the risk of malignancy.

6.43   Answer: B

The incidence of ulcerative colitis is stable, whilst that of Crohn's is rising. Genetic factors, some related to human leukocyte antigen (HLA), appear to be important, but environmental factors are also of great importance.

6.44   Answer: D

Crohn's disease is much more common in smokers, whilst ulcerative colitis is less common. Nicotine protects against flare-ups in patients with ulcerative colitis. IBD patients might have increased cardiovascular risk due to longstanding corticosteroid use.

6.45   Answer: E

COX-2 selective NSAIDs appear to increase the frequency of disease relapse. The role of probiotics in IBD is not fully established, but they appear effective for pouchitis in Crohn's disease.

6.46 Which of the following statements is correct regarding the extra-gastrointestinal features of inflammatory bowel disease (IBD)?

A Ankylosing spondylitis occurs in 20% of patients with ulcerative colitis

B Cholelithiasis is common in ulcerative colitis

C Erythema nodosum is more common in ulcerative colitis than Crohn's

D Ocular complications occur in around 10% of IBD patients

E Ureteric calculi complicate ulcerative colitis but not Crohn's disease

6.47 A 31-year-old woman has been admitted for investigation of diarrhoea and abdominal pain. A presumptive diagnosis of inflammatory bowel disease has been made. Which of the following features would most strongly suggest Crohn's disease rather than ulcerative colitis?

A Anal fissure

B Anorectal fistula

C Arthralgia

D Fever symptoms

E Pyoderma gangrenosum

6.48 A middle-aged woman is undergoing outpatient investigation of diarrhoea, weight loss and abdominal pain. Which of the following barium enema findings would most strongly suggest a diagnosis of ulcerative colitis?

A Cobblestone appearance on barium enema

B Deep mucosal ulceration

C Loss of normal colonic features and superficial ulceration

D Narrowing and stricturing around the terminal ileum

E Obscuration of the psoas muscle outline

6.46 Answer: D

Including uveitis, episcleritis and conjunctivitis. Erythema nodosum and pyoderma gangrenosum, gall stones and ureteric stones are more common in Crohn's disease than ulcerative colitis.

6.47 Answer: B

Anal fissure and fistulae are more specific to Crohn's disease, particularly the latter. Arthralgia and pyoderma are more common but not specific to Crohn's disease.

6.48 Answer: C

Cobblestone appearance, with deep ulceration and stricturing is indicative of Crohn's disease. Loss of the psoas shadow on an adequately penetrated abdominal film suggests retroperitoneal fluid, and can be seen in acute flare-ups of colitis or proctitis.

6.49 A 38-year-old man attends the Gastroenterology Outpatient Clinic for review. He has had inflammatory bowel disease for 6 years, and is currently asymptomatic. Which of the following investigations is most useful in assessing disease activity?

- [ ] A ESR
- [ ] B IgA
- [ ] C Iron studies
- [ ] D p-ANCA
- [ ] E Serum calcium

6.50 Which of the following interventions is *least* likely to be of value in the management of Crohn's disease?

- [ ] A Acetaminophen
- [ ] B Codeine phosphate
- [ ] C Rectal hydrocortisone
- [ ] D Smoking cessation
- [ ] E Sulfasalazine

6.51 A 40-year-old man is admitted to hospital for assessment of his ulcerative colitis. Which of the following features most strongly suggests a severe attack?

- [ ] A 3–5 stools per day
- [ ] B Albumin 36 g/l
- [ ] C ESR 40 mm/h
- [ ] D Haemoglobin 10.9 g/dl
- [ ] E Temperature 37.3°C

6.52 A 29-year-old man has had ulcerative colitis for the past 3 years, usually maintained on balsalazide. He has been admitted with a severe attack, having had two recent hospital admissions for high dose corticosteroid treatment. Which of the following factors would most strongly indicate the need to consider surgical intervention?

- [ ] A Allergy to sulfasalazine
- [ ] B Excessive corticosteroid requirement
- [ ] C Failure of medical therapy to control sepsis
- [ ] D Number of previous hospital admissions
- [ ] E Patient preference

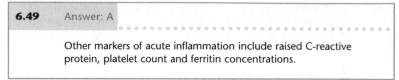

6.49   Answer: A

Other markers of acute inflammation include raised C-reactive protein, platelet count and ferritin concentrations.

6.50   Answer: A

Codeine can help reduce stool frequency; smoking cessation reduces the frequency of relapses.

6.51   Answer: C

Others include temperature > 37.5°C, haemoglobin < 10 g/dl and > 6 stools per day.

6.52   Answer: C

Other factors are active gastrointestinal haemorrhage, perforation or toxic bowel dilatation. Excess corticosteroid requirements, frequent admissions and patient choice are important considerations in chronic management.

6.53   A 41-year-old woman has been admitted for a relapse of Crohn's colitis. She has failed to respond to treatment with systemic high-dose corticosteroids and azathioprine. Which of the following is the most appropriate treatment to consider next?

☐ **A** Amoxicillin

☐ **B** Ciprofloxacin

☐ **C** Cyclophosphamide

☐ **D** Ciprofloxacin

☐ **E** Infliximab

6.54   A 27-year-old man has a 2-year history of ulcerative colitis. Over the past 5 days, he has experienced tenesmus and diarrhoea with blood and mucus. His GP had commenced him on oral sulfasalazine 2 days ago, but the frequency of his diarrhoea has worsened and he refers the patient to you for advice. Which of the following would be the most appropriate initial step in his management?

☐ **A** Add oral azathioprine and rectal budesonide

☐ **B** Commence intravenous hydrocortisone

☐ **C** Commence oral prednisolone

☐ **D** Commence rectal hydrocortisone

☐ **E** Substitute rectal mesalazine

6.55   A 54-year-old woman attends her GP requesting laxative treatment for constipation. She is taking a number of medications. Which of the following is most likely to be responsible for her symptoms?

☐ **A** Digoxin

☐ **B** Diltiazem

☐ **C** Furosemide

☐ **D** Lansoprazole

☐ **E** Simvastatin

6.53   Answer: E

Other treatment options are methotrexate or ciclosporin.

6.54   Answer: D

Appropriate for proctitis and left-sided proctocolitis. If patient fails to respond or moderate to severe symptoms, then oral prednisolone appropriate before considering other treatments.

6.55   Answer: B

Other possible causes include other calcium channel blockers, opiates and drugs with anticholinergic properties, eg amitriptyline. Lansoprazole is an important cause of diarrhoea.

6.56 Which of the following metabolic disturbances Is most likely to cause constipation?

- [ ] **A** Hyperkalaemia
- [ ] **B** Hypercalcaemia
- [ ] **C** Hyperglycaemia
- [ ] **D** Hyponatraemia
- [ ] **E** Hyperthyroidism

6.57 A 51-year-old woman complains of longstanding constipation. She is taking no regular medications, and is otherwise in good health. You decide to prescribe treatment for symptomatic relief. Which of the following statements is most accurate regarding the mechanism of action of laxative treatments?

- [ ] **A** Bisacodyl is a bulking agent
- [ ] **B** Ispaghula husk is a stimulant laxative
- [ ] **C** Magnesium sulphate is an osmotic laxative
- [ ] **D** Methylcellulose is an osmotic laxative
- [ ] **E** Senna suppositories are effective for slow-transit constipation

6.58 A 49-year-old man has regularly been taking over-the-counter laxative preparations for constipation. Which of the following is the most commonly recognised adverse effect of treatment?

- [ ] **A** Diarrhoea
- [ ] **B** Dry mouth
- [ ] **C** Hyperkalaemia
- [ ] **D** Postural hypotension
- [ ] **E** Toxic megacolon

6.56   Answer: B

Other possible causes include: hypothyroidism, hypokalaemia, porphyria, diabetes mellitus, spinal cord lesions and parkinsonism.

6.57   Answer: C

Other osmotic laxatives include lactulose. Stimulant laxatives include bisacodyl and senna, and bulking agents include methylcellulose and ispaghula husk. Bisacodyl and glycerol can be given rectally.

6.58   Answer: A

Long-term use of stimulant laxatives can cause colonic atonia.

6.59 A 65-year-old woman is admitted via the Emergency Department with abdominal pain, fever and constipation. On examination, there is tenderness overlying the left iliac fossa. Which of the following should be considered the most likely diagnosis?

☐ **A** Acute diverticulitis

☐ **B** Acute proctocolitis

☐ **C** Crohn's colitis

☐ **D** Diverticular disease of the descending colon

☐ **E** Ulcerative colitis

6.60 A 67-year-old man presents with abdominal pain, fever, nausea and vomiting He has previously been investigated for abdominal pain, and found to have diverticular disease. On examination, heart rate is 108 per min and blood pressure 98/64 mmHg, and his abdomen is rigid with absent bowel sounds. Which of the following complications of diverticular disease is most likely to have occurred?

☐ **A** Acute diverticulitis

☐ **B** Acute intestinal haemorrhage

☐ **C** Colo-vesical fistula formation

☐ **D** Intestinal obstruction due to adhesions

☐ **E** Perforation of the descending colon

6.61 A 52-year-old woman is being investigated for chronic abdominal pain, and her GP arranged for a plain abdominal X-ray. The report indicates the presence of multiple gaseous cysts, suggesting the diagnosis of *pneumatosis cystoides intestinalis*. Which of the following is a recognised treatment of this condition?

☐ **A** Cephalosporin

☐ **B** Oxygen administration

☐ **C** Prednisolone

☐ **D** Segmental colonic resection

☐ **E** Transabdominal ultrasonography

6.59 Answer: A

Diverticulosis affects around half of people over 50 years of age, and is asymptomatic. Constipation is a common feature, unlike colitis, where diarrhoea often predominates.

6.60 Answer: E

The clinical features suggest peritonitis. The other stems are all recognised complications of diverticular disease.

6.61 Answer: B

Treatment is often unnecessary. Oxygen can help disperse the cysts, which have a high nitrogen content.

6.62   A 45-year-old man undergoes barium enema for investigation of altered bowel habit and is found to have multiple colonic polyps. Which of the following statements most strongly indicates a risk of malignancy?

☐ A   Histology shows mild dysplasia

☐ B   Multiple rather than single polyp

☐ C   Pedunculated polyp rather than flat

☐ D   Squamous metaplasia

☐ E   Tubular architecture on microscopy

6.63   A 48-year-old man with longstanding Crohn's disease presents to the Gastroenterology Outpatient Clinic for investigation of chronic watery diarrhoea. ESR is 18 mm/h, C-reactive protein is < 10 g/dl and clinical examination is normal. Which of the following is the most likely explanation for his symptoms?

☐ A   Crohn's colitis

☐ B   Laxative abuse

☐ C   Malabsorption of bile salts

☐ D   Psychogenic polydipsia

☐ E   Terminal ileal inflammation

6.64   A 42-year-old woman attends the Medical Outpatient Department. She has recently undergone sigmoidoscopy and barium enema investigations of altered bowel habit, which are both normal. You suspect a diagnosis of IBS. Which of the following is a recognised diagnostic criteria?

☐ A   Abdominal bloating

☐ B   Abdominal pain for 12 consecutive weeks in the past year

☐ C   Abdominal pain relieved by defecation

☐ D   Altered stool frequency

☐ E   Change in form or appearance of stool

6.62 Answer: D

Multiple versus single polyp is, to a lesser extent, associated with increased risk, along with severe dysplasia, sessile or flat polyp shape, villous architecture and large polyps > 1.5 cm.

6.63 Answer: C

Often underdiagnosed, caused by ileal disease in coeliac disease, cystic fibrosis and post-infective gastroenteritis. Bile salts in colon cause water secretion, and increase oxylate absorption, and ureteric calculi can occur.

6.64 Answer: B

Alternatively, at least two of C, D or E are required for diagnosis (Rome II criteria). Other features often include bloating, urgency, straining, sensation of incomplete defecation and passage of mucus.

6.65 A 52-year-old woman presents with progressive jaundice over a 3–4 month period. Which of the following antibody tests would best confirm a diagnosis of primary biliary cirrhosis?

- A Anti-basement membrane antibody
- B Anti-kidney microsomal antibody
- C Antimitochondrial antibody
- D Antinuclear antibody
- E Antinuclear cytoplasmic antibodies (ANCA)

6.66 A 47-year-old man is referred to hospital for assessment of deranged liver biochemistry detected during a routine screen. Investigations show bilirubin 48 mmol/l, ALT 43 IU/l, ALP 198 IU/l, GGT 192 mmol/l, and albumin 38 g/l. He is asymptomatic, and ultrasound examination of the liver is normal. Which of the following is the most likely explanation for these findings?

- A Cholelithiasis
- B Cholestasis due to co-amoxiclav
- C Chronic autoimmune hepatitis
- D Pancreatic carcinoma
- E Resolving hepatitis after recent paracetamol overdose

6.67 A 52-year-old man presents with nausea and anorexia for the past 5 weeks. He has recently returned from a holiday in Paris. Investigations show bilirubin 55 mmol/l, ALT 256 IU/l, ALP 98 IU/l and GGT 62 mmol/l. Which of the following statements is correct in relation to further management?

- A Abdominal ultrasound is the most appropriate next step
- B Anti-hepatitis A virus (HAV) IgG antibodies confirm acute hepatitis A infection
- C Corticosteroids are indicated in proven cases of hepatitis A infection
- D Hepatitis A can be prevented by immunoglobulin administration
- E Post-hepatitis A syndrome is due to recurrent viral infection

6.65   Answer: C

Positive in over 95% of patients. Antinuclear and anti-smooth muscle antibody titres are typically raised in autoimmune chronic active hepatitis.

6.66   Answer: B

The raised ALP and GGT suggest biliary obstruction or cholestasis. Lack of biliary dilatation on ultrasound make cholestasis more likely. Gall stones are highly unlikely given the lack of symptoms.

6.67   Answer: D

Hepatitis A can be controlled by good hygiene. Infection can also be prevented when travelling to endemic areas by live inactivated HAV vaccine. Post-hepatitis A syndrome can cause debility for several months after infection, and is a functional disorder.

6.68   A 36-year-old doctor is referred to the Liver Unit with a 6-week history of jaundice. You are arranging a number of investigations, including screening for hepatitis B infection. Which of the following tests would be most helpful for confirming acute hepatitis B infection?

☐ **A** HBcAg positive

☐ **B** HBsAg positive

☐ **C** Anti-HBc IgG antibody positive

☐ **D** Anti-HBs IgM antibody positive

☐ **E** Antimitochondrial antibody positive

6.69   A 22-year-old woman is transferred to the Liver Unit from the local Medical Assessment Unit. She had been admitted 2 days earlier, having alleged to have taken a paracetamol overdose. Investigations show that her liver function has been deteriorating with ALT 25,500 IU/l and bilirubin 134 mmol/l. Which of the following most strongly suggests a need for liver transplantation?

☐ **A** Aged less than 30 years

☐ **B** Arterial pH 7.2

☐ **C** Grade II encephalopathy

☐ **D** Prothrombin time 58 s

☐ **E** Serum creatinine 180 µmol/l

6.70   A 90 kg woman attends the Medical Outpatient Clinic for assessment of deranged liver biochemistry detected on a routine test, which shows bilirubin 14 mmol/l, ALT 124 IU/l, ALP 76 IU/l and GGT 64 mmol/l. She denies alcohol intake and is taking no regular medications. Hepatitis viral serological tests are negative. Which is the most likely explanation for these findings?

☐ **A** Chronic autoimmune hepatitis

☐ **B** Non-alcoholic steatohepatitis

☐ **C** Primary biliary cirrhosis

☐ **D** Recurrent gallstones

☐ **E** Undisclosed paracetamol use

6.68   Answer: B

Also HBV DNA, suggesting active viral replication. HBsAg appears from about 6–12 months after infection, then disappears (persistence indicates chronic infection). Anti-HBc IgM appears early, and persists after HBsAg has disappeared. Anti-HBc IgG indicates past infection. Anti-HBs antibodies appear late and indicate immunity.

6.69   Answer: B

King's criteria are pH < 7.3 despite resuscitation, or serum creatinine > 300 µmol/l and prothrombin time > 100 s and grade III–IV encephalopathy.

6.70   Answer: B

Other possible causes should be considered including chronic autoimmune hepatitis (less likely), Wilson's disease and haemochromatosis. Non-alcoholic steatohepatitis is associated with fatty infiltration and inflammation of the liver, more common in patients with diabetes or obesity.

6.71 Which of the following disorders is most likely to cause cirrhosis without a preceding hepatitis?

- ☐ **A** Alcoholism
- ☐ **B** Autoimmune hepatitis
- ☐ **C** Paracetamol overdose
- ☐ **D** Primary biliary cirrhosis
- ☐ **E** Wilson's disease

6.72 A 56-year-old woman with alcohol-induced cirrhosis is regularly admitted to the Liver Unit. On this occasion, she is admitted after an episode of haematemesis, and has heart rate 98 per min and blood pressure 96/54 mmHg. She is transfused 2 units of packed red cells and given fluid resuscitation. Which of the following is the most appropriate initial step in her management?

- ☐ **A** Administration of oral propranolol
- ☐ **B** Infusion of somatostatin
- ☐ **C** Intravenous administration of terlipressin
- ☐ **D** Intravenous omeprazole
- ☐ **E** Urgent upper GI endoscopy

6.73 A 65-year-old patient is found to be jaundiced. His investigations show bilirubin 78 mmol/l, ALT 86 IU/l, ALP 176 IU/l and albumin 39 mmol/l. He is taking a number of different medications. Which of these is most likely to account for his jaundice?

- ☐ **A** Atorvastatin
- ☐ **B** Nifedipine
- ☐ **C** Methotrexate
- ☐ **D** α-Methyldopa
- ☐ **E** Rifampicin

6.71   Answer: D

In most other cases, cirrhosis is a late consequence of liver inflammation. Paracetamol overdose is notable for its ability to cause hepatitis but not cirrhosis. Hepatic fibrosis is a recognised adverse effect of methotrexate.

6.72   Answer: E

This will allow bleeding varices to be sclerosed or banded, and identify other potential sources of upper GI blood loss, eg peptic ulcer. Propranolol, somatostatin and terlipressin reduce bleeding risk (terlipressin improves survival).

6.73   Answer: B

Can cause cholestasis and hepatitis. The others may cause hepatitis (α-methyldopa is antibody-mediated). Other causes of cholestasis are co-amoxiclav, erythromycin and chlorpromazine.

6.74 A 38-year-old man is admitted via the Emergency Department with a short history of abdominal pain and vomiting. Which of the following would most strongly suggest a diagnosis of acute pancreatitis?

- ☐ **A** Epigastric pain radiating to the back
- ☐ **B** Haemoglobin concentration 9.6 g/dl
- ☐ **C** Serum amylase 192 IU/l (normal range 60–80 IU/l)
- ☐ **D** Serum calcium 1.94 mmol/l
- ☐ **E** Serum triglycerides 1.8 mmol/l

6.75 A 23-year-old man has been admitted with a recurrent episode of acute pancreatitis. Liver ultrasonography is normal, and he denies excess alcohol intake. Which of the following is most likely to increase the risk of a further episode?

- ☐ **A** Corticosteroid treatment
- ☐ **B** Hypercholesterolaemia
- ☐ **C** Hyperglycaemia
- ☐ **D** Hypocalcaemia
- ☐ **E** Thiazide diuretic use

6.74   Answer: D

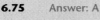

Amylase may be elevated in peptic ulcer perforation, biliary peritonitis, intestinal ischaemia and renal impairment. Pain characteristically radiates to the back in posterior duodenal ulceration.

6.75   Answer: A

Other provoking factors include alcohol, gallstones, viral infection, hypertriglyceridaemia and hypercalcaemia.

7. HAEMATOLOGY and ONCOLOGY

7.1   An 18-year-old man attends his GP with symptoms of fatigue and lethargy. He has been a strict vegan for the past 2 years, and is concerned that he may have become anaemic. Investigations show: Hb 108 g/l, MCV 118 fl, WBC 6.5 × 10⁹/l, platelets 212 × 10⁹/l. What is the most likely explanation for these findings?

   ☐ **A**   Coeliac disease

   ☐ **B**   Folate deficiency

   ☐ **C**   Hypothyroidism

   ☐ **D**   Iron deficiency

   ☐ **E**   Vitamin B$_{12}$ deficiency

7.2   A 79-year-old man lives alone, and is referred to clinic for investigation of anaemia. Investigations show: Hb 104 g/l, MCV 92 fl, WBC 4.5 × 10⁹/l, platelets 212 × 10⁹/l. What is the most likely explanation for these findings?

   ☐ **A**   Bone marrow infiltration

   ☐ **B**   Folate deficiency

   ☐ **C**   Iron deficiency

   ☐ **D**   Mixed iron and vitamin B$_{12}$ deficiency

   ☐ **E**   Subclinical inflammatory bowel disease

7.3   You are investigating a 53-year-old woman with anaemia in the Outpatient Department. Which of the following features most strongly suggests underlying vitamin B$_{12}$ deficiency?

   ☐ **A**   Haemoglobin less than 80 g/l

   ☐ **B**   MCV 104 fl

   ☐ **C**   Megaloblastic cells seen in peripheral blood film

   ☐ **D**   Poor diet

   ☐ **E**   Vitamin B$_{12}$ causes haemoglobin to increase by more than 20 g/l in 2 months

7.1   Answer: E

Macrocytic anaemia in a young vegan strongly suggests vitamin B_{12} deficiency; supplements are recommended, along with calcium, vitamin D, iron and zinc. Note coeliac disease typically causes iron deficiency anaemia, and low MCV.

7.2   Answer: D

Normal MCV can also suggest anaemia of chronic disease, but lack of clinical history makes IBD unlikely.

7.3   Answer: E

Although this does not always occur, eg pernicious anaemia due to lack of intrinsic factor. Usually, MCV is more than 115 fl. Poor diet might contribute, but usually occurs due to terminal ileal disease.

7.4 You request a peripheral blood film on one of your patients with unexplained anaemia. Which of the following features would most strongly suggest an underlying diagnosis of iron deficiency?

- [ ] **A** Elliptocytes
- [ ] **B** Howell–Jolly bodies
- [ ] **C** Red cell inclusion bodies
- [ ] **D** Target cells
- [ ] **E** Tear-drop cells

7.5 You are asked to review a 19-year-old woman in the Emergency Department. She has recently arrived in the UK from Cyprus, and presents with a short history of fever and productive cough. Investigations show: Hb 94 g/l, MCV 58 fl, WBC 16.5 × 10⁹/l, platelets 342 × 10⁹/l, and a chest X-ray shows bilateral patchy infiltration. What is the most likely explanation for her anaemia?

- [ ] **A** Bone marrow suppression
- [ ] **B** Pulmonary haemorrhage
- [ ] **C** Splenomegaly
- [ ] **D** Thalassaemia trait
- [ ] **E** Wegener's granulomatosis

7.6 A 36-year-old man with sickle cell anaemia is admitted to hospital with progressively worsening breathlessness over the past few days. He is found to have Hb 56 g/l, having been 87 g/l 2 months earlier, and you suspect that an aplastic crisis has precipitated his current admission. Which of the following infections is most likely to have been responsible?

- [ ] **A** Adenovirus
- [ ] **B** Coronavirus
- [ ] **C** Paramyxovirus
- [ ] **D** Parvovirus
- [ ] **E** Rhinovirus

7.4 Answer: D

Also seen in liver disease, post-splenectomy and haemoglobinopathies.

7.5 Answer: D

Defect of β-chain manufacture, gives microcytic anaemia with very low MCV. The high WBC is due to underlying pneumonia.

7.6 Answer: D

Parvovirus B19 causes short-term suppression of marrow red cell production, which is usually of no clinical consequence in healthy people. It can cause an aplastic crisis in patients with high rates of red cell turnover.

7.7 Which of the following statements is most accurate regarding the abnormal haemoglobin (HbS) found in patients with sickle cell disease compared to normal?

- [ ] **A** Binds oxygen more avidly
- [ ] **B** Has similar survival time to normal haemoglobin
- [ ] **C** It has no carbon dioxide carrying capacity
- [ ] **D** More susceptible to infection by malarial parasites
- [ ] **E** Oxygen dissociation curve is shifted to the right

7.8 Which of the following statements best describes iron metabolism and haemoglobin synthesis in humans?

- [ ] **A** Iron absorption is enhanced in the reduced state
- [ ] **B** Iron absorption rate is constant regardless of intake
- [ ] **C** Iron deficiency results from prolonged dietary intake < 100 mg per day
- [ ] **D** Iron excretion can increase greatly to prevent overload
- [ ] **E** Most iron in the body is found in the bone marrow

7.9 A 48-year-old man is attending the Medical Outpatient Department. His full blood count shows Hb 100 g/l, MCV 72 fl, WBC 5.1 × 10⁹/l, platelets 184 × 10⁹/l. You suspect iron deficiency anaemia. Which of the following findings would most strongly support this diagnosis?

- [ ] **A** Low serum ferritin
- [ ] **B** High serum folate concentration
- [ ] **C** Low serum iron concentration
- [ ] **D** Low serum transferrin saturation
- [ ] **E** Total iron binding capacity is increased

7.10 A 51-year-old woman is found to have anaemia during a routine check-up recently. Which of the following additional tests would most strongly suggest haemolysis as an underlying explanation for her anaemia?

- [ ] **A** Microcytic cells on blood film
- [ ] **B** Mildly elevated bilirubin
- [ ] **C** Red cell fragments on peripheral blood film
- [ ] **D** Reticulocyte count of 1%
- [ ] **E** Urine strongly positive for bilirubin

7.7   Answer: E

Therefore, oxygen dissociates more readily to tissues, and anaemia can be well tolerated.

7.8   Answer: A

Ferrous (Fe^{2+}) iron is absorbed better than the ferric (Fe^{3+}) state. Around 1 mg daily is required, although replacement doses are significantly higher. Most iron in the body is found in red cells.

7.9   Answer: D

Serum iron can be reduced and serum ferritin increased in patients with inflammatory disorders. TIBC is generally increased. Transferrin saturation is more reliable than serum iron or TIBC alone.

7.10   Answer: C

Slightly elevated bilirubin and/or mild jaundice is a recognised feature, but often associated with other causes. Red cell fragments suggest microangiopathic haemolytic anaemia.

7.11 You are currently investigating a 43-year-old man in clinic for unexplained anaemia. Which of the following statements best describes the direct Coombs' test?

- [ ] A Detects antibody on patient's red cells
- [ ] B Detects anti-RBC antibody in patient's serum
- [ ] C False positive test often arises in sepsis
- [ ] D Involves incubation of patient serum with test red cells
- [ ] E Positive test indicates extravascular haemolysis

7.12 Which of the following is most closely involved in the early development of thrombotic thrombocytopenic purpura (TTP)?

- [ ] A Abnormally high affinity for platelet adhesion to vascular endothelium
- [ ] B Coagulation factor depletion is often severe
- [ ] C Excessive platelet–platelet adhesions
- [ ] D Low circulating concentrations of von Willebrand factor
- [ ] E Overproduction of platelets by bone marrow

7.13 A 56-year-old woman is admitted to hospital with fever, confusion and renal impairment. Investigations show: Hb 96 g/l, MCV 98 fl, WBC 8.5 × 10^9/l, platelets 103 × 10^9/l, and peripheral blood film shows red cell fragments and polychromasia. Which of the following is the most likely explanation for these features?

- [ ] A Chronic alcohol excess
- [ ] B Meningococcal septicaemia
- [ ] C Penicillin-induced haemolytic anaemia
- [ ] D TTP
- [ ] E von Willebrand disease

7.11   Answer: A

The indirect test detects antibodies in the patient's serum against a number of red cell surface antigens.

7.12   Answer: A

Due to expression of high molecular weight (uncleaved) von Willebrand factor, which leads to excess platelet–endothelium adhesion and, therefore, platelet consumption and small vessel occlusion.

7.13   Answer: D

Similar to haemolytic uraemic syndrome (HUS) where renal failure and fever are the predominant features, whereas in TTP neurological features predominate. Due to excessive endothelium–platelet adhesiveness.

7.14 You are asked to see a 56-year-old man in the resuscitation area of the Emergency Department, who is found to have Hb 110 g/l, MCV 96 fl, WBC 6.0 × 10⁹/l, platelets 114 × 10⁹/l, and creatinine 186 μmol/l. You suspect a diagnosis of HUS as an underlying cause of his renal impairment. Which of the following initial treatments is likely to be most helpful?

    A Aspirin

    B Cryoprecipitate

    C Factor VIII concentrate

    D Fresh frozen plasma (FFP)

    E Haemodialysis

7.15 Which of the following mechanisms is most strongly linked to the pathophysiology of paroxysmal nocturnal haematuria (PNH)?

    A Can be diagnosed by immunophenotyping

    B Caused by excessive RBC transmembrane glycoprotein expression

    C Involvement is specific to red blood cells only

    D Erythrocytes prone to excess lysis only in vivo

    E There is increased risk of acute lymphocytic leukaemia

7.16 A 46-year-old woman who is taking a number of different medications is referred to the General Medical Outpatient Department for further assessment of raised white cell count. Her full blood count shows WBC 12.4 × 10⁹/l with 85% neutrophils. Which of the following medications is most likely to be responsible?

    A Chloramphenicol

    B Furosemide

    C Lithium

    D Propranolol

    E Topical betnovate ointment

7.14 Answer: D

In HUS, von Willebrand factor (vWF) expressed by endothelium is uncleaved due to plasma protease deficiency, which triggers excess platelet adhesion and vascular occlusion. FFP contains protease. Cryoprecipitate-poor FFP (vWF removed) and plasma exchange can be helpful.

7.15 Answer: A

Deficiency of a transmembrane glycoprotein (RBCs, white cells and platelets) that is normally associated with factors that inhibit complement. Excess lysis ex vivo is the basis of Ham's test. Increased prevalence of acute myeloid leukaemia.

7.16 Answer: C

A number of non-inflammatory conditions are associated with neutrophilia. Drugs such as corticosteroids and lithium decrease peripheral margination of WBCs (normally around 50% of the circulating pool).

7.17   During routine investigation of a 27-year-old man before elective orchidopexy, full blood count investigation shows eosinophils 1.6 × 10⁹/l. Which of the following is the most likely explanation for this finding?

⬜ A   Asthma

⬜ B   Corticosteroid treatment

⬜ C   Eosinophilic leukaemia

⬜ D   Recreational drug use

⬜ E   Tropical eosinophilia

7.18   Which one of the following statements is true with respect to compatibility testing of blood for transfusion?

⬜ A   ABO and Rhesus compatibility prevents transmission of infection

⬜ B   Both direct and indirect haemagglutination tests are used in screening

⬜ C   Full crossmatch procedures are always used except for emergencies

⬜ D   Group O-negative blood can be safely transfused in all patients

⬜ E   Rhesus group is determined only if the recipient is Rhesus negative

7.19   A 42-year-old man is admitted with abdominal pain thought due to acute haemorrhagic pancreatitis, and a blood sample is sent to the local transfusion service for 'Group and Save'. Which of the following best explains how the sample will be processed?

⬜ A   A unit of ABO and Rhesus-matched blood will be set aside

⬜ B   If antibody screening is negative, serum will be held and crossmatched later if blood is needed

⬜ C   Normally 2–3 units of matched whole blood are set aside

⬜ D   The sample will be held and examined only when blood is required

⬜ E   Two units of group O Rhesus-negative blood will be forwarded urgently

7.17   Answer: A

Other common causes include hay fever and eczema. Less common causes also include parasitic infection, Hodgkin's disease, sarcoidosis, polyarteritis nodosa and dermatitis herpetiformis.

7.18   Answer: B

Only ABO and Rhesus compatible blood should always be used. If antibody screening is negative, immediate spin crossmatch is normally sufficient so that full crossmatch would not be required.

7.19   Answer: B

Rapid crossmatching can be undertaken using spin crossmatch. If atypical antibodies are detected, then compatible blood may need to be crossmatched and held.

7.20 A 62-year-old man is admitted with lassitude and fatigue due to severe anaemia, and is being transfused with 4 units of packed red cells. You are asked to review him because he has developed fever and tachycardia 30 min after commencing transfusion of the second unit. What is the most likely explanation?

- ☐ **A** ABO incompatibility
- ☐ **B** Hepatitis C
- ☐ **C** Immediate transfusion reaction
- ☐ **D** Iron overload
- ☐ **E** Leukocyte-based transfusion reaction

7.21 The presence of atypical red cell antibodies increases the risk of severe transfusion reactions. In what percentage of the United Kingdom population are clinically significant atypical antibodies present?

- ☐ **A** 0.02%
- ☐ **B** 0.1%
- ☐ **C** 2%
- ☐ **D** 10%
- ☐ **E** 25%

7.22 A 52-year-old woman has undergone hysterectomy, and has required transfusion with 3 units of packed red cells. Around 6 h after commencing transfusion, she develops rigors, tachycardia and fever. Which of the following statements is correct regarding febrile transfusion reactions?

- ☐ **A** Aspirin is contraindicated due to the risk of Reye's syndrome
- ☐ **B** Commonest in patients who have never had blood transfusion before
- ☐ **C** More common in multiparous than nulliparous women
- ☐ **D** More likely after transfusion of leukocyte-depleted blood
- ☐ **E** Most cases are due to viral infection

7.20   Answer: E

Non-haemolytic transfusion reaction, delayed haemolytic reaction or urticarial or anaphylactic reactions.

7.21   Answer: C

Around 10% of the population test positive during antibody screening, but a clinically significant red cell antibody is only found in around 20–25% of these after more detailed screening.

7.22   Answer: C

Due to development of leukocyte antibodies; also more common if previously transfused. Aspirin or paracetamol can reduce fever.

7.23   Which of the following is most likely to give rise to neutropenia in a previously healthy adult?

☐ **A**   Acute gout

☐ **B**   Bacterial skin infection

☐ **C**   Oral prednisolone treatment

☐ **D**   Respiratory viral illness

☐ **E**   Vitamin B_{12} deficiency

7.24   You are asked to see a previously healthy 26-year-old woman in the Outpatient Department. She has been referred for investigation of easy bruising of her limbs after relatively minor trauma. Which of the following diagnoses is most likely?

☐ **A**   Aplastic anaemia

☐ **B**   Easy bruising syndrome

☐ **C**   Hereditary haemorrhagic telangiectasia

☐ **D**   Primary biliary cirrhosis

☐ **E**   von Willebrand's disease

7.25   You have been investigating a 54-year-old man in the Haematology Outpatient Department for unexplained bleeding and easy bruising. Investigations show that his bleeding time is abnormally prolonged. Which of the following disorders is most likely to be responsible?

☐ **A**   Autoimmune thrombocytopenic purpura

☐ **B**   Henoch–Schönlein purpura

☐ **C**   Hereditary haemorrhagic telangiectasia

☐ **D**   Multiple myeloma

☐ **E**   Scurvy

7.26   Which of the following statements best describes the pathophysiology of haemophilia A?

☐ **A**   Around one-third of cases are sporadic with no family history

☐ **B**   Inheritance in an autosomal recessive manner

☐ **C**   It is an autoimmune disorder

☐ **D**   Low levels of von Willebrand's factor

☐ **E**   Low levels of factor IX

7.23 Answer: D

Viral illnesses in general, also severe bacterial infections, overwhelming sepsis, bone marrow suppression and autoimmune disease.

7.24 Answer: B

Benign disorder characterised by increased small vessel fragility.

7.25 Answer: A

Prolonged bleeding time indicated reduced platelet function: reduced platelet numbers (eg AIP) or reduced platelet activity (eg aspirin).

7.26 Answer: A

Due to gene mutation, rather than non-paternity. Usually inherited in X-linked manner, and due to low levels of factor VIII:C.

7.27 Which one of the following statements most accurately describes the mechanisms involved in von Willebrand's disease?

- [ ] A Abnormally high levels of vWF
- [ ] B Deficiency of factor VIII:C
- [ ] C Excessive platelet adhesiveness
- [ ] D Inheritance is X-linked recessive
- [ ] E Profound thrombocytopenia is a common feature

7.28 A 61-year-old man is admitted as an emergency after a suspected upper gastrointestinal bleed. He has background chronic liver disease due to alcohol excess, and is found to have INR 1.6. Which of the following factors is most likely to be responsible for his increased bleeding risk?

- [ ] A Artefact due to sample dilution
- [ ] B Aspirin
- [ ] C Reduced synthesis of coagulation factors
- [ ] D Thrombocytopenia
- [ ] E Vitamin K deficiency

7.29 A 51-year-old man required transfusion of 10 units of packed red cells after a motorcycle accident and emergency orthopaedic surgery. A coagulation screen on arrival at hospital was normal, but now shows PT 15 s and APPT 54 s. Which of the following is most likely to be responsible for his abnormal coagulation?

- [ ] A Acute liver failure
- [ ] B Factor V and VIII deficiency
- [ ] C Immediate transfusion reaction
- [ ] D Thrombocytopenia
- [ ] E von Willebrand's disease

7.27 Answer: B

Deficiency of vWF causes low factor VIII:C levels, endothelial dysfunction and impaired platelet function. Mild thrombocytopenia can occur. Usually, autosomal dominant inheritance pattern.

7.28 Answer: C

Thrombocytopenia (due to hypersplenism) and vitamin K deficiency (due to malabsorption or poor diet) might also contribute.

7.29 Answer: B

Factors V and VIII are depleted in stored blood and FFP or platelet transfusion should be considered after massive blood transfusion.

7.30 You are asked to review a 45-year-old woman who was referred to the Emergency DVT Clinic by her GP. She had noted swelling of her left calf that morning. Which of the following factors most strongly increases the risk of deep vein thrombosis?

◻ **A** Anti-β_2 glycoprotein I antibody

◻ **B** Excess prothrombin activity

◻ **C** Lupus anticoagulant

◻ **D** Systemic lupus erythematosus

◻ **E** Total cholesterol > 10 mmol/l

7.31 A 58-year-old woman has recently undergone right hemicolectomy for colonic carcinoma. She required 4 units of packed red cells to be transfused for correction of peri-operative blood loss. Several hours after transfusion, she became breathless and hypoxic, and you suspect a clinical diagnosis of transfusion-related acute lung injury (TRALI). Which one of the following is a characteristic feature of this condition?

◻ **A** Men are more commonly affected than women

◻ **B** Mortality is around 50–75%

◻ **C** Most commonly occurs after administration of pooled plasma products

◻ **D** Onset 18–24 h after transfusion was commenced

◻ **E** Pulmonary infiltrates are seen on plain chest X-ray

7.32 A 34-year-old woman is commencing chemotherapy treatment for acute lymphoblastic leukaemia, and you are considering prevention of tumour lysis syndrome. Which of the following prophylactic treatments would be most effective in preserving renal function?

◻ **A** Cyclophosphamide

◻ **B** Intravenous oxypurinol

◻ **C** Oral allopurinol

◻ **D** Loop diuretic administration

◻ **E** Urate oxidase

7.30   Answer: A

Lupus anticoagulant also contributes, but poses greatest risks when present in addition to antibody against β_2 glycoprotein I or antiprothrombin antibody.

7.31   Answer: E

Often mimics adult respiratory distress syndrome (ARDS) but outcome is generally better, with mortality around 10–15%. Multiparous women and previously transfused people are at greatest risk. Most common after blood transfusion; rare after pooled products.

7.32   Answer: E

This causes lysis of uric acid to more soluble products including allantoin, and can cause very substantial lowering of serum uric acid concentrations. Allopurinol and its active metabolite oxypurinol lower uric acid by 30–40%. Pre-hydration is very important.

7.33 With respect to the ABO blood grouping system, which of the following statements is correct regarding a patient who is 'blood group A'?

- A Genotype must be 'AA'
- B Group A or group AB blood can safely be transfused
- C The group is inherited in an X-linked manner
- D They will have circulating anti-B antibodies
- E This accounts for 5–10% of the UK population

7.34 You review a 61-year-old woman with anaemia, and note her blood film report showing irregular red blood cells, target cells and the presence of Howell–Jolly bodies. Which of the following underlying diagnoses is most likely?

- A Acute myeloid leukaemia
- B Chronic lymphocytic leukaemia
- C Diabetes mellitus
- D Essential thrombocythaemia
- E Felty's syndrome

7.35 A 48-year-old woman is referred for assessment of anaemia associated with mild jaundice. Which of the following features most strongly suggests haemolysis as an underlying cause?

- A High conjugated serum bilirubin
- B Positive urine bilirubin test
- C Raised serum haptoglobin concentrations
- D Red cell polymorphism
- E Reticulocytosis

7.36 A 68-year-old man is referred for investigation of weight loss and fatigue, and a chest X-ray shows an abnormality suggestive of lung carcinoma affecting the right mid-zone. Initial investigations show serum calcium 2.64 mmol/l and albumin 28 mmol/l. What is the most likely diagnosis?

- A Dehydration
- B Lung carcinoma with bony metastases
- C Medullary carcinoma of the thyroid
- D Small cell lung carcinoma
- E Squamous carcinoma of the lung

7.33   Answer: D

In the UK, 45% are group A, 44% group O, 8% group B and 3% group AB. Genotype could be 'AA' or 'AO', and only group O or A can be transfused safely.

7.34   Answer: D

The appearance suggests splenic atrophy which is also seen in sickle cell disease, ulcerative colitis, coeliac disease and dermatitis herpetiformis.

7.35   Answer: E

High unconjugated serum bilirubin, high urinary urobilinogen and diminished serum haptoglobin concentrations are typical findings. Red cell fragments and abnormal morphology are also recognised features.

7.36   Answer: E

Although it would be important to exclude dehydration. Medullary thyroid carcinoma can cause hypocalcaemia due to calcitonin secretion.

7.37   A 58-year-old lifelong smoker is referred for investigation of
breathlessness, and a chest X-ray shows an abnormality in the left
perihilar region. Other investigations show Na+ 134 mmol/l,
K+ 3.4 mmol/l, urea 4.5 mmol/l, and serum and urine osmolalities of
258 mOsm and 324 mOsm, respectively. What is the most likely
underlying diagnosis?

- [ ] A   Adenocarcinoma of the lung
- [ ] B   Adrenal carcinoma with metastases
- [ ] C   Carcinoid
- [ ] D   Small cell lung carcinoma
- [ ] E   Squamous cell lung carcinoma

7.38   A 35-year-old woman is being investigated for vague abdominal
symptoms, and a CT scan reveals a small nodule in the head of
pancreas. Which of the following most strongly suggests a diagnosis
of insulinoma?

- [ ] A   Fasting plasma glucose 2.8 mmol/l
- [ ] B   Progressive weight loss
- [ ] C   Recurrent blackouts after standing upright from a seated position
- [ ] D   Random plasma glucose 2.5 mmol/l
- [ ] E   Sweating, tremor and personality change after a prolonged fast

7.39   A 58-year-old man is referred to the outpatient department for
investigation of progressive weight loss and fatigue. He is a lifelong
smoker, and there is marked clubbing of fingers and toes. Which of
the following diagnoses is most likely to account for these findings?

- [ ] A   Gastric carcinoma
- [ ] B   Nasopharyngeal carcinoma
- [ ] C   Non-small cell lung carcinoma
- [ ] D   Oesophageal adenocarcinoma
- [ ] E   Squamous lung carcinoma

7.37   Answer: D

Associated with SIADH. May also be associated with ectopic adrenocorticotrophic hormone (ACTH) secretion and Cushing's syndrome.

7.38   Answer: E

Prolonged fasting will provoke the typical symptoms of hypoglycaemia, which can be confirmed by biochemical testing. Frequent snacks to prevent symptoms, and the effects of insulin on carbohydrate storage encourage weight gain.

7.39   Answer: C

Tobacco use probably increases the likelihood of all of the above, however, finger clubbing is more typically associated with this cancer than the others.

7.40 A 43-year-old man with established small cell lung cancer is referred for investigation of progressive ataxia, unsteady gait and dysarthria. Examination shows bilateral impairment of coordination in upper and lower limbs, but there is no nystagmus. What is the most likely explanation for these findings?

- **A** Eaton–Lambert syndrome
- **B** Midline cerebellar metastases
- **C** Non-infiltrative cerebellar degeneration
- **D** Polymyositis
- **E** Raised intracranial pressure

7.41 A 76-year-old man is admitted for palliative care. He has widespread metastases involving his thoracic spine, which is causing significant back pain. Routine investigations show Hb 174 g/l, which is thought to be a paraneoplastic phenomenon. Which of the following disorders is *least* likely to be associated with erythrocytosis?

- **A** Cerebellar haemangioblastoma
- **B** Hepatoma
- **C** Renal cell carcinoma
- **D** Thyroid carcinoma
- **E** Wilm's tumour

7.42 You are asked to review the results of 56-year-old woman who was admitted to the oncology ward as an emergency earlier in the week due to haemoptysis and fever. Her coagulation screen shows prothrombin time 18 s, APPT 44 s, fibrinogen 0.8 g/l and D-dimer 652 IU/l, suggesting possible disseminated intravascular coagulation. Which of the following underlying diagnoses is most likely to account for this?

- **A** Acute lymphocytic leukaemia
- **B** Acute promyelocytic leukaemia
- **C** Chronic lymphocytic leukaemia
- **D** Multiple myeloma
- **E** Streptococcal pneumonia

7.40 Answer: C

Paraneoplastic phenomenon thought to be antibody mediated, relative lack of nystagmus, can also occur with other tumours (eg breast, thyroid). Eaton–Lambert and polymyositis are recognised complications, but give muscle weakness.

7.41 Answer: D

The others are associated with an increased risk of erythrocytosis, which can increase likelihood of complications due to vascular occlusion.

7.42 Answer: B

Associated with disseminated intravascular coagulation (DIC), although sepsis and pneumonia can also (less commonly) be associated with DIC.

7.43 You review a rather anxious 33-year-old woman in the General Medical Outpatient Department, who is seeking advice about genetic screening. Which of the following might most strongly suggest a need for breast cancer genetic screening tests?

- [ ] **A** History of oral contraceptive pill use for 16 years
- [ ] **B** Large breasts that are difficult to self-examine
- [ ] **C** One first-degree relative with male breast cancer
- [ ] **D** Second-degree relative with bilateral breast cancer
- [ ] **E** Two first-degree relatives diagnosed with breast cancer aged 70 years

7.44 Which one of the following statements is true regarding breast cancer screening programmes utilising mammography?

- [ ] **A** Cancer is advanced or fungating at presentation in 75% of patients in developing countries that do not have screening programmes
- [ ] **B** Cost per life saved is around £5000 in the UK
- [ ] **C** Diagnostic yield is around 0.7% in the UK
- [ ] **D** Postal invitations for screening can breach patient confidentiality
- [ ] **E** Uptake for screening invitations is around 15–20% in Western Societies

7.45 A 45-year-old woman is undergoing chemotherapy treatment for advanced breast cancer. You are asked to review her because she has developed progressive breathlessness and a chest X-ray now shows evidence of diffuse pulmonary oedema. Which of the following chemotherapeutic agents is most likely to cause cardiomyopathy?

- [ ] **A** Busulphan
- [ ] **B** Daunorubicin
- [ ] **C** Etoposide
- [ ] **D** Mitomycin C
- [ ] **E** Vincristine

7.43   Answer: C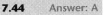

Potential for paternal inheritance. Other factors include a first-degree relative with bilateral breast cancer or onset < 40 years, two or more relatives diagnosed at < 60 years, or three or more relatives diagnosed at any age.

7.44   Answer: A

A number of factors contribute in addition to lack of mammographic screening, including poor education, lack of general surgical facilities and cultural factors. Diagnostic yield is less than 0.01% and is said to cost between £0.5 and 1.5 million per life saved.

7.45   Answer: B

This can be an immediate or delayed reaction to anthracyclines, including doxorubicin. Limiting the cumulative total drug exposure reduces long-term risk of chronic cardiomyopathy.

7.46 A 38-year-old premenopausal woman has recently been diagnosed with breast cancer. Which of the following statements is most accurate regarding hormonal treatment in this case?

☐ **A** Endometrial hyperplasia is a recognised adverse effect of tamoxifen

☐ **B** Fulvestrant blocks oestrogen receptors less effectively than tamoxifen

☐ **C** Letrozole is likely to be a useful adjunctive treatment in this patient

☐ **D** Response rate to tamoxifen is greater in oestrogen receptor-positive disease

☐ **E** Tamoxifen is an oestrogen antagonist

7.47 A 64-year-old man attends the Urology Outpatient Department with a progressive 6-month history of symptoms suggestive of prostatic hypertrophy. Which one of the following features would most strongly suggest prostate carcinoma, rather than benign hyperplasia?

☐ **A** Hard enlarged prostate palpable on rectal examination

☐ **B** History of low back pain

☐ **C** Prostate specific antigen 5.2 µg/l

☐ **D** Serum calcium 2.52 mmol/l

☐ **E** Strong family history

7.48 You are asked to review the analgesia prescription of a 62-year-old man with metastatic lung carcinoma, who is complaining of chest wall and back pain. Which of the following statements best describes the effects of palliative analgesics in this patient?

☐ **A** Agitation is a characteristic adverse effect of baclofen

☐ **B** Amitriptyline is effective in 75% of patients with neuropathic pain

☐ **C** Carbamazepine can reduce the effects of other existing treatments

☐ **D** Dexamethasone is effective only for cerebral metastases

☐ **E** High doses of ibuprofen should be avoided due to the risks of gastrointestinal haemorrhage

7.46   Answer: A

Tamoxifen is a partial oestrogen receptor agonist, whereas fulvestrant is an oestrogen receptor antagonist used if tamoxifen is ineffective. Letrozole is an aromatase inhibitor used in post-menopausal women.

7.47   Answer: A

Raised PSA > 4 µg/l is suggestive, but false positive results can occur.

7.48   Answer: C

Enzyme inducer, so other drugs metabolised more readily, eg corticosteroids. Dexamethasone can be useful for visceral pain. Treatments for neuropathic pain are only effective in around 20% of patients.

7.49 A 56-year-old woman is found to have Hb 98 g/l and MCV 72 fl. You suspect iron deficiency as the cause of her anaemia. Which of the following is most likely to have contributed to the development of this condition?

- [ ] **A** Corticosteroid treatment
- [ ] **B** Diverticulitis
- [ ] **C** Omeprazole treatment
- [ ] **D** Terminal ileitis secondary to inflammatory bowel disease
- [ ] **E** Vitamin C tablets

7.50 You are asked for general advice regarding the potential benefits or harm of iron supplementation in pregnancy. Which of the following statements is most accurate?

- [ ] **A** Ferrous sulphate is teratogenic and should be avoided in the first trimester
- [ ] **B** High antenatal body mass index carries a 2- to 3-fold increased risk of post-partum iron deficiency
- [ ] **C** Iron deficiency is uncommon among pregnant women in Western societies
- [ ] **D** Post-partum iron deficiency can cause psychosis
- [ ] **E** Post-partum iron stores return to normal before haemoglobin is restored

7.51 A 58-year-old man is being investigated for early-onset dementia, and is found to have Hb 97 g/l and MCV 118 fl. Which one of the following statements is most accurate with respect to folate or vitamin B$_{12}$ deficiency?

- [ ] **A** Depression is more common in patients with folate deficiency
- [ ] **B** High serum homocysteine concentrations improve vascular function
- [ ] **C** Thiamine is an important co-factor for folate absorption
- [ ] **D** Vitamin B$_{12}$ alkylates methionine to homocysteine
- [ ] **E** Vitamin B$_{12}$ supplementation is required in suspected Wernicke's encephalopathy

7.49   Answer: C

Iron absorption occurs in the proximal small intestine, and is greatest for haem rather than non-haem iron, and enhanced in the ferrous (Fe^{2+}) state. Gastric acid and ascorbic acid prevent conversion to ferric iron (Fe^{3+}) and enhance gastrointestinal absorption.

7.50   Answer: C

Post-partum anaemia impairs physical work capacity, contributes to cognitive and mood problems. Haemoglobin may appear normal, although iron stores are depleted. Iron requirements are high during pregnancy, and the incidence of iron-deficiency increases 5-fold.

7.51   Answer: A

Neuropsychiatric disorders are associated with both folate and vitamin B$_{12}$ deficiency. Vitamin B$_{12}$ is a methyl donor in the conversion of methionine to homocysteine.

7.52 Which of the following statements is correct regarding vitamin B_{12} absorption in humans?

☐ **A** Absorption is enhanced in presence of vitamin B_{12} deficiency

☐ **B** Intrinsic factor is synthesized by the liver and secreted in bile

☐ **C** Intrinsic factor–vitamin B_{12} complexes bind to enterocyte receptors

☐ **D** Vitamin B_{12} is synthesised de novo from cobalt and essential amino acids

☐ **E** Transcobalamin is found only in extracellular fluids

7.53 A 61-year-old man is admitted in extremis after collapsing at home. He has been taking warfarin for atrial fibrillation, and describes a short history of melaena. His INR is found to be 8.5, and you suspect that he has had a large gastrointestinal haemorrhage. Which of the following would be the most appropriate means of reversing his anticoagulation?

☐ **A** Administration of clotting factor concentrates

☐ **B** Fresh frozen plasma

☐ **C** Intravenous vitamin K 1–2 mg

☐ **D** Intravenous vitamin K 10 mg

☐ **E** Pooled platelet administration

7.54 A 56-year-old man with established chronic liver disease presents with a 12-h history of upper gastrointestinal bleeding. Which of the following factors would most strongly support administration of platelet concentrate?

☐ **A** Activated partial thromboplastin time 53 s

☐ **B** Bleeding time 13 s

☐ **C** Platelet count $18 \times 10^9/l$

☐ **D** Preceding aspirin therapy

☐ **E** Prothrombin ratio 2.4

7.55 A 42-year-old woman in the Intensive Care Unit is receiving transfusion with platelet concentrate. Which one of the following features is most characteristically associated with platelet therapy?

☐ **A** Alloimmunisation can diminish the effectiveness of treatment

☐ **B** Clotting of peripheral veins occurs due to local thrombocytosis

☐ **C** Fresh frozen plasma contains both platelets and clotting factors

☐ **D** Haemopoietic growth factors do not stimulate platelet synthesis

☐ **E** Transfusion reactions less likely than after blood transfusion due to the absence of leukocytes

7.52   Answer: C

Intrinsic factor is a gastric glycoprotein; complexes bind to receptors before endocytosis. Vitamin B_{12} cannot be formed de novo in people. Transcobalamin (transport protein) is also found in the gut.

7.53   Answer: A

In life or limb-threatening haemorrhage, the priority is rapid reversal of anticoagulation. Fresh frozen plasma (FFP) has comparatively low concentrations of factor IX, and is less good. Low dose vitamin K should only be used for low-risk bleeding for reversal towards therapeutic anticoagulation.

7.54   Answer: C

Platelet administration should be considered if count is very low, eg $< 10 \times 10^9/l$, or at levels $< 25 \times 10^9/l$ if the patient is actively bleeding.

7.55   Answer: A

Antibodies are generated by recipient. Local clotting is not typically encountered, presumably due to low background platelet numbers. Haemopoietic growth factors stimulate red cell, white cell and platelet lineages to a variable extent.

7.56 A 57-year-old woman is due to undergo combination chemotherapy for breast carcinoma. Which of the following treatments is most likely to be effective in preventing neutropenic sepsis as a complication?

- ☐ **A** Corticosteroids
- ☐ **B** Factor VIII administration
- ☐ **C** Granulocyte transfusion
- ☐ **D** Granulocyte colony stimulating factor
- ☐ **E** Treatment administered in a quiet ward side-room

7.57 A 60-year-old man is diagnosed with non-Hodgkin lymphoma, and is due to undergo autologous stem cell transplantation (ASCT). Which of the following statements best describes the role of ASCT in this patient?

- ☐ **A** Disease relapse is comparatively rare
- ☐ **B** Rituximab reduces the risk of disease recurrence
- ☐ **C** Shorter courses of chemotherapy are needed but morbidity is higher
- ☐ **D** Stem cells are transfused from a matched donor first-degree relative
- ☐ **E** Transplant rejection is a common limitation of this technique

7.58 A 58-year-old woman undergoes renal biopsy for unexplained proteinuria, which shows diffuse fibrillary protein deposition that shows green birefringence with polarised light. Which one of the following is the most characteristic feature of light-chain amyloidosis?

- ☐ **A** Cardiomegaly
- ☐ **B** Leukocytoclastic vasculitic rash
- ☐ **C** Nephritic syndrome
- ☐ **D** Peripheral neuropathy
- ☐ **E** Psoriatic arthropathy

7.56 Answer: D

Granulocyte CSF and granulocyte–macrophage CSF administration enhances circulating neutrophil counts and reduces the prevalence and severity of neutropenic sepsis. Granulocyte transfusion has been studied, but the potential benefits remain unproven.

7.57 Answer: B

Stem cells are harvested from the patient and used to repopulate the haemopoietic system after high-dose chemotherapy. The risk of relapse is lower for allogenic transplantation, but rejection is a problem. Rituximab is a monoclonal antibody to CD20.

7.58 Answer: A

Cardiomegaly is present in around 50% of patients, and peripheral neuropathy is present in 10–15%. It is also associated with nephrotic syndrome and hepatosplenomegaly.

7.59 A 51-year-old woman is referred to the Outpatient Department for investigation of anaemia, which was detected during a routine medical assessment. She has had no significant past illnesses, and is taking no regular medications. Investigations show Hb 87 g/l, MCV 82 g/l, red cell distribution width 24%. Which one of these is the most likely explanation?

- [ ] A Anaemia of chronic disease
- [ ] B Mixed folate and vitamin B_{12} deficiency
- [ ] C Mixed iron and vitamin B_{12} deficiency
- [ ] D Myelodysplasia
- [ ] E Thalassaemia

7.60 A 19-year-old man is admitted via the Emergency Department in the early hours of Saturday morning with drowsiness and confusion. He appears markedly cyanosed and an arterial blood gas shows pH 7.31, PaO_2 14.5 kPa, $PaCO_2$ 4.0 kPa and lactate 3.8 mmol/l. Which of the following diagnoses should be considered most strongly?

- [ ] A Methaemoglobinaemia
- [ ] B Pulmonary embolism
- [ ] C Sickle cell anaemia
- [ ] D Tension pneumothorax
- [ ] E Thalassaemia

7.61 A 62-year-old woman has suffered progressively worsening angina over the past 3 days, and has been using increasingly large amounts of sublingual and buccal nitrate therapy for symptom control. On arrival in the Emergency Department she is noted to be heavily cyanosed and is found to have PaO_2 12.3 kPa, $PaCO_2$ 3.9 kPa, and methaemoglobin concentration of 45%. Which of the following is the most appropriate course of action?

- [ ] A Administer high-flow oxygen
- [ ] B Arrange for urgent exchange transfusion
- [ ] C Give intravenous methylene blue
- [ ] D Give intravenous glyceryl trinitrate to maintain systolic BP at 100 mmHg
- [ ] E Observe only and recheck arterial gases in 12 h

7.59   Answer: C

Normal MCV and high RDW could also suggest anaemia of chronic disease or sideroblastic anaemia; normal MCV and normal RDW found in anaemia of chronic disease or haemoglobinopathy.

7.60   Answer: A

Common causes include nitrate excess (including recreational use of amyl nitrate). Features are due to tissue hypoxia despite apparently normal PaO_2 and $PaCO_2$, and can be treated with methylene blue if methaemoglobin > 30%.

7.61   Answer: C

Given if methaemoglobin > 30%. Exchange transfusion is used for severe, life-threatening methaemoglobinaemia (> 80%), including haemolysis, or if methylene blue is likely to be ineffective (eg G6PD deficiency).

7.62 A 42-year-old man is admitted to the Emergency Department late on a Friday evening complaining of vague chest pain. Physical examination, resting ECG and chest X-ray are normal. Full blood count shows Hb 121 g/l, MCV 103 fl and platelet count 80×10^9/l. What is the most likely explanation for these haematology findings?

- A Chronic alcohol excess
- B Folate deficiency
- C Hyperthyroidism
- D Iron deficiency
- E Sideroblastic anaemia

7.63 A 58-year-old woman is referred to the General Medical Outpatient Department for investigation of weight loss and abdominal bloating for the past 10 months. Investigations show Hb 102 g/l, MCV 76 fl and peripheral blood film shows hypochromic, microcytic cells and occasional Howell–Jolly bodies. What is the most likely underlying diagnosis?

- A Caecal carcinoma
- B Coeliac disease
- C Hypothyroidism
- D Ovarian carcinoma
- E Pernicious anaemia

7.64 Which of the following factors is most useful as a prognostic indicator in patients with systemic amyloidosis?

- A Circulating lymphocyte count
- B Serum β_2 microglobulin
- C Renal size on ultrasound scan
- D Serum calcium
- E Weight loss

7.65 Which of the following is a recognised feature of vitamin B_{12} deficiency in elderly patients?

- A Can be due to inability to release cobalamin from food
- B Is diagnosed by Schilling's test
- C Is due to intrinsic factor deficiency in most cases
- D Prevalent in 0.5–1.0% of patients
- E Rarely causes neuropsychiatric complications

7.62 Answer: A

The blood results suggest a simple macrocytosis, rather than a megaloblastic anaemia (in the latter Hb is usually low and MCV often > 115 fl). Typical causes also include hypothyroidism and liver disease.

7.63 Answer: B

Coeliac disease is a common cause of iron-deficiency anaemia in middle-aged patients, and is often overlooked.

7.64 Answer: B

Marker of overall disease burden and linked to survival; cardiac mass is also important.

7.65 Answer: A

Probably the commonest cause, or deficiency of intestinal cobalamin transport proteins; intrinsic factor deficiency accounts for fewer than one in five cases. Neuropsychiatric and haematological complications are common, and deficiency is present in around 20% of elderly patients.

7.66 Which of the following conditions most strongly indicates a need to perform thrombophilia screening?

☐ **A** Cerebral vein thrombosis

☐ **B** Family history of lower limb deep venous thrombosis

☐ **C** Ischaemic stroke in 47-year-old woman

☐ **D** Microcytic anaemia

☐ **E** Peripheral vascular disease in a 56-year-old man

7.67 You are asked to perform a thrombophilia screen in a 32-year-old woman who has had a number of recurrent spontaneous deep vein thromboses. Which of the following blood tests is most likely to be helpful?

☐ **A** Anti-protein C antibody

☐ **B** Anti-Scl antibody

☐ **C** Cysteine

☐ **D** Factor II Leiden

☐ **E** Factor IX

7.68 Which of the following features is most strongly suggestive of HELLP syndrome?

☐ **A** Alanine transaminase 142 IU/l

☐ **B** Microscopic haematuria

☐ **C** Platelet count 165×10^9/l

☐ **D** Raised serum haptoglobin concentrations

☐ **E** Reticulocytes 0.8%

7.69 A 56-year-old woman with chronic alcoholic liver disease is admitted with general malaise. She is deeply jaundiced, and her full blood count shows Hb 64 g/l, MCV 88 fl. Which of the following findings most strongly suggests haemolysis as an explanation for her anaemia?

☐ **A** Dipstick urinalysis positive for bilirubin

☐ **B** Raised serum haptoglobin concentrations

☐ **C** Red cell fragments on blood film

☐ **D** Serum bilirubin 148 mmol/l

☐ **E** Serum lactate dehydrogenase 586 IU/l

7.66   Answer: A

Venous thrombosis in unusual site, including hepatic or portal veins, recurrent venous thrombosis, strong family history, or if there is both arterial and venous occlusion.

7.67   Answer: D

Others include antithrombin, protein C, protein S, factor V Leiden, homocysteine, lupus anticoagulant and anti-cardiolipin antibody.

7.68   Answer: A

Features are haemolysis, elevated liver enzymes, low platelets (HELLP); it is seen as a subset of the antiphospholipid syndrome, which is often characterised by recurrent spontaneous abortions.

7.69   Answer: C

Also associated with low or undetectable haptoglobin concentrations and urinalysis positive for urobilinogen. Raised bilirubin and lactate dehydrogenase (LDH) can be features of liver disease or haemolysis.

7.70 A 34-year-old woman has undergone allogenic bone marrow transplantation for chronic myeloid leukaemia. Which of the following conditions is correct regarding graft-versus-host disease (GVHD)?

◻ **A** Acute GVHD usually appears within 6–12 hours

◻ **B** Can be prevented using high-dose corticosteroids

◻ **C** Rash is uncommon

◻ **D** Risks are less than autologous bone marrow transplantation

◻ **E** Thrombocythaemia is a common feature

7.71 A 62-year-old man is admitted to the Acute Medical Receiving Unit with progressive breathlessness. On examination, he is found to have widespread lymphadenopathy and hepatomegaly. Chest X-ray shows diffuse interstitial opacification and increased lung markings. Which of the following is the most likely diagnosis?

◻ **A** Acute lymphocytic leukaemia

◻ **B** Chronic lymphocytic leukaemia

◻ **C** Chronic myeloid leukaemia

◻ **D** Hodgkin's disease

◻ **E** Non-Hodgkin's lymphoma

7.72 A 21-year-old man is referred to the Haematology Clinic for investigation of night-sweats and fever. He is noted to have enlarged non-tender cervical, inguinal and axillary lymph nodes, and a palpable liver edge. A lymph node biopsy is performed. Which of the following features most strongly suggests an underlying diagnosis of Hodgkin's disease?

◻ **A** Howell–Jolly body

◻ **B** Green birefringence under polarised light

◻ **C** Multiple non-caseating granulomata

◻ **D** Reed–Sternberg cells

◻ **E** Tear-drop cells

7.70 Answer: B

Although this can increase infection risk. Acute disease usually presents within 2–3 weeks. Rash and thrombocytopenia are recognised features of chronic GVHD.

7.71 Answer: B

Although difficult to distinguish from non-Hodgkin's lymphoma, the patient's age, insidious onset and pulmonary involvement make chronic lymphocytic leukaemia more likely.

7.72 Answer: D

These are large lymphoid cells, often surrounded by normal lymphocytes and plasma cells, and are pathognomonic for the disease.

7.73 Which of the following statements most correctly applies to non-Hodgkin's lymphoma?

- A 75% are derived from T-lymphocytes
- B Bone marrow aspiration should normally be avoided
- C Prevalence is higher in patients with impaired cellular immunity
- D There is less extranodal involvement than in Hodgkin's disease
- E Women are more commonly affected than men

7.74 A 73-year-old woman is referred to the Medical Outpatient Department for investigation of weight loss and fatigue. She is found to have Hb 95 g/l, MCV 82 fl, and ESR 98 mm/h. Which of the following would most strongly suggest an underlying diagnosis of malignant myeloma?

- A High serum β_2 microglobin concentration
- B Normal serum IgG concentration
- C Raised serum calcium
- D Serum alkaline phophatase is elevated
- E Stool is negative for faecal occult blood

7.75 A 74-year-old woman is admitted for investigation of confusion associated with mild anaemia. Which of the following features most strongly suggests an underlying diagnosis of Waldenström's macroglobulinaemia?

- A Cervical lymphadenopathy
- B ESR is 54 mm/h
- C High IgG concentration
- D Impaired vision
- E Leukocyte infiltration on bone marrow aspiration

7.73 Answer: C

Most are B-cell in origin, and men are more often affected. Unlike Hodgkin's disease, bone marrow aspirate and trephine are often performed, and cell surface immunotyping.

7.74 Answer: A

Normally, immunoglobulin concentrations are reduced (immune paresis) in association with high paraprotein or light chain levels. Alkaline phosphatase is usually normal in the absence of fractures.

7.75 Answer: D

Due to IgM paraproteinaemia. Other features due to hyperviscosity include bruising or nosebleeds. Lymphadenopathy and splenomegaly are recognised, and bone marrow shows lymphoid cell infiltration.

8. INFECTIOUS DISEASES

8.1 A previously healthy 31-year-old aid worker has returned to the UK from Sudan in Africa. He presents with sudden onset of fever, severe myalgia and diarrhoea. On examination, there is non-suppurative pharyngitis, generalised lymphadenopathy and an erythematous rash over the trunk and limbs. Which of the following organisms is most likely to cause these features?

- A Adenovirus
- B Ebola virus
- C *Haemophilus influenzae*
- D Influenza type A virus
- E *Neisseria meningitides*

8.2 Which of the following haemorrhagic fevers is caused by a non-viral organism?

- A Dengue fever
- B Lassa fever
- C Marburg disease
- D Rocky Mountain spotted fever
- E Yellow fever

8.3 A 27-year-old woman has recently returned from a rural camp in West Africa, and complains of fever, nausea, backache and headache. She has facial flushing and conjunctiva are injected. What is the most likely diagnosis?

- A Malaria
- B Meningococcal meningitis
- C Systemic lupus erythematosus
- D Trichomoniasis
- E Yellow fever

8.1 Answer: B

Recognised cause of viral haemorrhagic fever. Sporadic cases and outbreaks have been reported in Africa. There is an unknown animal reservoir, and incubation period of 5–9 days. Treatment is supportive, and mortality is high.

8.2 Answer: D

Caused by rickettsial infection; dengue (flavivirus), lassa fever (arenavirus), Marburg disease (filovirus), and yellow fever (flavivirus).

8.3 Answer: E

Later phase characterised by petechial haemorrhages and liver failure. Zoonosis caused by a flavivirus; tropical rainforests of West and Central Africa, South and Central America. Monkey pool and *Aedes* mosquito vectors.

8.4 A 23-year-old man has returned to the UK from Southeast Asia, where a fever epidemic had broken out. He has suffered from malaise and headache for 3 days, and now complains of fever, arthralgia, muscle cramps and backache. Temperature is 38.1°C, there is generalised lymphadenopathy, pulse rate 68 per min and blood pressure 122/68 mmHg. What is the most likely diagnosis?

- ☐ **A** Dengue fever
- ☐ **B** Epstein–Barr viraemia
- ☐ **C** HIV seroconversion illness
- ☐ **D** Respiratory syncytial virus infection
- ☐ **E** Schistosomiasis

8.5 A 7-year-old boy has developed a fever associated with nasal catarrh. His younger sister is recovering from measles infection. Which of the following is correct regarding measles?

- ☐ **A** Children are non-infectious until rash appears
- ☐ **B** Infection is most severe in young children
- ☐ **C** Koplik's spots are a pathognomonic feature
- ☐ **D** MMR vaccination is effective but increases risk of autism
- ☐ **E** Morbilliform rash typically persists for 2–3 weeks

8.6 For the past 3 days, a 6-year-old boy has suffered a febrile illness with upper respiratory tract symptoms. He has now developed a maculo-papular rash over the face, head and neck. Which of the following features would most strongly suggest a diagnosis of measles?

- ☐ **A** Consolidation on plain chest X-ray
- ☐ **B** Photophobia
- ☐ **C** Previous measles infection
- ☐ **D** Recent infectious measles contact
- ☐ **E** Recent treatment with corticosteroids

8.4 Answer: A

Flavivirus viral haemorrhagic fever transmitted by *Aedes* mosquito vector in tropical and subtropical countries. Incubation period 2–7 days, often epidemic. May be associated with leukopenia and thrombocytopenia.

8.5 Answer: C

In the early 'catarrhal' stage (days 1–2), the patient is highly infectious. More severe in older children and adults. Koplik's spots in mucous membranes are seen early. In the 'exanthematous' stage (days 3–6), a maculo-papular rash develops and fades to pale brown discoloration.

8.6 Answer: D

Highly infectious during the early catarrhal phase (day 1–2). Previous infection is associated with immunity. MMR vaccination is highly effective active immunisation. Photophobia is a non-specific feature. Pneumonia can occur due to secondary bacterial infection.

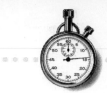

8.7 An 8-year-old girl is suspected of having measles infection. Which of the following is correct regarding the risk of this infection?

- A Incubation period is 12–24 h
- B Infection is usually via faeco-oral route
- C Measles is caused by a paramyxovirus
- D MMR offers passive immunity against infection
- E Risk of infection greatest after morbilliform rash has developed

8.8 A 24-year-old man presents with a 2-day history of fever, malaise and painful swelling of the left parotid gland. He is suspected of having mumps. Which of the following statements is correct regarding this infection?

- A Encephalitis is a common complication
- B Infection spread by droplet transmission
- C Infectivity rate is > 90% of contacts
- D More than 95% of infections have clinical features
- E Orchitis occurs in 1–2% of post-pubescent men

8.9 Which of the following statements is correct about HIV infection?

- A Commonest global cause of death across all ages
- B Heterosexual transmission rates are increasing in Western society
- C Intravenous drug use is the commonest global means of transmission
- D The virus arose through genetic mutation in 1979
- E Prevalence is up to 90% in rural African towns

8.10 You are asked to counsel a 47-year-old woman who has had HIV infection for 4 years. She is expecting her first child and is 8 months pregnant. Which of these is the most appropriate advice?

- A Anti-retroviral treatments should be withheld in the peri-partum period
- B Breast-feeding does not increase transmission risk
- C Delivery by Caesarean section reduces transmission risk
- D Maternal viral titres do not influence transmission likelihood
- E Vaginal delivery has transmission rate of 80–90%

8.7   Answer: C

Measles (rubeola) transmitted by droplets, with incubation period of 10 days. Early catarrhal stages are more infectious than when rash has developed. MMR is a highly effective live attenuated vaccine.

8.8   Answer: B

Mumps is a paramyxovirus with low infectivity, and infection is unapparent in around a third. Orchitis affects around 25% of post-pubescent men and can cause infertility if bilateral. Viral meningitis is a recognised feature.

8.9   Answer: B

Origins obscure, but HIV confirmed present in Africa in 1940s or earlier. Vaginal and anal intercourse predominant route. Cardiovascular and cerebrovascular disease commonest global cause of death. Rural and urban prevalence as high as 10% and 20% in parts of Africa.

8.10   Answer: C

There is a 15–55% risk of transmission (in utero, during parturition and breast-feeding), especially with high maternal viral load, hence prenatal screening important. Pre-partum and peri-partum anti-retrovirals reduce transmission.

8.11 What is the risk that a single unit of packed red blood cells available for transfusion in the UK will transmit HIV infection?

☐ **A** 1 in 1000

☐ **B** 1 in 1000 if blood collected before 1992

☐ **C** 1 in 1,000,000

☐ **D** None due to heat-treatment and irradiation of all donated blood

☐ **E** None due to screening of all donated blood

8.12 You are working as an SHO in the Infectious Diseases Unit. One of your colleagues asks you for advice following a recent needlestick injury when drawing blood from an HIV-positive patient. Which of the following is correct regarding potential transmission of HIV infection?

☐ **A** Anti-retrovirals should be taken within 1–2 h for greatest efficacy

☐ **B** Gloves do not reduce transmission after needlestick injury

☐ **C** Overall transmission risk is around 10%

☐ **D** Negative HIV antibody serology at 1 month is highly reassuring

☐ **E** Stage of HIV infection of the patient is irrelevant

8.13 A 39-year-old woman has been diagnosed with HIV infection 18 months earlier. Which one of the following disorders most strongly indicates progression to AIDS?

☐ **A** Basal cell carcinoma overlying the nasal bridge

☐ **B** Cytomegalovirus retinitis

☐ **C** Oral candida

☐ **D** Pulmonary tuberculosis

☐ **E** Right basal pneumonia

8.14 A 26-year-old man presents with a 4-week history of night sweats, fever and malaise. There is generalised lymphadenopathy. Full blood count shows WBC 1.2×10^9/ml and platelets 56×10^9/ml, and a plain chest X-ray shows bilateral diffuse interstitial perihilar shadowing. What is the most likely diagnosis?

☐ **A** AIDS

☐ **B** Disseminated CMV infection

☐ **C** HIV seroconversion illness

☐ **D** Progressive generalised lymphadenopathy

☐ **E** Sarcoidosis

8.11   Answer: C

Estimated as negligibly small but not zero. Volunteers with strong HIV risk factors are discouraged from donating, and screening involves serodiagnosis: this can be negative in early infection before seroconversion.

8.12   Answer: A

Zidovudine reduces seroconversion rate by > 75%; current recommendation is for triple anti-retroviral therapy for 1 month, started as soon as possible after exposure, eg zidovudine, lamivudine and indinavir.

8.13   Answer: B

Pulmonary TB may be an AIDS-defining condition if associated with a low CD4 count (< 200/mm^3). Oesophageal or pulmonary candida infection is also AIDS-defining, as per the WHO case definition for AIDS (1987).

8.14   Answer: A

The chest X-ray appearance strongly suggests *Pneumocystis* pneumonia, an AIDS-defining illness.

8.15 A 41-year-old woman has been diagnosed with HIV infection for 8 years. During a routine clinic appointment, she is noted to have retinitis with an appearance suggestive of CMV infection. Which of the following is true of CMV retinitis?

   A Characteristically caused by droplet transmission

   B Disseminated infection may involve the adrenal glands

   C Rarely associated with perivascular exudates

   D Typically develops despite CD4 count > 200/mm^3

   E Vision is normally preserved

8.16 A 31-year-old man has recently developed AIDS. Recently, he has suffered from deteriorating vision and is diagnosed with CMV retinitis. What is the most appropriate treatment for this condition?

   A Intravenous aciclovir

   B Intravenous ganciclovir

   C Intravenous hydrocortisone

   D Oral foscarnet

   E Topical ganciclovir

8.17 For the past 4 weeks, an HIV-positive man has suffered fever, weight loss and fatigue. Plain chest X-ray shows consolidation and cavitation in the right mid-zone accompanied by a small pleural effusion. Which of the following infections is most likely?

   A *Candida albicans*

   B *Mycobacterium bovis*

   C *Mycobacterium tuberculosis*

   D *Pneumocystis carinii*

   E *Streptococcus pneumoniae*

8.15 Answer: B

Uncommon unless CD4 count < 50/mm^3, can lead to rapid blindness. Perivascular exudates are typical feature, with haemorrhages in severe cases. Infection due to reactivation of latent CMV.

8.16 Answer: B

Ganciclovir or foscarnet are the treatments of choice, usually intravenous administration via a central vein. Oral and intra-ocular ganciclovir preparations are now available.

8.17 Answer: C

Can occur at any stage in TB, and often associated with cavitation and systemic features. *Pneumocystis carinii* pneumonia very rarely associated with effusion.

8.18 A 51-year-old woman has had AIDS for 18 months. She complains of fever, malaise, weight loss and breathlessness. She is found to have hepatomegaly and widespread lymphadenopathy. CD4 count is < 30/mm³, plain chest X-ray shows patchy consolidation and sputum contains numerous acid-fast bacilli. What is the most likely causative organism?

☐ A *Candida albicans*

☐ B *Chlamydia pneumoniae*

☐ C Cytomegalovirus

☐ D *Mycobacterium avium intracellulare*

☐ E *Mycobacterium tuberculosis*

8.19 A 28-year-old man is admitted to the Emergency Department with seizures. He had been diagnosed with HIV infection 7 years earlier, and has suffered headaches, fever and malaise for the past 6 weeks. CT head scan shows a ring-enhancing mass lesion in the right cerebral hemisphere, with a rim of surrounding oedema. What is the most likely diagnosis?

☐ A Cryptococcal meningitis

☐ B Pneumococcal abscess

☐ C Staphylococcal infection

☐ D *Toxoplasma gondii* infection

☐ E Tuberculous meningitis

8.20 A 21-year-old woman has been diagnosed with HIV infection for 7 years. She has recently noticed the development of raised, well circumscribed dark-red lesions over the lower legs and nose. What is the most likely cause of these abnormalities?

☐ A Cryoglobulinaemia

☐ B Erythema nodosum

☐ C Kaposi's sarcoma

☐ D *Mycobacterium bovis* infection

☐ E Small-vessel vasculitis

8.18 Answer: D

Usually low virulence, causes disease with very low CD4 counts. Treatment is with combinations of clarithromycin, azithromycin, rifabutin, ethambutol and amikacin.

8.19 Answer: D

Serological tests often unreliable. Diagnosis often depends on characteristic CT or MRI appearances, and brain biopsy in certain cases. Treatment is with pyrimethamine and sulfadiazine.

8.20 Answer: C

Typical distribution. This and other secondary neoplasms, eg non-Hodgkin's lymphoma, indicated disseminated disease in AIDS.

8.21 A 34-year-old woman has been diagnosed HIV-positive for 9 years, and recently diagnosed with Kaposi's sarcoma. Which of the following is most characteristic of this disorder?

A Arises from arterial endothelium

B Associated with herpesvirus 8 (HHV 8) infection

C Common feature in transfusion-acquired HIV infection

D Preferentially affects the trunk and back

E Skin involvement heralds poorer prognosis than lymph node infiltration

8.22 A 48-year-old man has suffered AIDS for 2 years and, over the past 4 months, has developed fever, weight loss, profuse night sweats and hepatomegaly. What is the most likely diagnosis?

A B-cell lymphoma

B Disseminated cytomegalovirus (CMV) infection

C Kaposi's sarcoma

D Systemic candidiasis

E Toxoplasmosis

8.23 You are asked to review a 36-year-old patient in the Infectious Diseases Unit. He has developed white plaques on his tongue, and the nursing staff have queried whether he may have developed oral candida infection. Which of the following features most strongly suggest an alternative diagnosis?

A Plaques mainly affecting the upper part of the tongue

B Plaques adherent and cannot be removed with spatula

C Poor response to 3 days of oral nystatin

D Previously treated oral candidiasis

E Recent course of oral co-amoxiclav

8.21   Answer: B

AIDS-defining. HHV 8 infection appears sexually transmitted, and Kaposi's sarcoma is uncommon in transfusion-acquired HIV infection. Arises from venules, typically involves skin on nose, penis and lower legs, mouth and hard palate.

8.22   Answer: A

Non-Hodgkin's lymphoma typically presents with 'B symptoms', and extra-reticular involvement is more common than in non-HIV patients, eg gastrointestinal or bone marrow involvement. CMV less likely to cause hepatomegaly.

8.23   Answer: B

Suggests oral hairy leukoplakia: usually painless, adherent plaques on the sides of the tongue. Caused by Epstein–Barr virus and responds to aciclovir and ganciclovir.

8.24 A 14-year-old boy presents with pink macular rash over the head, neck and trunk. He is otherwise well, with no constitutional symptoms. A diagnosis of rubella is suspected. Which of the following is most likely to be a feature of this infection?

- A   Diagnosis can be confirmed by serological testing
- B   Fever and respiratory symptoms usually predominate
- C   Incubation period is around 1–2 days
- D   Lymphadenopathy suggests an alternative diagnosis
- E   Recurrent rubella infection occurs in 5–10% of patients

8.25 An adult female presents with headache and fever symptoms. She is found to have a non-blanching purpuric rash overlying her trunk, neck and limbs. Which of the following infections is most likely to cause this appearance?

- A   Enterovirus
- B   Epstein–Barr virus
- C   Parvovirus B19
- D   Rubivirus
- E   Varicella zoster virus

8.26 Which of the following statements regarding herpes simplex virus infection is correct?

- A   Encephalitis complicates primary or recurrent infection
- B   HSV type-2 causes only genital infection
- C   Recurrent infection is caused by repeated viral exposure
- D   Serology is the most useful means of diagnosis
- E   Ulcerative stomatitis is a rare complication

8.27 Which of the following statements is most accurate with regard to HSV infection?

- A   Aciclovir resistance is common
- B   Genital herpes rarely recurs
- C   Herpes labialis may be provoked by menstruation
- D   Prolonged aciclovir eradicates latent HSV from dorsal root ganglia
- E   Valciclovir has direct anti-viral action against HSV-1 and HSV-2

8.24   Answer: A

Rash most common presenting feature; children have no/mild symptoms, including sub-occipital lymphadenopathy. Adults may have complications including polyarthropathy and encephalitis. Infection or MMR confer high immunity.

8.25   Answer: D

The typical rash of rubella is a pink, erythematous blanching rash. Adult infection can be complicated by thrombocytopenic purpura in some cases. The other infections listed are characteristically associated with an erythematous rash.

8.26   Answer: A

Primary infection can be diagnosed by serology, but many people have positive serology due to asymptomatic childhood infection. Recurrence is due to reactivation of virus latent in sensory ganglia. Can be diagnosed by viral culture and PCR of CSF.

8.27   Answer: C

Oral or genital infections can be caused by HSV-1 or HSV-2, and often recur. Recurrence risk is reduced by regular aciclovir administration. Valciclovir is a prodrug.

8.28 A 12-year-old boy presents with a morbilliform rash, and IgM antibody to parvovirus B19 is found to be positive. Which of the following is the most likely diagnosis?

◻ **A** Erysipelas

◻ **B** Erythema infectiosum

◻ **C** Erythema multiforme

◻ **D** Erythema nodosum

◻ **E** Systemic lupus erythematosus

8.29 A 42-year-old man with longstanding sickle cell disease presents with fever and morbilliform rash overlying his trunk, face and neck. He is found to have a symmetrical polyarthritis, and his haemoglobin has fallen from 9.8 g/dl to 6.6 g/dl during the past month. Which of the following is the most likely explanation for his anaemia?

◻ **A** Anaemia of chronic renal failure

◻ **B** Blast cell crisis

◻ **C** Blood loss due to multiple haemarthroses

◻ **D** Parvovirus B19 infection

◻ **E** Tuberculous bone marrow infiltration

8.30 Which of the following is most likely to be a characteristic feature of molluscum contagiosum?

◻ **A** Less common in immunocompromised patients

◻ **B** Parvovirus

◻ **C** Rarely resolve spontaneously

◻ **D** Should generally be excised to prevent malignant transformation

◻ **E** Transmitted via infected towelling

8.28   Answer: B

Also known a 'fifth disease', characterised by fever and erythematous rash ('slapped cheek'). Parvovirus B19 infection in adults often associated with arthropathy and red cell aplasia.

8.29   Answer: D

B19 infection causes erythroid arrest, usually of little consequence in previously healthy, but causes aplastic crises in those with high red cell turnover. Infection in immunocompromised patients can cause chronic anaemia. May be treated by administration of neutralising antibody.

8.30   Answer: E

Poxvirus transmitted by direct contact or infected clothing. More common in atopic and immunocompromised individuals (incubation period 2–5 weeks). Often resolve spontaneously, but can also be treated with cryotherapy.

8.31 You review a 31-year-old visiting student in the Medical Outpatient Department. He is noted to have hyperaemia affecting the conjunctiva of his left eye, which shows numerous pale follicles. The right eye does not appear inflamed, but there is a marked entropion. Which of the following is the most likely infective organism in this condition?

A *Chlamydia trachomatis*

B Epstein–Barr virus

C Herpes simplex virus

D *Mycoplasma pneumoniae*

E *Staphylococcus aureus*

8.32 Trachoma is the leading preventable cause of blindness worldwide. Which of the following statements is most likely to be true regarding this infectious disease?

A *Chlamydia trachomatis* cannot be demonstrated on culture

B Commonly spread by nasal droplet transmission

C Infection may be latent for many years

D The cornea is typically spared

E Typically endemic spread occurs close to lakes and rivers

8.33 Which of the following diseases is caused by rickettsial infection in humans?

A Dengue fever

B Endemic typhus fever

C Lassa fever

D Marburg disease

E Yellow fever

8.31   Answer: A

Trachoma is commonest cause of blindness. Caused by direct contact with fomites and often presents insidiously. Treated with prolonged topical or oral tetracycline. May cause scarring and entropion.

8.32   Answer: C

Endemic, often in dry and dusty climates, and spread by direct contact or via infected fomites. Upper eyelid conjunctiva involved first, can lead to scarring and entropion. Vascularisation and opacification of the cornea cause blindness.

8.33   Answer: B

Caused by *Rickettsia mooseri*. Others include epidemic typhus fever (*R. prowazekii*), Rocky Mountain spotted fever (*R. rickettsii*), scrub typhus fever (*R. tsutsugamushi*), rickettsialpox and trench fever. Stems A, C, D and E are recognised causes of viral haemorrhagic fever.

8.34 A 47-year-old farmer presents to the Medical Outpatient Department with flu-like symptoms, arthralgia, fever and headaches for around 4 weeks. He is found to have a soft systolic cardiac murmur. Three sets of blood cultures are negative. Which of the following organisms is the most likely to have caused his symptoms?

- [ ] **A** *Chlamydia pneumoniae*
- [ ] **B** *Coxiella burnetii*
- [ ] **C** *Haemophilus influenzae*
- [ ] **D** *Mycobacterium bovis*
- [ ] **E** *Streptococcus faecalis*

8.35 A 40-year-old woman presents to the Emergency Department with a short history of fever symptoms and a facial rash. On examination, there is well-defined, raised erythematous patch of skin overlying her left cheek, and there are a number of slightly enlarged, tender cervical lymph nodes. Which of the following is the most likely explanation?

- [ ] **A** Erythema infectiosum
- [ ] **B** Erysipelas
- [ ] **C** Kaposi's sarcoma
- [ ] **D** Staphylococcal cellulitis
- [ ] **E** Subcutaneous lymphoma

8.36 A 52-year-old woman complains of pain and redness affecting her left ankle and lower leg. On examination, there is erythema and swelling. Which of the following features would most strongly indicate bacterial cellulitis, rather than an alternative diagnosis?

- [ ] **A** Knee-joint swelling bilaterally
- [ ] **B** Lymphadenitis of the left inguinal region
- [ ] **C** Pain on weight-bearing
- [ ] **D** Superficial skin veins appear dilated
- [ ] **E** Temperature 37.5°C

8.34   Answer: B

Q-fever is a rickettsia-like organism, spread by airborne transmission from infected cattle hide, animal products or infected (unpasteurised) milk. Diagnosed by rising antibody titres, and treated with tetracycline.

8.35   Answer: B

Streptococcal in majority of cases. Often spread from the nose and, therefore, involves face. Raised, oedematous lesions and well-defined margin distinguishes from common bacterial cellulitis. Responds well to penicillin.

8.36   Answer: B

Lymphangitis (erythema tracking proximally from the infection site) and lymphadenitis (involving nodes that drain the infected region) are strong indicators of cellulitis. DVT and ruptured Baker's cyst may also be associated with the other features listed.

8.37 A 54-year-old patient with diabetes mellitus is admitted for treatment of an infected skin ulcer. Culture of wound swab demonstrates multiple colony forming units of *Staphylococcus aureus*. Which of the following would be most appropriate treatment?

- A Benzylpenicillin
- B Ciprofloxacin
- C Erythromycin
- D Flucloxacillin
- E Vancomycin

8.38 A 32-year-old woman is admitted for investigation of chronic fever symptoms, recent weight loss and a murmur that fluctuates in its site and intensity. *Staphylococcus epidermidis* is grown from blood culture bottles taken on two separate occasions. Which of the following statements is most likely to be true?

- A Culture findings are likely to be due to skin contamination
- B Endocarditis may be eradicated with short courses of antibiotics
- C Skin colonisation requires antibiotic treatment for eradication
- D *Staphylococcus epidermidis* may be resistant to flucloxacillin
- E This bacterium characteristically causes acne

8.39 A 13-year-old boy attends the Infectious Diseases Unit for assessment of laryngitis, mild fever and nasal discharge. On examination, he is found to have diffuse neck swelling, an injected throat and tonsils, with an overlying grey membrane. Which of the following diagnoses requires most urgent consideration?

- A Acute Epstein–Barr virus infection
- B Diphtheria
- C Epiglottitis
- D Peri-tonsillar abscess
- E Primary herpes simplex infection

8.37 Answer: D

More than 90% of *S. aureus* are resistant to penicillin (eg amoxicillin). Most are sensitive to flucloxacillin, but an increasing proportion are resistant to this and other antimicrobials (methicillin-resistant *S. aureus*, MRSA) and may necessitate vancomycin treatment.

8.38 Answer: D

Methicillin-resistant strains are now recognised. Common skin commensal that can cause endocarditis in patients with valvular lesions or immunocompromise. Notoriously difficult to eradicate.

8.39 Answer: B

Incubation period 2–4 days. Early symptoms may be mild. May be followed by exotoxin-mediated neuropathy, laryngeal paralysis and myocarditis. Requires urgent antitoxin administration and intravenous benzylpenicillin whist confirmation is awaited.

8.40 Which of the following statements is correct in relation to infection with *Corynebacterium diphtheriae*?

- [ ] **A** Erythromycin is ineffective treatment
- [ ] **B** Is becoming less prevalent due to passive immunity
- [ ] **C** Nasal infection does not require treatment
- [ ] **D** Only exotoxin-positive cases require public health notification
- [ ] **E** Serum sickness is a recognised complication of antiserum treatment

8.41 Which of the following clinical features is most likely to be a feature of infection by *Bordetella pertussis*?

- [ ] **A** Bouts of coughing followed by vomiting
- [ ] **B** Commonly associated with neurological complications
- [ ] **C** Diagnosis is by electron microscopy of nasopharyngeal secretions
- [ ] **D** Lymphopenia on full blood count
- [ ] **E** Onset between 10 and 20 years of age

8.42 A medical student has returned from a 2-month elective in India, where there had been an outbreak of a febrile illness. He complains of headache, fever and muscle aches for 10 days, and has developed diarrhoea over the past 24 h. Which of the following infectious organisms is most likely to be responsible for his symptoms?

- [ ] **A** *Bacillus anthracis*
- [ ] **B** *Bacillus cereus*
- [ ] **C** Hepatitis A virus
- [ ] **D** *Rickettsia mooseri*
- [ ] **E** *Salmonella typhi*

8.43 Which of the following organisms characteristically causes food poisoning mediated by toxin production?

- [ ] **A** *Bacillus cereus*
- [ ] **B** *Campylobacter jejuni*
- [ ] **C** Norwalk virus
- [ ] **D** *Staphylococcus aureus*
- [ ] **E** Wootbot virus

8.40   Answer: E

Erythromycin eradicates organisms in carriers. Intravenous benzylpenicillin is given in acute infection; antiserum is used to prevent life-threatening exotoxin-mediated complications (myocarditis and neuropathy). All cases should be reported to the Public Health Department.

8.41   Answer: A

Pathognomonic of the paroxysmal stage. Most infectious during the earlier catarrhal stage. Typically occurs in young children. Diagnosis is established by demonstration culture of nasopharyngeal swabs, and treatment is with erythromycin.

8.42   Answer: E

Salmonella typhi and *S. paratyphi* cause typhoid and paratyphoid enteric fevers respectively, associated with faeco–oral spread and outbreaks in areas with poor sanitation. *Bacillus cereus* is a recognised cause of food poisoning, often short-lived and characterised by rapid onset of vomiting.

8.43   Answer: D

Wootbot does not cause human disease. The others are recognised causes of non-toxin-mediated gastroenteritis. Other toxin-mediated food poisoning causes are *E. coli* 0157, *Clostridium botulinum* and *Clostridium perfringens*.

8.44 Which one of the following organisms is believed to cause gastroenteritis due to local infection, ie non-toxin-mediated infection?

☐ A   *Campylobacter jejuni*

☐ B   Ciguatoxin

☐ C   *Clostridium botulinum*

☐ D   *Clostridium perfringens*

☐ E   *E. coli* 0157

8.45 A 26-year-old woman is admitted with a 48-h history of severe vomiting and profuse watery diarrhoea. She is dehydrated, tachycardic and temperature is 38.6°C. Which one of the following steps is most appropriate in her initial management?

☐ A   High dose corticosteroids intravenously for at least 48 h

☐ B   Intravenous ciprofloxacin is indicated

☐ C   Paracetamol should be given to reduce pyrexia

☐ D   Rapid intravenous hydration with 0.9% saline

☐ E   Restrict fluid intake until diarrhoea settling

8.46 A 23-year-old aid worker returns to the UK complaining of diarrhoea, colicky abdominal pain and fever. Abdomen is generally tender and rectal examination shows loose, blood-stained stool. Infection with which organism is most likely to cause these symptoms?

☐ A   Bagel virus

☐ B   *Campylobacter jejuni*

☐ C   *Shigella flexneri*

☐ D   *Staphylococcus aureus*

☐ E   Varicella zoster reactivation

8.44   Answer: A

Ciguatoxin is a recognised cause of non-infective gastroenteritis, sourced from tropical fish. The others listed in stems C, D and E are recognised causes of toxin-mediated food poisoning.

8.45   Answer: D

In the absence of heart failure, very rapid hydration can be tolerated. This should aim to quickly restore normal hydration status, and meet the requirements of on-going fluid loss. In hydration, saline interferes less with potassium homeostasis than, for example, 5% dextrose administration.

8.46   Answer: C

Shigella (*S. sonnei*, *S. flexneri*, *S. boydii* and *S. dysenteriae*) cause bacillary dysentery (shigellosis). It is endemic worldwide, particularly in areas of poor sanitation and overcrowding.

8.47 A 28-year-old traveller presents to the Emergency Department with persistent fever, sweating, headache and muscle cramps for 2 weeks. On examination, he is found to have a palpable spleen and temperature is 38.1°C. Which of the following is most likely to account for his symptoms?

- [ ] A Bacterial meningitis
- [ ] B Brucellosis
- [ ] C Leptospirosis
- [ ] D Scurvy
- [ ] E Tuberculosis

8.48 A 28-year-old nurse has returned from a 3-week trip to Asia. She has suffered 3 days of fever, profuse watery diarrhoea and colicky abdominal pain. Over the past 24 h she has started vomiting, and is becoming increasingly dehydrated. Which of the following infections is most likely to account for these symptoms?

- [ ] A Brucellosis
- [ ] B Cholera
- [ ] C HIV seroconversion illness
- [ ] D Malaria
- [ ] E Primary tuberculosis

8.49 You are working in a first-aid hospital in India during a special relief project, and a cholera epidemic has broken out. Which of the following statements is most accurate in relation to this condition?

- [ ] A Chronic carriage of *V. cholerae* is common
- [ ] B Death results from high fever and seizures
- [ ] C Pandemics have occurred due to *V. cholerae* 'El Tor' biotype
- [ ] D *V. cholerae* organisms readily traverse the intestinal wall
- [ ] E *V. cholerae* organisms survive for 20–30 min in salt water

8.50 Which of the following measures is most likely to be effective in limiting the spread of a cholera epidemic?

- [ ] A Antiserum administration
- [ ] B Bed-rest and avoidance of swimming pools
- [ ] C Ensuring good sanitation and hygiene
- [ ] D Oral co-trimoxazole administration
- [ ] E Oral tetracycline administration

8.47   Answer: B

Now uncommon in UK, and can be spread via unpasteurised milk. More common in farmers and animal workers. In Mediterranean and Far East is transmitted from infected goats and sheep. Treated with tetracycline plus rifampicin, or tetracycline plus streptomycin.

8.48   Answer: B

Vibrio cholerae causes severe acute gastrointestinal infection. Faeco–oral transmission is through contaminated water, unwashed hands or infection of food via flies.

8.49   Answer: C

Chronic carriage is rare. The organism survives for several weeks in salt or fresh water. It is minimally invasive, and features are due to exotoxin-mediated gut secretion, profound fluid loss and electrolyte disturbance.

8.50   Answer: C

The major route of spread is through contamination of drinking supplies by vomit and/or stool from infected patients. Tetracycline or co-trimoxazole treatment shortens the duration of *Vibrio* excretion, but are less effective than measures to improve personal hygiene.

8.51 Which of the following clinical features is most strongly indicative of lepromatous leprosy?

☐ **A** Absence of *Mycobacterium leprae* on tissue biopsy

☐ **B** Involvement of nasopharyngeal mucosa

☐ **C** Loss of sensation overlying skin lesions

☐ **D** Marked skin hypopigmentation

☐ **E** Prominent involvement of peripheral nerves

8.52 Which of the following treatments is most likely to be useful in the treatment of leprosy?

☐ **A** Amoxicillin

☐ **B** Clarithromycin and amoxicillin

☐ **C** Dapsone

☐ **D** Rifampicin

☐ **E** Rifampicin, clofazimine and dapsone

8.53 A 49-year-old farmer is admitted with headache, fever and myalgia. He is jaundiced, and has an enlarged tender liver, conjunctivitis and multiple petechiae overlying his trunk and limbs. Infection with which organism is most likely to account for these features?

☐ **A** *Borrelia burgdorferi*

☐ **B** *Leptospirosis icterohaemorrhagiae*

☐ **C** *Mycobacterium tuberculosis*

☐ **D** *Plasmodium falciparum*

☐ **E** *Treponema pallidum*

8.54 A 43-year-old veterinary surgeon is admitted with sudden onset of fever, jaundice and hepatitis. A diagnosis of Weil's disease is suspected. Which of the following is the most useful diagnostic test in this condition?

☐ **A** Blood cultures

☐ **B** CSF microscopy and culture

☐ **C** Liver biopsy

☐ **D** Rising specific leptospiral antibody titres

☐ **E** Urine microscopy

8.51 Answer: B

In lepromatous leprosy, there is widely disseminated skin and nerve involvement, with poorly demarcated skin lesions; nerve enlargement is a late feature. The natural outcome is progression, and other tissues and organs may be involved. Immune-complex-mediated reactions are a recognised feature.

8.52 Answer: E

Rifampicin is the most effective, and need be given only 1 day per month because of the slow *M. leprae* turnover. Clofazimine and dapsone are given daily in combination to reduce resistance, and treatment is usually for 2 years.

8.53 Answer: B

Weil's disease is transmitted from infected rat urine via contaminated water supply, or via penetration of mucous membranes or broken skin. Liver, kidney and heart involvement can be severe, and mortality is as high as 10–20%.

8.54 Answer: D

Liver function tests often indicate a hepatitis (high AST and ALT), often with some degree of biliary obstruction (high GGT and ALP). Renal involvement is signified by raised serum creatinine and red cells and granular casts on urine microscopy. Treatment is with high-dose intravenous penicillin or macrolide antibiotics.

8.55　A 56-year-old forestry worker presents with a 4-week history of fever, erythematous rash overlying trunk and limbs, neck stiffness and photophobia. There is tenderness and mild swelling affecting the small joints of both ankles, wrists and hands. Which of the following is the most likely diagnosis?

- A　Brucellosis
- B　Echovirus infection
- C　Leptospirosis
- D　Lyme disease
- E　Primary tuberculosis

8.56　A 23-year-old student is referred by her GP with a scaly erythematous rash over her left forearm. The appearance is strongly suggestive of ringworm. Which of these factors is most likely to have predisposed to ringworm infection in this patient?

- A　Eczema
- B　History of hay fever
- C　Inhaled corticosteroids
- D　Menstruation
- E　Recent course of amoxicillin

8.57　A 24-year-old woman with a history of asthma presents to the Emergency Department with fever and breathlessness. A plain chest X-ray shows diffuse interstitial opacification in both lung fields. Which of the following is the most probable diagnosis?

- A　Acute exacerbation of asthma
- B　Acute pulmonary oedema
- C　Allergic bronchopulmonary aspergillosis
- D　Corticosteroid-induced cardiomyopathy
- E　Fibrosing alveolitis

8.55   Answer: D

Around one in four forestry workers are seropositive. Caused by *Borrelia burgdorferi*, a spirochaete transmitted by the *Ixodes ricinus* tick from infested sheep and deer. Erythema chronicum migrans is an early feature, followed by neurological and cardiac involvement. Late features are arthropathy and neuropathy.

8.56   Answer: A

Due to loss of skin integrity. Other factors include diabetes, pregnancy, malignancy, topical or systemic corticosteroids and HIV infection.

8.57   Answer: C

Commonest systemic fungal infection in UK, more common in patients with asthma. Treatment includes anti-fungal therapy (eg amphotericin) but often this cannot be given long term. Corticosteroids are used to suppress local inflammation, and physiotherapy aids expectoration and prevents collapse.

8.58 A 34-year-old man with longstanding asthma suffers an exacerbation of his respiratory symptoms. A chest X-ray shows diffuse pulmonary infiltration, and a diagnosis of allergic bronchopulmonary aspergillosis is suspected. Which of these findings would be most helpful in establishing the diagnosis?

- **A** Allergic response to amoxicillin administration
- **B** Demonstration of *A. fumigatus* on sputum microscopy
- **C** Elevated serum IgE concentrations
- **D** High peripheral blood eosinophil count
- **E** Skin hypersensitivity to *A. fumigatus* extract

8.59 A 32-year-old man with HIV infection presents with a short history of fever, photophobia and neck stiffness. Meningitis is suspected, and a lumbar puncture shows mildly turbid CSF with spores seen on microscopy. What is the most likely infective organism?

- **A** *Candida albicans*
- **B** *Chlamydia trachomatis*
- **C** *Cryptococcus neoformans*
- **D** *Cryptosporidium parvum*
- **E** Cytomegalovirus

8.60 A 31-year-old man has recently returned to the UK from a 4-week holiday in Kenya. He is complaining of headache, nausea and fever. Investigations show haemoglobin 8.9 g/dl. Examination shows icteric sclera and temperature 38.3°C. A diagnosis of malaria is suspected. What is the most likely explanation for anaemia in this patient?

- **A** Acute haemolysis of infected red blood cells
- **B** Autoimmune anaemia
- **C** Bone marrow suppression
- **D** Hepatomegaly and red cell sequestration
- **E** Vitamin B_{12} depletion

8.58   Answer: B

C, D and E are associated features, but less specific. Additionally, the presence of serum precipitating antibodies to *A. fumigatus* helps confirm the diagnosis.

8.59   Answer: C

Cryptococcal meningitis is much more common in immunocompromised patients. Diagnosis is made by demonstration of spores in CSF, or demonstration of serum cryptococcal antigen.

8.60   Answer: A

Haemolysis of infected red cells and, to a lesser extent, non-infected red cells is the major cause. Other contributing factors include impaired erythropoiesis, splenic sequestration and folate depletion. Jaundice is a common feature due to haemolysis and hepatic involvement.

8.61 A 36-year-old woman has recently been in Tanzania and is complaining of headache, fever and rigors. On examination, she is mildly jaundiced, and temperature is 38.6°C. Which of these most strongly suggests a diagnosis of malaria?

A Anaemia

B Haemoglobinuria

C Raised serum alanine transaminase

D Ring forms seen on peripheral blood film

E Splenomegaly

8.62 A 48-year-old previously healthy businessman has returned from a 4-week trip to Indonesia. He is admitted via the Emergency Department after a witnessed generalised seizure. He is mildly jaundiced, there is palpable splenomegaly, and temperature is 39.2°C. What organism is most likely to be responsible?

A *Entamoeba histolytica*

B *Mycobacterium tuberculosis*

C *Plasmodium falciparum*

D *Plasmodium malariae*

E *Treponema pallidum*

8.63 A 34-year-old woman has recently returned to the UK after a vacation in Egypt. She is complaining of abdominal cramps and fever, associated with intermittent constipation and diarrhoea with offensive-smelling stool. What is the most likely diagnosis?

A Amoebic dysentery

B *Campylobacter* infection

C *Clostridium difficile* gastroenteritis

D Malaria

E Schistosomiasis

8.61   Answer: D

Feature of early *Plasmodium falciparum* infection; direct visualisation
of parasites is pathognomonic. A, B, C and E are characteristic
findings in malaria, but less specific.

8.62   Answer: C

The features are consistent with malaria infection; the *falciparum*
strain is more likely to be associated with severe anaemia,
intravascular haemolysis, shock and organ damage than others.
Plasmodium malariae is usually associated with mild fever every 3rd
day, and fewer systemic complications.

8.63   Answer: A

Caused by ingestion of *Entamoeba histolytica* cysts in contaminated
water, or food contamination by infected faeces. Often runs a
chronic course, responds quickly to oral metronidazole or tinidazole.
Diloxanide furoate eliminates intestinal cysts.

8.64 A 41-year-old man presents to the Emergency Department with a history of intermittent fever, malaise and right upper quadrant pain for 6 weeks after returning to the UK from India. On examination, temperature is 37.7°C and a tender, enlarged liver is palpable. Which of the following is the most likely explanation for these findings?

A Bacterial overgrowth syndrome

B Chronic cholecystitis

C Crohn's disease with secondary abscess

D Hepatic amoebiasis

E Tropical sprue

8.65 A 24-year-old medical student has recently returned from a medical elective in India. He is complaining of persistent diarrhoea, vomiting and abdominal pain, and 8 kg weight loss over the past 4 weeks. Which of the following diagnoses is most likely?

A Amoebic dysentery

B Campylobacter gastroenteritis

C Giardiasis

D Schistosomiasis

E Typhoid

8.66 Which of the following features is most closely associated with schistosomiasis?

A Cercariae are unable to penetrate skin or mucous membranes

B Larval migration can cause myositis and hepatitis

C Peripheral blood neutrophil count is usually raised

D Sheep and goats are the natural host for this infection

E Typically spread by ixodes mosquito vector

8.64 Answer: D

Symptoms are often vague. Large abscesses can rupture and cause secondary complications in the pleural or abdominal cavities. Treatment is with metronidazole or tinidazole.

8.65 Answer: C

Caused by the parasite *G. lamblia*, common in the tropics, spread by contaminated water supplies. Cysts remain viable in water for several months. Symptoms last between several days and months, and can be associated with malabsorption and steatorrhoea. Treated with metronidazole or tinidazole.

8.66 Answer: B

The helminiths *S. mansoni*, *S. japonicum* and *S. haematobium* can also cause pneumonitis, serum sickness and eosinophilia. Egg deposition in the bladder causes cystitis and haematuria; cysts passed into water by urine or faeces multiply in fresh-water snails that release cercariae into water; these cause infection after penetrating skin. Praziquantel is effective treatment.

8.67 A 58-year-old Asian farmworker is visiting his daughter in the UK. He attends the Emergency Department after sustaining a fall when climbing a set of stairs. Pelvic X-rays show two discreet calcified cystic lesions of the left quadriceps muscle. Which of the following is most likely to account for these?

- A Amyloidosis
- B Cysticercosis
- C Haemarthrosis
- D Tuberculosis
- E Weil's disease

8.68 A 43-year-old man complains of abdominal pain and intermittent diarrhoea. He is found to have a raised peripheral blood eosinophil count. Which of the following is the most likely explanation?

- A Cysticercosis
- B Cryptosporidiosis
- C Giardiasis
- D Oropharyngeal candidiasis
- E Strongyloidiasis

8.69 A 16-year-old boy had unsuccessfully attempted to pierce his own ear using a long pin. Twelve hours later he is admitted to hospital with fever, reduced conscious level and rash. Temperature is 39.9°C, blood pressure 88/60 mmHg and heart rate 146 per minute in sinus rhythm. Several sets of blood cultures are negative. What is the most likely diagnosis?

- A Anaphylaxis
- B MRSA infection
- C Staphylococcal septicaemia
- D Streptococcal sepsis
- E Toxic shock syndrome

8.67   Answer: B

Taenia solium (pork tapeworm) is common in Central Europe, Asia and S. America, often acquired by ingesting undercooked pork. Cysts can eventually die and become calcified. Neurological involvement can cause seizures, abnormal gait and raised intracranial pressure.

8.68   Answer: E

Other conditions associated with eosinophilia are trichinosis (myositis), onchocerciasis (skin involvement) and cysticercosis (muscle and CNS involvement).

8.69   Answer: E

Diagnosis can be confirmed by demonstration of TSS-1 toxin in serum. *Staphylococcus aureus* is the most likely causal organism, which can be a localised rather than systemic infection. More commonly associated with staphylococcal infection introduced via tampons in young females.

8.70   Which of the following is most commonly recognised as a feature of gonorrhoea infection?

☐ **A** > 98% of organisms are sensitive to penicillin

☐ **B** Bacteraemia is a more common complication in men

☐ **C** Ceftriaxone is a recognised effective treatment

☐ **D** Pharyngeal or rectal infection is rarely asymptomatic

☐ **E** Organism responsible is a spirochaete

8.71   Which of the following statements is most correct with respect to syphilis?

☐ **A** Blood transfusion is not recognised as a mode of transmission

☐ **B** Diagnosis can be made by serology

☐ **C** HIV-positive patients are less likely to develop CNS complications

☐ **D** Penicillin treatment is curative for tertiary complications

☐ **E** Urine microscopy is a highly sensitive diagnostic technique

8.72   A 34-year-old woman is undergoing investigation because she and her husband have been unsuccessful in their attempts to conceive over the past 2 years. Which of the following organisms is most likely to be responsible for infertility?

☐ **A** Adenovirus

☐ **B** *Chlamydia trachomatis*

☐ **C** Herpes simplex

☐ **D** Recurrent *E. coli* urinary tract infections

☐ **E** *Treponema pallidum*

8.70   Answer: C

Caused by *Neisseria gonorrhoeae*, most strains (90%) sensitive to penicillin; third-generation cephalosporins and ciprofloxacin are alternative agents. Bacteraemia is more common in women, and the disease is often asymptomatic.

8.71   Answer: B

Either ELISA or EIA tests can be confirmatory. Dark ground microscopy can allow direct demonstration of spirochaetes in chancre or rash biopsy specimens. HIV patients have a higher risk of neurosyphilis as a complication.

8.72   Answer: B

This is the commonest cause of pelvic inflammatory disease in the UK, and is often asymptomatic in women. It is often asymptomatic in men but is a recognised cause of prostatitis and epididymitis. Treatment is with a macrolide or tetracycline.

8.73   Which of the following statements is most correct with respect to current methods of HIV testing employed in the United Kingdom?

   A   Antibody tests can now detect infection within 2 weeks of inoculation

   B   Antibody titre is a good indicator of overall viral load

   C   Detection of p24 antigen can allow an earlier diagnosis

   D   HIV-1 but not HIV-2 can be detected

   E   Seroconversion illness makes the test redundant

8.74   Which of the following features most strongly supports a clinical diagnosis of *Pneumocystis carinii* pneumonia?

   A   Bilateral lower zone shadows on plain chest X-ray

   B   Clinical response to co-trimoxazole treatment

   C   Hypoxia at rest

   D   Identification of sputum cysts that are positive after silver staining

   E   Positive HIV antibody test.

8.73   Answer: C

Seroconversion can take several months after infection, and antibody tests are unreliable before then. Seroconversion illness consists of non-specific features (fever, diarrhoea, sore throat, lymphadenitis, sore throat) and affects around two-thirds of patients. HIV PCR can also be positive before seroconversion takes place.

8.74   Answer: D

Usually requires specimen to be obtained by broncho-alveolar lavage for positive confirmation. Treatment is with high-dose oral co-trimoxazole, or intravenous pentamidine (alternatively: clindamycin and primaquine, dapsone and trimethoprim). Prophylactic treatment may be needed if CD4 count < 200/mm^3.

9. NEPHROLOGY

9.1 In which of the following conditions is plasma exchange recognised as an effective treatment?

- [ ] **A** Acute interstitial nephritis
- [ ] **B** Goodpasture's syndrome
- [ ] **B** Idiopathic thrombocytopenia
- [ ] **C** Nephrotic syndrome
- [ ] **D** Non-steroidal induced nephritis

9.2 A 41-year-old woman is referred to the Renal Outpatient Department for investigation of polyuria. She reports passing large volumes of dilute urine, and drinks around 3 l per day to avoid thirst. Which of the following conditions might account for her symptoms?

- [ ] **A** Adverse effect of sertraline
- [ ] **B** Addison's disease
- [ ] **C** Cranial diabetes insipidus
- [ ] **D** Hypocalcaemia
- [ ] **E** SIADH

9.3 In which one of the following situations would renal biopsy be most helpful in establishing the underlying cause of presumed kidney disease?

- [ ] **A** c-ANCA positive
- [ ] **B** Chronic renal failure with normal-sized kidneys
- [ ] **C** Recurrent proteinuria on dipstick urinalysis
- [ ] **D** Severe hypertension and renal impairment
- [ ] **E** Strong family history of nephrotic syndrome

9.1 Answer: B

Others include hyperviscosity syndrome, myasthenia gravis and sickle cell crisis.

9.2 Answer: C

Diabetes insipidus is associated with polyuria and polydipsia. Other causes include nephrogenic diabetes insipidus, psychogenic polydipsia and drugs (eg lithium).

9.3 Answer: B

Note that severe hypertension is a contraindication to renal biopsy.

9.4 A 45-year-old man undergoes renal biopsy during investigation of unexplained chronic renal failure. Which of the following is not a typical early complication of the procedure and would most strongly suggest an alternative diagnosis?

- A Bladder tenderness
- B Colicky back pain
- C Epigastric pain and vomiting
- D Haematuria with clots
- E Hypotension

9.5 You are asked to 'check over' a 36-year-old man who has been admitted for renal biopsy later in the day. Which of the following would be most strongly associated with an increased risk of complications?

- A Creatinine > 300 μmol/l
- B INR 2.5
- C Persistent haematuria
- D Proteinuria +++ on dipstick urinalysis
- E Systolic BP 146 mmHg

9.6 A 26-year-old man complains of dusky discoloration of his urine. Dipstick urinalysis shows blood ++, but urine microscopy is clear. Which of these options offers the most likely explanation for these findings?

- A Alkaptonuria
- B Myoglobinuria
- C Mild haematuria
- D Porphyria
- E Rifampicin treatment

9.7 A 19-year-old man has noticed occasional dark urine, and is concerned that he may be suffering from haematuria. Dipstick urinalysis is negative. Which of the following statements is correct?

- A A renal ultrasound should be considered
- B Cystoscopy should be performed irrespective of urinalysis result
- C Dipstick urinalysis has a high false negative rate
- D Test should be repeated
- E The patient should be reassured

9.4   Answer: C

Recognised complications include local pain, external bleeding, haematuria and clots, which can lead to ureteric colic and bladder outflow obstruction.

9.5   Answer: B

Due to increased bleeding risk. Normally deferred until INR ≤ 1.5 in most cases.

9.6   Answer: B

Urinalysis dipstick tests detect haemoglobin, and often cross-react with myoglobin. The absence of red cells on microscopy makes haemoglobinuria or myoglobinuria more likely than haematuria. The other options are recognised causes of dipstick-negative dark urine.

9.7   Answer: E

There are a number of innocent causes of dark urine. Dipstick urinalysis is highly sensitive, and a negative result is very reassuring. Occasional haematuria does not mandate investigation, whereas persistent haematuria may do.

9.8   A 24-year-old woman is found to have blood +++ and protein + on
dipstick urinalysis. Urine microscopy shows 14,000 neutrophils/mm³,
but no organisms are seen. Blood pressure is 118/62 mmHg, and
serum urea, creatinine and electrolytes are normal. Which of the
following offers the most likely explanation for these findings?

  A Acute tubular necrosis

  B Cystitis

  C Early glomerulonephritis

  D Renal carcinoma

  E Systemic lupus erythematosus

9.9   A 42-year-old woman has been aware of passing dark urine over the
past few weeks. Dipstick urinalysis shows blood +++ and protein +,
and urine microscopy shows numerous dysmorphic red blood cells
and red cell casts. Which of the following is the most likely
explanation for her symptoms?

  A Acute tubular necrosis

  B Amyloidosis

  C Cystitis

  D Glomerulonephritis

  E Pyelonephritis

9.10   A 23-year-old man is found to have microscopic haematuria during a
routine medical screen. There is no proteinuria, and blood pressure
and renal function are normal. Which of the following underlying
disorders should be considered?

  A Acute nephritis

  B IgA nephropathy

  C Mesangioproliferative glomerulonephritis

  D Renal cell carcinoma

  E Renal tubular acidosis

9.8   Answer: B

Despite lack of demonstrable organisms, recent or current infection is the most likely explanation. Culture may identify organisms.

9.9   Answer: D

Red cell casts and dysmorphic red cells are indicative of glomerular bleeding. RBC morphology is altered as they leak through the dysfunctional glomerular basement membrane.

9.10   Answer: B

In the vast majority of cases, there will be no underlying significant pathology and observation is sufficient. Haematuria may be an early marker of IgA nephropathy, which is also associated with recurrent respiratory infections.

9.11 A 22-year-old woman is found to have proteinuria ++ during a routine medical screening. Subsequent 24-h urine collection showed total protein amount of 2.6 g. Which of these is the most likely site of the renal abnormality to account for these findings?

- [ ] **A** Bladder mucosa
- [ ] **B** Distal convoluted tubule
- [ ] **C** Glomerulus
- [ ] **D** Loop of Henlé
- [ ] **E** Proximal convoluted tubule

9.12 A 56-year-old patient is found to have dipstick urinalysis protein + and haemoglobin negative. Which one of the following conditions is *least* likely to cause proteinuria, and therefore most suggestive of the need for further investigation?

- [ ] **A** Chronic heart failure
- [ ] **B** Diabetes mellitus
- [ ] **C** Febrile illness
- [ ] **D** Severe asthma
- [ ] **E** Vigorous exercise

9.13 Biochemical urine analysis reveals the presence of Bence–Jones protein. Which of the following statements is most accurate regarding this protein?

- [ ] **A** Arises from production of excess immunoglobulin light chains
- [ ] **B** Characteristically is toxic to the renal glomerulus
- [ ] **C** Is also known as β_2-microglobin
- [ ] **D** Presence in urine signifies glomerular dysfunction
- [ ] **E** Results in positive urinalysis dipstick test

9.14 A 56-year-old woman is undergoing assessment for unexplained weight loss and fever symptoms. Investigations show the presence of Bence–Jones protein in the urine. Which of the following is most likely to account for this?

- [ ] **A** Amyloidosis
- [ ] **B** Chronic bronchitis
- [ ] **C** Chronic lymphocytic leukaemia
- [ ] **D** Nephrotic syndrome
- [ ] **E** Sarcoidosis

9.11 Answer: C

Heavy proteinuria is pathognomonic of glomerular dysfunction, particularly if albumin content is high.

9.12 Answer: D

The other conditions can be associated with mild, transient proteinuria, which disappears on resolution of the provoking condition.

9.13 Answer: A

Often due to overproduction of light chains by B-lymphocytes, which are freely filtered by the glomerulus (around 25 kDa) and can be toxic to the renal tubules. Characteristically, urinalysis dipsticks are insensitive to Bence–Jones protein.

9.14 Answer: A

Other causes include plasma cell dyscrasias and, most importantly, myeloma.

9.15 A 61-year-old woman complains of weight loss, fever and generalised malaise for around 3 months. Clinical examination is normal. Haemoglobin is 9.5 g/dl, mean cell volume 84 fl and ESR 88 mm/h, and you suspect a diagnosis of multiple myeloma. Which of the following findings on urinalysis would most strongly support this diagnosis?

- [ ] **A** Albuminuria > 1.5 g/24 h
- [ ] **B** Bence–Jones protein
- [ ] **C** Dipstick urinalysis protein +++ and haemoglobin –
- [ ] **D** Red cell casts on microscopy
- [ ] **E** Tamm–Horsfall protein

9.16 Which of the following provides the most sensitive means of assessing renal protein loss?

- [ ] **A** 24-h urinary albumin measurement
- [ ] **B** 24-h urinary protein : creatinine ratio
- [ ] **C** 24-h urinary protein measurement
- [ ] **D** Dipstick urinalysis
- [ ] **E** Serum albumin : protein ratio

9.17 A 43-year-old woman attends the Renal Outpatient Department for assessment of unexplained chronic renal impairment. She has diabetes mellitus, and her most recent HbA1c is 6.9% and blood pressure 138/88 mmHg. Twenty-four-hour urine collection shows albumin excretion is 250 mg/24 h. Which of the following fits best with these findings?

- [ ] **A** Acute interstitial nephritis
- [ ] **B** Microalbuminuria
- [ ] **C** Minimal-change glomerulonephritis
- [ ] **D** Nephritic syndrome
- [ ] **E** Nephrotic syndrome

9.15   Answer: B

Found in plasma cell dyscrasia and systemic amyloidosis. Urinalysis dipstick tests are characteristically insensitive to Bence–Jones proteins and laboratory quantification is required.

9.16   Answer: B

This allows variation in dilution to be taken into account, although will be subject to variability in creatinine generation (eg muscle bulk, diet and exercise).

9.17   Answer: B

Normal albumin excretion < 30 mg/24 h, microalbuminuria 30–300 mg/24 h and overt proteinuria > 300 mg/24 h.

9.18 A 38-year-old man is found to have hypoalbuminaemia, fluid retention and peripheral oedema, and a diagnosis of nephrotic syndrome is suspected. Which of the following would most strongly support this diagnosis?

   A   Urinary albumin excretion 500 mg/24 h

   B   Dipstick urinalysis shows protein +++

   C   Urinary 24-h protein : creatinine ratio 3 mg/mmol

   D   Urinary protein excretion 4 g/24 h

   E   Urine osmolality 282 mOsm/l

9.19 A 29-year-old man is found to have serum albumin 27 g/l, urinary protein excretion of 3.8 g/24 h. Which of the following is most likely to explain these abnormalities?

   A   Acute tubular necrosis

   B   Diabetic nephropathy

   C   Focal segmental glomerulosclerosis

   D   Renal cell carcinoma

   E   Type 2 renal tubular acidosis

9.20 A 31-year-old woman has proteinuria and hypoalbuminaemia, and a diagnosis of nephrotic syndrome is suspected. Which of the following features would strongly suggest an alternative diagnosis?

   A   Hypercholesterolaemia

   B   Hypogammaglobulinaemia

   C   Venous thromboembolism

   D   Pneumococcal infection

   E   Urinary protein excretion 1.2 g/24 h

9.21 A 28-year-old man is found to have serum albumin 24 g/l and urinary protein excretion of 4.4 g/24 h. Which of the following steps is most appropriate in his management?

   A   Azathioprine

   B   High-dose prednisolone

   C   Renal biopsy

   D   Renal ultrasound scan

   E   Serum electrophoresis

9.18   Answer: D

Typically, nephrotic syndrome is associated with protein excretion of > 3.5 g/24 h, and serum albumin < 30 g/l.

9.19   Answer: C

Other causes of nephrotic syndrome are minimal-change nephropathy, membranous nephropathy, mesangiocapillary glomerulonephritis, SLE, diabetic nephropathy (less common) and amyloidosis.

9.20   Answer: E

Nephrotic syndrome is characteristically associated with urinary protein excretion of > 3.5 g/24 h.

9.21   Answer: C

Biopsy is important to establish the cause of nephrotic syndrome because treatment will vary according to the morphological category.

9.22   A 27-year-old woman attending the Renal Outpatient Department for investigation of proteinuria and oedema is diagnosed with nephrotic syndrome. Which of the following is *least* likely to be useful in her subsequent management?

- [ ] **A**   Amiloride
- [ ] **B**   Atenolol
- [ ] **C**   Furosemide
- [ ] **D**   Simvastatin
- [ ] **E**   Warfarin

9.23   Which of the following mechanisms is most likely to influence glomerular filtration pressure in an elderly patient?

- [ ] **A**   Afferent arteriolar constriction by prostaglandin E_2
- [ ] **B**   Angiotensin II-mediated vasoconstriction of the efferent arteriole
- [ ] **C**   Baroreceptor reflex insensitivity
- [ ] **D**   Increased permeability of the loop of Henlé
- [ ] **E**   Relaxation of bladder tone

9.24   A 49-year-old woman is complaining of general malaise and lethargy. She is found to have serum urea 28.5 mmol/l and creatinine 348 µmol/l. Which of the following would most strongly indicate 'pre-renal' acute renal impairment?

- [ ] **A**   Blood pressure 107/65 mmHg
- [ ] **B**   Dipstick urinalysis shows blood +++
- [ ] **C**   Urine osmolality < 280 mOsm/kg
- [ ] **D**   Urinary sodium < 20 mmol/l
- [ ] **E**   Urine : plasma urea ratio < 5:1

9.25   A 56-year-old woman is admitted with lethargy and non-specific malaise. On examination, she appears dehydrated and cachectic. Serum urea is 24 mmol/l, creatinine 288 µmol/l and potassium 6.9 mmol/l. Which is the most appropriate step in her immediate management?

- [ ] **A**   Intravenous 10% calcium gluconate 10 ml over 10 min
- [ ] **B**   Intravenous 5% dextrose at 250 ml/h
- [ ] **C**   Intravenous 0.9% saline at 500 ml/h
- [ ] **D**   Oral calcium resonium
- [ ] **E**   Urgent haemodialysis

9.22 Answer: B

Nephrotic syndrome is less likely to cause hypertension than most other chronic renal disease. Hypercholesterolaemia and increased risk of venous thromboembolism are recognised features. The mainstay of treatment is diuretics and salt restriction; hypotension is often a complication.

9.23 Answer: B

This is an important mechanism for maintaining glomerular filtration rate (GFR) in the setting of reduced afferent arteriolar pressure; hence, blockade by ACE inhibitors or angiotensin II receptor blockers can precipitate acute renal failure.

9.24 Answer: D

Hypotension is suggestive but not specific. Typically, concentrated urine is produced in small quantities. Osmolality is > 600 mOsm/kg and urine : plasma urea ratio > 10:1.

9.25 Answer: A

This will protect against arrhythmia. Administration of 50 ml of 50% dextrose (equivalent to 500 ml of 5%) stimulates insulin secretion, which facilitates intracellular movement of potassium. Haemodialysis should be considered in anuric patients.

9.26 Which of the following treatments is most appropriate for preventing osteodystrophy in patients with chronic renal failure?

A   1-α-hydroxycholecalciferol

B   25-α-hydroxycholecalciferol

C   Calcium carbonate

D   Cholecalciferol

E   Magnesium silicate

9.27 Which of the following strategies is most likely to prevent or delay the progression of renal osteodystrophy?

A   Aluminium silicate

B   Aluminium hydroxide

C   Calcium chloride

D   High phosphate diet

E   Thyroid replacement therapy

9.28 Which of the following statements is correct regarding renal replacement therapy in chronic renal failure?

A   Continuous ambulatory peritoneal dialysis (CAPD) is used in fewer than 5% of patients with end-stage renal failure

B   Haemodialysis has been available to NHS patients for 15 years

C   Home dialysis has increased in prevalence in the past 10 years

D   Number of haemodialysis patients has fallen over the past 5 years

E   Renal transplantation rates are progressively increasing

9.29 A 47-year-old man has had deteriorating renal function for the past 8 months. Which of the following factors would most strongly indicate the need for renal replacement therapy, eg haemodialysis?

A   Blood pressure 186/98 mmHg despite two anti-hypertensive drugs

B   Pulmonary oedema despite fluid restriction

C   Serum calcium 2.45 mmol/l

D   Serum potassium 5.8 mmol/

E   Serum urea 32 mmol/l

9.26   Answer: A

Vitamin D normally undergoes 1-α-hydroxylation by the kidney and 25-α-hydroxylation by the liver to its biologically active form 1,25-dihydroxycholecalciferol.

9.27   Answer: B

Calcium carbonate and aluminium hydroxide have phosphate-binding properties so as to reduce gut absorption, coupled with a low-phosphate diet.

9.28   Answer: E

CAPD is used in around 20% of patients with end-stage renal failure (ESRF). Haemodialysis has been available for more than 40 years, and the number of patients receiving regular treatment is progressively increasing.

9.29   Answer: B

Serum urea > 30 mmol/l and creatinine > 600 μmol/l are relative indications (> 50 mmol/l and > 1000 μmol/l are definite indications). Severe hyperkalaemia, not controlled by other measures, may also necessitate dialysis.

9.30 A 52-year-old woman is transferred to the Renal Unit for haemodialysis for acute renal failure. Which of the following is most accurate in relation to haemodialysis?

- A Can be performed using single-lumen femoral catheter
- B Causes less cardiovascular instability than continuous haemofiltration
- C Effectiveness may be assessed by the urea reduction ratio
- D Heparin must be infused to reduce thrombosis risk
- E Treatment should be administered for 3–4 h every day

9.31 Which of the following statements is correct regarding the use of peritoneal dialysis in end-stage renal failure?

- A Causes less haemodynamic disturbance than haemodialysis
- B Fluid exchange must be performed manually
- C Dialysis fluid is normally instilled and drained 1–2 times per day
- D Patients should switch to haemodialysis if peritonitis occurs
- E Sterile dialysis fluid is normally hypertonic

9.32 A 45-year-old woman has had dialysis-dependent end-stage renal failure for the past 2 years, and is being considered for renal transplantation. Which of the following factors is most important in identifying a suitable donor match?

- A ABO blood group
- B Age of the donor
- C HLA MHC matching
- D Smoking status of the donor
- E Size of the donor kidney

9.33 A 56-year-old man has developed acute renal failure 3 days after initiation of enalapril treatment for hypertension. Which underlying condition is most likely to have caused acute renal failure?

- A Bladder outflow obstruction
- B Extensive renal artery atherosclerosis
- C Previous nephrectomy
- D Renal sarcoidosis
- E Retroperitoneal fibrosis

9.30   Answer: C
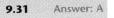

A double-lumen catheter is used. Daily treatment is reserved for catabolic patients, otherwise, treatment on alternate days is normally adequate. Prostacyclin is an alternative to heparin and may be associated with lower bleeding risk.

9.31   Answer: A

Isotonic dialysate is instilled for around 6 h then drained, 3–4 times per day. Automated peritoneal devices allow dialysis exchange to take place overnight.

9.32   Answer: A
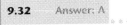

This must be matched, and ideally the graft should be MHC matched as far as possible to improve graft survival. Age, smoking status and health factors may influence graft survival.

9.33   Answer: B

ACE inhibitors and angiotensin receptor antagonists can precipitate acute renal failure where there is reduced renal blood flow because angiotensin II constricts the efferent arteriole to maintain GFR. They should be used only with great caution in patients who have undergone previous nephrectomy.

9.34 You are considering introducing an ACE inhibitor for blood pressure control in a patient with uncontrolled hypertension and mild renal impairment. In which of the following situations is treatment most likely to be associated with worsening of renal function?

    A Already receiving nifedipine

    B Anaphylactic reaction to contrast media in the past

    C Associated haematuria ++ on urinalysis

    D Asymmetric kidneys on ultrasound examination

    E Atrial fibrillation

9.35 A 51-year-old woman is found to have serum urea 18 mmol/l and creatinine 344 μmol/l. Full blood count shows haemoglobin 9.8 g/dl, MCV 82 fl and red cell fragments are seen on the peripheral blood film. Which of these is the most likely cause of her renal impairment?

    A Acute pyelonephritis

    B Acute tubular necrosis

    C Microscopic polyangiitis

    D Scleroderma

    E Tuberculosis

9.36 A 68-year-old patient develops pain and dusky discoloration of several toes of both feet. Serum urea is 18 mmol/l and creatinine 348 μmol/l. He underwent coronary angiography 3 days ago, and renal function was normal before the procedure. Which is the most likely cause of his renal impairment?

    A ACE inhibitor-induced nephritis

    B Cholesterol atheroembolism

    C Contrast-mediated nephropathy

    D Disseminated intravascular coagulation

    E Excess furosemide administration

9.34   Answer: D

This is strongly suggestive of renovascular disease, which is often asymmetrical.

9.35   Answer: C

The features suggest small-vessel disease, which can be caused by DIC, systemic sclerosis, accelerated hypertension, cholesterol embolism, thrombotic microangiopathy and small-vessel vasculitis (eg microscopic polyangiitis).

9.36   Answer: B

Very common in patients with extensive atherosclerosis, usually after invasive vascular procedures although spontaneous atheroembolism has been described. Contrast-mediated nephropathy would not cause distal embolic phenomena.

9.37 Which of the following statements is correct in relation to Alport's syndrome?

   A Associated with conductive hearing loss

   B Autosomal dominant inheritance

   C End-stage renal failure usually develops in late teens or twenties

   D Contra-indication to renal transplantation

   E Renal impairment due to anti-GBM antibodies

9.38 A 24-year-old patient with Alport's syndrome has been receiving haemodialysis treatment for 3 years. He is being considered for renal transplantation. Which complication of transplantation occurs more commonly in Alport's syndrome than other types of end-stage renal failure?

   A Acute graft artery occlusion

   B Anti-GBM disease

   C Ciclosporin toxicity

   D Pyelonephritis

   E Graft ureteric occlusion

9.39 A 38-year-old woman has had fever symptoms and malaise for 6 weeks. She is found to have impaired renal function, low C3 complement, and red cell casts on urine microscopy. Which is the most likely cause of these findings?

   A Acute tubular necrosis

   B Drug-induced nephritis

   C Mesangiocapillary glomerulonephritis

   D Systemic sclerosis

   E Tuberculosis

9.40 Renal histopathology in a 31-year-old man with unexplained acute renal failure shows the presence of multiple glomerular 'crescents'. Which is the most likely cause of his renal failure?

   A IgA nephropathy

   B Hypertensive nephropathy

   C Nephrotic syndrome

   D Obstructive uropathy

   E SLE

9.37   Answer: C

X-linked and autosomal recessive patterns. Abnormalities of basement membrane collagen (type IV), hence renal GBM abnormalities, sensorineuronal deafness and ocular defects.

9.38   Answer: B

Some patients develop antibodies to normal type IV collagen in the donor kidney, which can cause anti-GBM disease in a small number.

9.39   Answer: C

Features suggest glomerular disease associated with low serum complement. Other causes are SLE, post-infective glomerulonephritis, SBE and cryoglobulinaemia.

9.40   Answer: A

Also seen in SLE (more common in women and often associated with other features), systemic vasculitis and Goodpasture's disease.

9.41 A 28-year-old man has suffered intermittent haematuria over the past 18 months. He has recently been treated with amoxicillin for a suspected chest infection, and found to have urea 19 mmol/l and creatinine 288 μmol/l, and dipstick urinalysis shows blood +++. Which is the most likely cause of his renal impairment?

   A Acute pyelonephritis

   B Alport's syndrome

   C Disseminated intravascular coagulation

   D Drug-induced SLE

   E IgA nephropathy

9.42 A renal biopsy is undertaken in a 37-year-old woman with unexplained chronic renal failure. Which appearance would most strongly suggest a diagnosis of membranous glomerulonephritis?

   A Deposition of amorphous fibrillary material in glomeruli

   B Disruption of epithelial cell architecture

   C Focal glomerulosclerosis

   D Immunoglobulin light-chains deposited in the glomerular basement membrane

   E Thickened glomerular basement membrane

9.43 A 34-year-old man with cystic fibrosis is found to have heavy proteinuria and hypoalbuminaemia associated with mild chronic renal impairment. Renal biopsy shows deposition of fibrillary material throughout the glomeruli which takes up Congo red stain. Which is the most likely cause of these findings?

   A Acute interstitial nephritis

   B Primary amyloidosis

   C Reactive amyloidosis

   D Retroperitoneal fibrosis

   E Tuberculosis

9.41   Answer: E

History also suggestive of acute post-infectious glomerulonephritis and Goodpasture's disease.

9.42   Answer: E

Focal glomerulosclerosis is a feature of diabetic nephropathy, Ig deposition in light-chain disease and amorphous fibrillary deposition suggests amyloidosis.

9.43   Answer: C

Primary amyloidosis involves deposition of immunoglobulin light-chains. In reactive amyloidosis there is deposition of amyloid A component (AA), which is an acute-phase protein, and occurs in chronic infectious or inflammatory disorders.

9.44   A renal biopsy from a 49-year-old man shows intense inflammatory changes with multiple neutrophils, lymphocytes and occasional eosinophils, predominantly around the tubules and blood vessels. Which is the most likely cause of these findings?

    A   Allopurinol-induced nephritis

    B   Auto-immune glomerulonephritis

    C   Bacterial pyelonephritis

    D   Corticosteroid-induced nephritis

    E   Sarcoidosis

9.45   A 56-year-old woman has recently commenced a new anti-hypertensive drug. She develops impaired renal function, which is thought due to acute interstitial nephritis. Which of the following would most strongly suggest an alternative diagnosis?

    A   Anuria

    B   Eosinophilia

    C   Fever

    D   Generalised erythematous rash

    E   Urine microscopy shows eosinophils

9.46   A 46-year-old man has developed acute renal failure shortly after initiation of lansoprazole therapy. There is associated fever and an erythematous rash over his trunk and arms, and peripheral blood shows an eosinophilia. What is the most likely explanation for these findings?

    A   Acute interstitial nephritis

    B   Acute pancreatitis

    C   Acute pyelonephritis

    D   Acute tubular necrosis

    E   Drug-induced urinary calculus formation

9.47   Which of the following statements is correct regarding adult polycystic kidney disease?

    A   Inherited in autosomal recessive manner

    B   Male : female prevalence is around 10:1

    C   PKD-1 gene is encoded on chromosome 1

    D   PKD-2 gene is associated with more aggressive form of the disease

    E   Polycystin appears to mediate pathological features

9.44   Answer: A

The morphological appearance suggests acute interstitial nephritis, and eosinophil infiltration favours a drug cause (also NSAIDs, furosemide, penicillins) rather than non-drug cause (sarcoid, myeloma, pyelonephritis, TB).

9.45   Answer: A

Acute interstitial nephritis may be associated with moderate to severe renal impairment, but oliguria is not a prominent feature. The other features listed are characteristic of drug-induced nephritis.

9.46   Answer: A

Other features include eosinophils in urine. Other causes include allopurinol, ciprofloxacin, penicillin, NSAIDs, diuretics, aciclovir, H_2-receptor blockers.

9.47   Answer: E

Autosomal dominant inheritance, hence men and women equally affected. PKD-1 gene on chromosome 16 encodes polycystin. PKD-2 gene on chromosome 4 associated with milder disease form.

9.48 A 34-year-old man presents with vague loin pain and haematuria. He is found to have blood pressure 168/94 mmHg, a ballotable right kidney and serum creatinine 424 µmol/l. Which is the most likely diagnosis?

- A Acute interstitial nephritis
- B Adult polycystic kidney disease
- C Hypertensive encephalopathy
- D NSAID-induced nephropathy
- E Renal cell carcinoma

9.49 A 24-year-old woman is found to have glucose ++ on dipstick urinalysis during a routine health check. What is the most likely cause?

- A Factitious glycosuria
- B False positive
- C Renal glycosuria
- D Type 1 diabetes
- E Type 2 diabetes

9.50 Which of the following is most likely to cause renal failure as a consequence of underlying malignancy?

- A Hypercalcaemia due to lung carcinoma
- B Hyperviscosity associated with myeloma
- C Interstitial nephritis due to methotrexate
- D Light-chain deposition in patients with colonic carcinoma
- E Obstructive uropathy immediately after chemotherapy

9.51 A 45-year-old woman has had SLE for 12 years, and is found to have heavy proteinuria and impaired renal function. Renal biopsy shows diffuse proliferative glomerulonephritis. Which of the following treatments has been shown to delay the progression to end-stage renal impairment?

- A Azathioprine
- B Ciclosporin A
- C Cyclophosphamide
- D Methotrexate
- E Prednisolone

9.48 Answer: B

Renal cell carcinoma should also be considered, and IgA nephropathy. The diagnosis can be confirmed by demonstration of multiple bilateral renal cysts.

9.49 Answer: C

This is the commonest cause of glycosuria detected by dipstick urinalysis in otherwise healthy individuals, accompanied by normal plasma glucose. Due to reduced renal threshold, which is subject to high inter-individual variablity.

9.50 Answer: E

Due to urate crystal deposition in tumour lysis syndrome. Methotrexate may cause interstitial and retroperitoneal fibrosis (obstructive nephropathy). Myeloma is associated with light-chain deposition.

9.51 Answer: C

More than 50% of SLE patients will have renal involvement more than 5 years after diagnosis. Over-reliance on corticosteroids leads to chronic adverse effects; azathioprine is often used as a 'steroid-sparing' agent.

9.52 A 33-year-old woman has suffered recurrent lower urinary tract infections. Which of the following steps would most effectively lower the risk of future infection?

- A Avoid excess fluid intake
- B Avoid passing small urine volumes
- C Emptying bladder before and after intercourse
- D Partial bladder voiding
- E Regular sodium bicarbonate intake

9.53 A 27-year-old woman has symptoms suggestive of urethritis, but mid-stream urine culture is negative. What is the most likely explanation of her symptoms?

- A Bladder carcinoma
- B Chlamydia urethritis
- C Klebsiella cystitis
- D Pregnancy
- E Trauma secondary to regular vigorous jogging

9.54 Culture of a mid-stream urine specimen from an apparently well 65-year-old woman shows growth of > 10^6 organisms/ml. Which is the correct statement?

- A Antibiotic treatment is indicated
- B Asymptomatic bacteriuria occurs in 2–5% of adult women
- C Is associated with acute pyelonephritis in 30% of cases
- D Renal ultrasound is indicated
- E This is diagnostic of bacterial cystourethritis

9.55 A 24-year-old woman is admitted via the Emergency Department with severe left loin pain radiating to the left iliac fossa. On examination, temperature is 37.3°C and there is tenderness overlying the left lumbar area. What is the most likely diagnosis?

- A Acute cystitis
- B Acute pyelonephritis
- C Dissection of the aorto–iliac vessels
- D Focal myositis
- E Ureteric colic

9.52 Answer: C

Other steps include oral fluid intake > 2.5 l/day, regular and complete bladder voiding and prophylactic oral antibiotics in some cases.

9.53 Answer: B

Infection due to organisms not easily grown by routine culture methods; klebsiella could usually be detected. Other causes include trauma associated with intercourse and chemical irritation.

9.54 Answer: B

Asymptomatic bacteriuria requires no further investigation or treatment unless found in infants or pregnant women (risk of scarring).

9.55 Answer: B

Other features include rigors, vomiting, septicaemia, leukocytosis, pyuria and bacteriuria.

9.56 A 22-year-old man is admitted with fever, rigors and right flank pain. On examination, there is tenderness overlying the right lumbar region and suprapubic area. Urinalysis reveals blood ++ and protein +. What is the most probable cause of his fever?

- [ ] A   Acute appendicitis
- [ ] B   Aortic dissection
- [ ] C   Cystitis
- [ ] D   Pyelonephritis
- [ ] E   Ureteric colic

9.57 A 25-year-old woman attends the Emergency Department with fever, sweating and right flank pain. She is very tender over the right lumbar area, temperature 37.9°C and dipstick urinalysis shows blood +++, protein ++ and nitrites +. What is the best initial treatment?

- [ ] A   Intravenous ceftriaxone
- [ ] B   Intravenous gentamicin
- [ ] C   Oral amoxicillin
- [ ] D   Oral ciprofloxacin
- [ ] E   Oral vancomycin

9.58 A 57-year-old man complains of loin pain, malaise and fever. An ultrasound scan shows left-sided hydronephrosis with dilatation of the left ureter, and normal bladder appearance. Which is the most likely diagnosis?

- [ ] A   Bladder outflow obstruction
- [ ] B   Pelvi-ureteric obstruction
- [ ] C   Prostatic encroachment on the urethral lumen
- [ ] D   Retroperitoneal fibrosis
- [ ] E   Vesico–ureteric junction obstruction

9.56   Answer: D

Suprapubic pain suggests additional cystitis (30% of cases), but this alone would be less likely to cause systemic features.

9.57   Answer: A

Oral amoxicillin or ciprofloxacin may be appropriate in some cases. In severe cases, with systemic features, intravenous treatment is indicated. Gentamicin is highly effective but relatively toxic and requires therapeutic drug monitoring. Subsequent treatment should be guided by urine culture and sensitivities.

9.58   Answer: E

Lack of dilatation of the right collecting system suggests the obstruction is proximal to the bladder. VUJ blockage will cause dilatation along the whole length of the ureter. Retroperitoneal fibrosis may cause stricturing of the ureter and obstruction at any level.

9.59 Ultrasonography of the renal tract indicates dilatation of both ureters and renal pelvises. Which statement regarding subsequent investigations is correct?

- A Antegrade pyelography should be avoided
- B Intravenous urography can distinguish the cause of the obstruction
- C Nephrostomy should be performed in acute renal failure
- D Retrograde pyelography can identify the cause of the obstruction
- E Transurethral cystoscopy should be performed

9.60 A 65-year-old man is admitted with back pain and acute renal failure. What is the correct initial treatment for this condition?

- A Finasteride if prostatic hypertrophy suspected
- B High dose furosemide
- C Intravenous hydrocortisone
- D Percutaneous nephrostomy if hydronephrosis present
- E Suprapubic catheter insertion if urethral blockage suspected

9.61 What is the commonest component of urinary calculi occurring in patients in the United Kingdom?

- A Calcium chloride
- B Calcium oxalate
- C Calcium pyruvate
- D Glycosaminoglycan
- E Urate

9.62 Which one of the following disorders is most strongly associated with an increased risk of ureteric calculus formation?

- A Alport's syndrome
- B Amiloride treatment
- C Chronic lymphocytic leukaemia
- D Hypoparathyroidism
- E Wegener's granulomatosis

9.59   Answer: C

Obstructive uropathy may be the cause of acute renal failure; nephrostomy insertion may restore renal function, and allow antegrade pyelography. The listed investigations identify the site, but not the cause of obstruction in most cases.

9.60   Answer: D

Treatment of suspected urethral blockage (eg prostatism) should be with transurethral catheter insertion in the first instance. Finasteride has no role in acute treatment.

9.61   Answer: B

Around one-third are predominantly calcium oxalate, and a further one-third involve predominantly calcium or magnesium salts (but not calcium pyruvate!).

9.62   Answer: C

Myeloproliferative disorders increase the risk of urate nephropathy and ureteric calculi due to tumour lysis syndrome. Hyperparathyroidism is associated with increased risk of calcium-based calculus formation.

9.63 A 61-year-old man presents with haematuria and loin pain, and is found to have a palpable mass in his left flank, and renal cell carcinoma is suspected. Which of these would most strongly suggest an alternative cause?

☐ **A** Anaemia

☐ **B** Hypertension

☐ **C** Raised ESR

☐ **D** Strong family history of dialysis-dependent renal failure

☐ **E** Weight loss

9.64 Which of the following disorders is most likely to be associated with hypercalcaemia and hypercalciuria?

☐ **A** Cushing's syndrome

☐ **B** Familial hypercalciuria

☐ **C** High dietary calcium intake

☐ **D** Renal tubular acidosis

☐ **E** Sarcoidosis

9.65 Which statement is correct in relation to renal stone formation?

☐ **A** Bile salt malabsorption is associated with urate stone formation

☐ **B** Dehydration predisposes to all types of ureteric calculi

☐ **C** Hypocalciuria predisposes to calcium oxalate stones

☐ **D** Urinary tract infection is associated with calcium oxalate stones

☐ **E** Xanthinuria is associated with urate stone formation

9.66 A 38-year-old male smoker presents with recurrent haemoptysis and progressive renal impairment. Anti-GBM antibody is detected. What is the most likely diagnosis?

☐ **A** Alport's syndrome

☐ **B** Goodpasture's syndrome

☐ **C** IgA nephropathy

☐ **D** SLE

☐ **E** Wegener's granulomatosis

9.63 Answer: D

This might suggest APKD instead. Other features of renal cell carcinoma include pyrexia, raised alkaline phosphatase, hypercalcaemia, polycythaemia and neuropathy.

9.64 Answer: E

Other causes include hyperparathyroidism, myeloma and vitamin D intoxication. The other listed stems are associated with hypercalciuria and normal serum calcium concentrations.

9.65 Answer: B

Bile salt malabsorption is associated with increased colonic oxalate absorption and calcium oxalate calculi formation; hypocitraturia and hypercalciuria also predispose to these. Xanthinuria and cystinuria associated with xanthine and cystine stones respectively.

9.66 Answer: B

Alport's syndrome is associated with defective type IV collagen. Renal transplantation can give rise to anti-GBM antibodies and, in some patients, features similar to Goodpasture's syndrome.

9.67 A 34-year-old man presents with recurrent haemoptysis and progressive renal failure. A diagnosis of Goodpasture's syndrome is suspected. Which treatment is the most likely to be effective?

- A Azathioprine
- B Ceftriaxone
- C Plasma exchange
- D Prednisolone
- E Smoking cessation

9.68 A 14-year-old boy presents with colicky abdominal pain and purpuric rash overlying the anterior aspect of both lower limbs. Investigations show serum urea 19 mmol/l and creatinine 236 μmol/l. What is the most likely diagnosis?

- A Acute appendicitis
- B Bacterial peritonitis
- C Henoch–Schoenlein purpura
- D Renal tuberculosis
- E Sarcoidosis

9.69 A 42-year-old woman presents with arthralgia, nail-fold infarcts and is found to have significantly impaired renal function. p-ANCA is positive. What is the most likely cause of renal impairment?

- A Cryoglobulinaemia
- B Microscopic polyangiitis
- C Polyarteritis nodosa
- D Sarcoidosis
- E Wegener's granulomatosis

9.70 A 67-year-old woman is recovering from a viral gastroenteritis, but is found to have rapidly declining renal function. Investigations show haemoglobin 9.7 g/dl and multiple red cell fragments on microscopy. What is the most likely cause of her renal impairment?

- A Ciprofloxacin-induced acute interstitial nephritis
- B Haemolytic–uraemic syndrome
- C Pseudomembranous colitis
- D Ulcerative colitis
- E Vancomycin-induced nephrotoxicity

9.67 Answer: C

Removes the anti-GBM antibody, often used in combination with immunosuppressive cytotoxics and high-dose corticosteroids. Haemoptysis is more common in smokers and cessation advice seems sensible.

9.68 Answer: C

Characteristic features also include raised serum IgA concentrations in some patients and focal segmental glomerulosclerosis.

9.69 Answer: B

ANCA is characteristically negative in polyarteritis nodosa; c-ANCA is positive in Wegener's granulomatosis.

9.70 Answer: B

Characterised by intravascular haemolysis, red cell fragmentation, thrombocytopenia and renal impairment. TTP has similar features, with more prominent neurological involvement.

9.71   A patient with loin pain and suspected ureteric colic is referred for intravenous urography. Which factor will most increase the likelihood of contrast-mediated nephropathy?

A   Asthma

B   Diabetes mellitus

C   Hypercholesterolaemia

D   Hypovolaemia

E   Male gender

9.72   Which of the following factors is most likely to cause chronic tubulointerstitial nephritis?

A   Amyloidosis

B   Diabetes

C   Heart failure

D   Hypertension

E   Tuberculosis

9.73   A 56-year-old woman undergoes abdominal X-ray for investigation of constipation, which shows diffuse calcification of both renal parenchyma. Which disorder is most likely to account for this appearance?

A   Chronic glomerulonephritis

B   Nephrotic syndrome

C   Osteomalacia

D   Osteoporosis

E   Renal tubular acidosis

9.71   Answer: D

Risk also enhanced by renal impairment, especially diabetic nephropathy (not diabetes alone). Risk reduced by intravenous hydration.

9.72   Answer: B

Others include NSAID use, sickle cell disease, reflux nephropathy and hyperuricaemic nephropathy.

9.73   Answer: E

This appearance is consistent with nephrocalcinosis, which can also be caused by hypercalcaemia, medullary sponge kidney and tuberculosis.

10. NEUROLOGY

10.1   A 48-year-old man is referred to the Neurology Clinic with a history of four blackout episodes in the past year. These start with a feeling that he is going to pass out, and he does so within a few seconds. The attacks are unrelated to postural change, and he is not aware of any change in his heart rate or breathing, or tongue biting or loss of continence. After the attacks, he usually sleeps for around 2 h then feels completely well. Which of the following is the most likely diagnosis?

- A   Absence attacks
- B   Autonomic neuropathy
- C   Cardiac arrhythmia
- D   Generalised seizures
- E   Recurrent hypoglycaemia

10.2   A 62-year-old man is admitted to the Medical Admissions Unit after a witnessed collapse episode. When queuing in a local shop 1 h ago, he had fallen to the ground unconscious. He is reported to have looked pale, and was shaking all four limbs for around 1 min. On assessment, he is slightly drowsy but is fully rousable and physical examination is entirely normal. Which of the following is the most likely diagnosis?

- A   Autonomic neuropathy
- B   Cardiac arrhythmia
- C   Generalised seizure
- D   Myocardial infarction
- E   Vasovagal syncope

10.3   A 68-year-old man attends the Emergency Department complaining of sudden onset of profound weakness affecting his right upper limb. On examination, there is a flaccid paresis and impaired sensation affecting his right upper limb. Physical examination is otherwise normal. Which of the following is the most likely diagnosis?

- A   Partial anterior circulation stroke
- B   Partial focal seizure
- C   Posterior circulation stroke
- D   Subacute combined degeneration of the cord
- E   Total anterior circulation stroke

10.1   Answer: D

Lack of cardio-respiratory symptoms and absence of any postural trigger make a cardiac cause of blackout less likely. Somnolence is consistent with a post-ictal state.

10.2   Answer: C

Transient cerebral ischaemia can provoke limb twitching, but these are not normally sustained. Drowsiness 1 h after the collapse favours epilepsy rather than cardiac syncope.

10.3   Answer: A

Depending on timing, the diagnosis might be stroke or transient ischaemic attack (TIA), but the clinical features suggest a left cerebral anterior circulation distribution. Total anterior circulation stroke would additionally involve dysphasia, visual field loss, cranial nerve and/or lower limb involvement.

10.4 A 72-year-old woman attends the Emergency Department after a fall in the street. She remembers feeling faint and dizzy, then losing consciousness for an uncertain duration. She now feels completely well. There is a laceration over the left side of her forehead, and examination is otherwise normal. Which of the following is the most likely explanation for her collapse?

A Episode of complete heart block

B Subarachnoid haemorrhage

C Subdural haematoma

D Total anterior circulation stroke

E Transient ischaemic attack

10.5 A 58-year-old man presents to the Emergency Department 4 h after sudden onset of severe dizziness, vomiting and occipital headache. He is found to have coarse nystagmus on left lateral gaze, and marked incoordination of all four limbs. Which of the following is the best explanation for his symptoms and signs?

A Bacterial meningitis

B Partial complex seizures

C Posterior circulation stroke

D Total anterior circulation stroke

E Viral encephalitis

10.6 An 18-year-old man attends the neurology outpatient department for investigation of recurrent blackouts. During these, he is aware of forced deviation of his eyes to the right and nausea, followed by loss of consciousness. His mother reports that on two occasions, she has found him collapsed, shaking his limbs violently for a few moments. Which of the following offers the best explanation for these attacks?

A Cardiac syncope

B Left frontal lobe tumour

C Partial seizures

D Temporal lobe epilepsy

E Vertebro-basilar insufficiency

10.4   Answer: A

Loss of consciousness is *not* a typical feature of TIA or stroke. Subdural haematoma does not cause collapse, but can complicate a head injury. Loss of consciousness and rapid recovery after syncope are characteristic of an underlying cardiac cause.

10.5   Answer: C

The symptom and sign clusters indicate a peripheral cerebellar lesion. The sudden onset suggests posterior circulation TIA or stroke; prominent headache suggests vertebrobasilar dissection.

10.6   Answer: B

Deviation of the eyes strongly suggests a left frontal focus, and the history indicates partial seizures with secondary generalisation.

10.7 A 72-year-old woman is admitted as an acute medical emergency after a sudden collapse and weakness affecting her left arm and leg. She does not report loss of consciousness, and her weakness is already beginning to improve 12 h after her collapse. Which of these is the best explanation for her limb weakness?

- ☐ A Compression of the cervical spine
- ☐ B Partial anterior circulation stroke (PACS)
- ☐ C Post-ictal phenomenon
- ☐ D Total anterior circulation stroke (TACS)
- ☐ E Vertebro-basilar ischaemia

10.8 A 65-year-old man is referred to the Medical Admissions Unit after a sudden collapse and right arm and leg weakness which has now resolved 8 h later. He has previously had a TIA and has been taking aspirin 75 mg and simvastatin 40 mg daily. Which of the following treatment options would be most appropriate?

- ☐ A Add clopidogrel 75 mg daily
- ☐ B Add dipyridamole MR 200 mg twice daily
- ☐ C Stop aspirin and introduce clopidogrel 75 mg daily
- ☐ D Stop aspirin and introduce dipyridamole MR 200 mg twice daily
- ☐ E Stop aspirin and introduce warfarin

10.9 A 60-year-old woman attends the Medical Outpatient Clinic for review. She had been discharged from hospital 8 weeks earlier, having suffered a stroke with mild right arm weakness and dysaesthesia. On examination, there is mild weakness of her right upper limb. Blood pressure is 146/72 mmHg. Serum cholesterol is 4.1 mmol/l and random glucose is 4.8 mmol/l. Which of the following measures would best reduce her risk of future stroke?

- ☐ A Low cholesterol diet
- ☐ B Nifedipine MR 20 mg daily
- ☐ C Pravastatin 20 mg nocte
- ☐ D Regular moderate aerobic exercise
- ☐ E Smoking cessation

10.7   Answer: D

Involvement of upper and lower limbs makes TACS more likely than PACS. It is unlikely that spine compression would manifest so suddenly, and resolve spontaneously. Seizure is unlikely, given no loss of consciousness.

10.8   Answer: B

There is good evidence that long-term aspirin reduces stroke incidence in high-risk patients, and clopidogrel appears at least as effective. Addition of dipyridamole to aspirin appears to be effective in recurrent stroke; substitution of clopidogrel might be effective in some patients, but evidence of this is less convincing.

10.9   Answer: B

Hypertension is the most important modifiable risk factor for stroke. Treatment of isolated systolic hypertension in elderly patients is particularly important, aiming for target SBP of ≤ 140 mmHg, or ≤ 130 mmHg in patients who have had a previous stroke. The other measures listed also contribute to cardiovascular risk reduction.

10.10   A 52-year-old woman presents to the Emergency Department with sudden onset of severe occipital headache. There is marked dysarthria and incoordination of her upper and lower limbs. Blood pressure is 168/102 mmHg, and examination is otherwise normal. Which of the following diagnoses would be most important to consider?

- [ ] **A**   Anterior circulation infarction
- [ ] **B**   Central pontine haemorrhage
- [ ] **C**   Parietal lobe haemorrhage
- [ ] **D**   Undisclosed phenytoin overdose
- [ ] **E**   Vertebral artery dissection

10.11   A 69-year-old man attends the Neurovascular Outpatient Clinic for assessment. He has experienced two short-lived episodes of right arm weakness and dysarthria, and his GP has commenced aspirin 75 mg daily and simvastatin 20 mg nocte. On examination, heart rate is regular and 82 bpm, and blood pressure is 172/86 mmHg. Which of the following statements is most accurate regarding cardiovascular risk reduction?

- [ ] **A**   Atenolol is the first-line antihypertensive of choice
- [ ] **B**   Calcium channel blockers reduce risk stroke in elderly patients
- [ ] **C**   Diastolic BP is a more important treatment target
- [ ] **D**   Dipyridamole should be added to aspirin in all patients
- [ ] **E**   Target systolic BP is 160 mmHg

10.12   A 56-year-old man attends the General Medical Outpatient Department with a 2-year history of recurrent dizzy spells associated with vertigo and falling to the left. On examination, he is found to have nystagmus that is pronounced on left lateral gaze, and impaired heel–shin coordination on the left side. Which of the following diagnoses is most likely?

- [ ] **A**   Acute cerebellar infarction
- [ ] **B**   Recurrent TIAs affecting the left cerebellar cortex
- [ ] **C**   Recurrent TIAs affecting the right cerebellar cortex
- [ ] **D**   Recurrent TIAs affecting the cerebellar vermis
- [ ] **E**   Subacute combined degeneration of the cord

10.10   Answer: E

Typically causes severe occipital headache, complicated by cerebellar ischaemia/infarction. Can be precipitated by cervical spine hyperextension, eg leaning head backwards into hair washbowl. Can be diagnosed by four-vessel neck Doppler scans, and CT or MR angiography.

10.11   Answer: B

Dihydropyridine calcium channel blockers (eg nifedipine) or a thiazide diuretic should be first-line treatment in patients > 60 years. Target systolic BP should be ≤130 mmHg in patients with established cerebrovascular disease.

10.12   Answer: B

Typically, lateral cerebellar lobe lesions cause ataxia and falls towards the side of the lesion, impaired coordination on the side of the lesion, nystagmus on gaze towards the lesion. Vermis lesions cause marked truncal and gait ataxia.

10.13 A 58-year-old woman presents to the Emergency Department with sudden onset of right-sided facial numbness and weakness affecting her left arm and leg. She is found to have nystagmus and ataxia affecting her right upper limb. Which of the following is the most likely diagnosis?

- A Acute infarction of the left cerebellar lobe
- B Acute infarction of the right cerebellar lobe
- C Acute infarction of the cerebellar vermis
- D Internal capsule infarction
- E Lateral medullary syndrome

10.14 A 71-year-old man attends the Emergency Department with sudden onset of visual impairment. On examination, there is a right homonomous hemianopia. Physical examination appears otherwise normal. Which of the following is the most likely explanation?

- A Lacunar infarction
- B Middle cerebral artery occlusion
- C Partial anterior circulation stroke
- D Posterior cerebral artery occlusion
- E Total anterior circulation infarction

10.15 You are asked to review a 65-year-old woman in the Emergency Department. She had presented with sudden onset of left arm and leg weakness. On examination, there is a partial right ptosis, diplopia and dilatation of the right pupil. Which of the following is the most likely anatomical site of the lesion responsible?

- A Hypothalamus
- B Left midbrain
- C Right midbrain
- D Left medulla
- E Right medulla

10.13   Answer: E

Also called Wallenberg's syndrome; caused by thrombosis of the posterior inferior cerebellar artery or vertebral artery.

10.14   Answer: C

Other features of anterior circulation stroke are hemiparesis, hemisensory loss and aphasia (dominant hemisphere). Posterior circulation strokes can cause hemianopia, but are typically associated with other features, eg diplopia, vertigo, ataxia and nystagmus.

10.15   Answer: C

Weber's syndrome, typically causing an ipsilateral third cranial nerve palsy and contralateral hemiparesis.

10.16 A 27-year-old woman is admitted to the Emergency Department with a short history of fever, headache and photophobia. A lumbar puncture is performed, and CSF shows 80 lymphocytes/mm³, protein 0.5 g/l and glucose 3.2 mmol/l (plasma glucose 5.1 mmol/l). Which of the following is the most likely diagnosis?

- A Cryptococcal meningitis
- B Herpes simplex virus (HSV) encephalitis
- C Enterovirus meningitis
- D Pneumococcal meningitis
- E Tuberculous meningitis

10.17 You are telephoned by the ward staff to tell you the results of CSF analyses of a patient admitted earlier in the day with headache. These show 168 neutrophils/mm³, protein 0.7 g/l and glucose 2.3 mmol/l (plasma glucose 4.9 mmol/l). Which one of the following is the most likely diagnosis?

- A *Cryptococcus neoformans* meningitis
- B Herpes simplex meningitis
- C *Mycobacterium tuberculosis* cerebral abscess
- D Sarcoidosis with neurological involvement
- E *Staphylococcus aureus* meningitis

10.18 A 21-year-old student is admitted to the Neurology Unit with a short history of headache, fever, and neck stiffness. On examination, there is photophobia and you note the presence of a petechial rash overlying the trunk and upper arms. Which of the following should be undertaken as the best initial management of this patient?

- A CT head scan
- B Intravenous benzylpenicillin
- C Intravenous hydrocortisone
- D Lumbar puncture
- E Venous blood sampling for culture

10.16 Answer: C

History indicates meningism, and modestly raised or normal protein, and glucose > 50% of plasma concentrations and lymphocytosis suggest a viral cause. Commonest causes are enteroviruses (eg echovirus and coxsackievirus), or mumps, HSV, HIV or Epstein–Barr virus.

10.17 Answer: E

Polymorph leukocytosis, raised protein concentration and CSF glucose < 50% plasma concentration strongly suggest bacterial infection. TB is typically associated with a higher protein concentration and lymphocytosis.

10.18 Answer: B

The scenario suggests meningococcal meningitis, which is a medical emergency. If the patient is known to be allergic to penicillin, high dose cephalosporin is an alternative. Lumbar puncture for CSF microscopy and culture, and blood cultures are important, but should never delay antibiotic treatment.

10.19 You are looking after a 23-year-old female who presented 3 days earlier with meningococcal meningitis. Which of the following prophylactic measures is most appropriate?

- [ ] **A** Amoxicillin should be offered to suspected contacts
- [ ] **B** Contacts with headache should undergo lumbar puncture
- [ ] **C** Public health department must be notified
- [ ] **D** Rifampicin treatment should be offered to all next of kin
- [ ] **E** Steps should be taken to prevent faeco-oral transmission

10.20 Which of the following meningitis infections can most effectively be prevented by the use of vaccines?

- [ ] **A** Epstein–Barr virus
- [ ] **B** *Listeria monocytogenes*
- [ ] **C** *Staphylococcus aureus*
- [ ] **D** *Streptococcus pneumoniae*
- [ ] **E** *Treponema pallidum*

10.21 A previously well 38-year-old man is admitted to the Acute Medical Assessment Unit with a 24 h history of fever and headache. On arrival in the unit, he has a generalised seizure terminated by diazepam. His wife reports that his behaviour and personality have been rather odd over the past 1–2 days. Which of the following diagnoses is most likely to explain his presenting features?

- [ ] **A** Acute alcohol withdrawal
- [ ] **B** Bacterial meningitis
- [ ] **C** Cerebral abscess
- [ ] **D** Mycoplasma pneumonia
- [ ] **E** Viral encephalitis

10.19   Answer: C

Potential contacts should be offered rifampicin, and vaccination with a meningococcal C conjugate should be considered.

10.20   Answer: D

Particularly in patients with recurrent pneumococcal meningitis, eg after a skull fracture and CSF leak. Other vaccines used to prevent meningitis include Hib (*Haemophilus influenzae*) and MenC (*Neisseria meningitidis*).

10.21   Answer: E

Other features are drowsiness, focal neurological signs, seizures and coma. HSV infection carries a 20% mortality. The others are important differential diagnoses.

10.22 A 39-year-old woman has recently returned to the UK from a holiday in the tropics. She presents with a short history of headache, neck stiffness and photophobia, and a diagnostic lumbar puncture is performed. Which of the following is most accurate regarding the differential diagnosis in this patient?

A Cryptococcal meningitis is diagnosed by direct microscopy

B Normal microscopy excludes bacterial meningitis

C Polymerase chain reaction (PCR) techniques are ineffective in detecting *N. meningitidis*

D Relief of headache after LP is characteristic of viral meningitis

E Ziehl–Nielsen staining is highly sensitive for tuberculous meningitis

10.23 A 52-year-old woman presents with a rapidly progressive history of lower limb weakness and urinary retention. MRI scan of the spine shows some white matter changes and diffuse swelling at the T12 level. Which of the following diagnoses offers the best explanation for these findings?

A HSV encephalitis

B Meningioma

C Neuroma with spinal cord compression

D Spinal abscess with cord infiltration

E Transverse myelitis due to varicella

10.24 A 69-year-old man is found to have a rash overlying the left side of his chest with early vesicle formation. Which of the following features is most strongly suggestive of shingles?

A Erythema surrounding the vesicles

B History of chickenpox earlier in life

C Recent contact with patient with chickenpox infection

D Recent treatment with oral prednisolone

E Tenderness overlying the rash

10.22   Answer: D

PCR is highly sensitive for detecting meningococcal and other
bacterial infections; microscopy alone can be insensitive.
Cryptococcal and other fungal infections can be detected using India
ink.

10.23   Answer: E

Transverse myelitis involves inflammation of the spinal cord, causing
paraparesis or tetraparesis depending on the level of involvement.
This occurs due to varicella zoster virus (VZV) or post-infective
encephalomyelitis (eg after measles, VZV, mumps or rubella).

10.24   Answer: D

Dorsal root ganglion VZV re-activation, often many years after
primary infection. Patients cannot acquire chickenpox from shingles
patients, but not the other way around.

10.25 Which of the following neurotransmitters is most likely to raise seizure threshold in adults?

☐ A Acetylcholine

☐ B Dopamine

☐ C Gamma-aminobutyric acid (GABA)

☐ D Glutamate

☐ E Norepinephrine

10.26 A 24-year-old man is referred for electroencephalography (EEG) for suspected generalised epilepsy. Which of these statements is correct in relation to the EEG?

☐ A Alpha rhythm is provoked by visual stimulation

☐ B Benzodiazepines increase β waveform activity

☐ C Is effective as a means of diagnosing epilepsy

☐ D Is less good than CT for identifying electrical focus in epilepsy

☐ E Scalp electrodes detect more than 90% of brain electrical activity

10.27 A 24-year-old woman with suspected epilepsy is referred for EEG. Which of the following statements regarding this investigation is correct?

☐ A Diagnostic sensitivity can be increased by hyperventilation

☐ B False positive rate is around 10%

☐ C Sensitivity for diagnosing epilepsy is around 90%

☐ D Spikes and sharp waveforms cannot be found between seizures

☐ E Total wave activity of > 50/s is diagnostic of epilepsy

10.28 A 32-year-old woman has complained of transient visual loss affecting the right eye, and is suspected of having suffered retrobulbar neuritis. Which of the following tests would most strongly confirm this diagnosis?

☐ A CT scan through the orbits

☐ B Delayed visual evoked responses

☐ C Diffuse cerebral white matter changes noted on MRI scan

☐ D Temporal lobe atrophy on CT scanning

☐ E Widened cerebral sulci

10.25   Answer: C

GABA is an inhibitory neurotransmitter whose effects are enhanced by a number of antiepileptic drugs (eg vigabatrin and gabapentin). The others are stimulatory neurotransmitters.

10.26   Answer: B

As with other sedative drugs. Resting β rhythms are abolished by eye opening. EEG can be useful in distinguishing the type of epilepsy and source of abnormal electrical activity. Scalp electrodes detect < 1% of all brain electrical activity.

10.27   Answer: A

Sensitivity is around 50%, and can be increased by stimuli (eg flickering lights). False positive rate is low, typically less than 0.1%. Spikes and sharp waveforms are 'epileptiform' abnormalities typically noted between seizures.

10.28   Answer: B

Delayed visual evoked responses can detect involvement of any part of the visual pathway from eye to occipital cortex. Often, the structural appearance on CT or even MRI scanning can be normal.

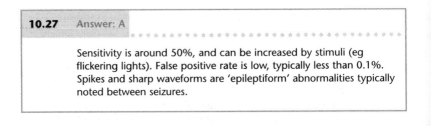

10.29 A 21-year-old man attends the Neurology Outpatient Clinic for investigation of chronic headache. Which of the following is correct regarding lumbar puncture investigation?

A A standard 20-gauge needle should routinely be used

B Bed-rest is important to prevent headache

C Fluid restriction is important in the first 24 h after the procedure

D May relieve headache in benign intracranial hypertension

E No more than 10 ml CSF should be withdrawn

10.30 A 32-year-old woman is admitted via the Emergency Department with sudden onset of headache. A lumbar puncture is performed, and CSF is clear and microscopy shows 1500/mm^3 lymphocytes and glucose 4.1 mmol/l. Plasma glucose is 5.3 mmol/l. What is the most likely diagnosis?

A Bacterial meningitis

B Multiple sclerosis

C Sarcoidosis

D Tuberculous meningitis

E Viral meningitis

10.31 A 19-year-old woman complains of headaches over the past 2 months, which are severe in the morning. She is suspected of having tension headaches. Which of the following symptoms most strongly suggests an alternative diagnosis?

A Constant pain

B Occipital pain radiating to the vertex

C Pain worsens with bending forward

D Relieved by analgesia

E Sensation of a tight band around the head

10.29   Answer: D

Also a characteristic feature in viral meningitis. Up to 100 ml CSF can leak over 24 h after lumbar puncture, and maintaining hydration can prevent post-lumbar puncture headache. Bed-rest can exacerbate headache on mobilising, and is not necessary.

10.30   Answer: E

Lymphocytosis, normal glucose (> 60% plasma glucose) and normal or slightly high protein (< 0.5 g/l).

10.31   Answer: C

Headache made worse with cough, straining or bending forward suggests raised intracranial pressure. Tension headache may be poorly relieved by analgesia in some patients.

10.32 A 29-year-old woman has suffered from headaches for the past 9 weeks, thought to be simple tension headaches. Which of the following would most strongly suggest an alternative underlying diagnosis?

- A Brisk plantar reflex responses
- B Local scalp tenderness
- C Photophobia
- D Poor response to analgesia
- E Urinary frequency

10.33 For the past 9 months, a 27-year-old woman has suffered from intermittent episodes of severe headache associated with vomiting and transient visual disturbance. Which of the following is the most likely diagnosis?

- A Benign intracranial hypertension
- B Glioblastoma multiforme
- C Migraine
- D Retinal detachment
- E Temporal arteritis

10.34 A 26-year-old woman has suffered intermittent headaches for the past year. These are characterised by a feeling of nausea and irritability followed by a severe throbbing left-sided headache which persists for several days accompanied by dysphasia. Which of these is the most likely diagnosis?

- A Benign intracranial hypertension
- B Cluster headache
- C Migraine
- D Temporal lobe epilepsy
- E Transient ischaemic attacks

10.35 Which of the following is correct with regard to migraine?

- A Attacks typically occur at times of intense emotional stress
- B May be provoked by dietary chocolate in some patients
- C Female : male prevalence is around 1.5:1
- D Headache phase is associated with extra-cranial vasoconstriction
- E Vomiting suggests an alternative diagnosis

10.32   Answer: C

Brisk, symmetrical reflexes are a common finding in healthy young women. Local scalp tenderness is a common feature of tension headache, and can also be found in trigeminal neuralgia and temporal arteritis.

10.33   Answer: C

Lifetime prevalence is 20% in women, 5% in men, and presents before age 40 years in > 90%.

10.34   Answer: C

Classical migraine is also associated with visual disturbance, including fortification spectra, sensory symptoms, and (rarely) weakness, ie hemiplegic migraine.

10.35   Answer: B

Migraine may occur *after* periods of stress. Female : male prevalence is around 4:1, and the headache phase is associated with vasodilatation of extracranial vessels.

10.36 Over the past 10 days, a 22-year-old man has suffered severe intermittent left-sided frontal headache associated with lacrimation of his left eye. He reports similar headaches occurring 1 year before. Which is the most likely diagnosis?

- [ ] A Allergic conjunctivitis
- [ ] B Cluster headache
- [ ] C Temporal lobe epilepsy
- [ ] D Tension headache
- [ ] E Viral meningitis

10.37 A previously well 45-year-old man presents to the Emergency Department with sudden onset of severe headache during sexual intercourse. The pain intensity gradually diminished over 45 min, and there are no residual neurological symptoms or signs. What is the most likely explanation?

- [ ] A Coital cephalalgia
- [ ] B Subarachnoid haemorrhage
- [ ] C Subdural haematoma
- [ ] D Temporal arteritis
- [ ] E Transient ischaemic attack

10.38 A 58-year-old woman complains of severe facial pain associated with involuntary facial twitching, and a diagnosis of trigeminal neuralgia is suspected. Which of the following treatments is most likely to be effective?

- [ ] A Co-codamol
- [ ] B Frontal lobectomy
- [ ] C Indomethacin
- [ ] D Phenol injection into the trigeminal nerve root ganglion
- [ ] E Phenytoin

10.36   Answer: B

Also known as migrainous neuralgia, this is uncommon and occurs mostly in men. Characteristically, pain is periorbital and can be associated with an ipsilateral Horner's syndrome and nasal congestion.

10.37   Answer: A

No vomiting, neck stiffness or photophobia. Unlikely to recur, but may be prevented with simple analgesia or treatments for migraine prophylaxis. Needs CT and lumbar puncture to distinguish from subarachnoid haemorrhage.

10.38   Answer: E

Carbamazepine is often preferred as first-line therapy. Phenol or alcohol injections into the trigeminal nerve branches, and vascular decompression of the nerve via posterior craniotomy may be effective.

10.39 A 61-year-old man complains of severe, sharp right-sided facial pain associated with facial twitching. The pain is exacerbated by chewing food. Which is the most likely diagnosis?

- [ ] **A** Cluster headache
- [ ] **B** Migraine
- [ ] **C** Tension headache
- [ ] **D** Toothache
- [ ] **E** Trigeminal neuralgia

10.40 A 38-year-old woman presents to the Emergency Department with an 18-h history of severe vertigo, ataxia and vomiting. Vertigo is exacerbated by sudden head movements. Tone, power and reflexes appear normal in upper and lower limbs. What is the most likely diagnosis?

- [ ] **A** Acute gastritis
- [ ] **B** Labyrinthitis
- [ ] **C** Meningioma
- [ ] **D** Otitis media
- [ ] **E** Transient ischaemic attack

10.41 A 51-year-old man presents with recurrent attacks of vertigo and a sensation of 'pressure' in his left ear. He has suffered from tinnitus for around 6 months. On examination, there is sensorineuronal deafness of his left ear. What is the likely underlying diagnosis?

- [ ] **A** Acoustic neuroma
- [ ] **B** Labyrinthitis
- [ ] **C** Ménière's disease
- [ ] **D** Salicylate toxicity
- [ ] **E** Transient ischaemic attacks involving the posterior cerebral circulation

10.39 Answer: E

Can also be precipitated by touching facial trigger zones.

10.40 Answer: B

Also known as vestibular neuronitis; assumed to be viral in origin, usually self-limiting. Can also be associated with nystagmus.

10.41 Answer: C

Classically, presents with tinnitus, distorted hearing and paroxysmal vertigo. Can be treated with cinnarizine, prochlorperazine and betahistine.

10.42   A 42-year-old heavy goods vehicle driver is admitted via the Emergency Department following a generalised seizure lasting < 2 min, terminated with rectal diazepam. There is no past history of seizures. Clinical examination and CT head scan are normal. What advice should he be given regarding driving?

A   Advise to inform DVLA and avoid all driving for 6 weeks

B   Advise to inform DVLA and avoid vocational driving for 1 year

C   Advise to inform DVLA and avoid vocational driving lifelong

D   Advise to inform DVLA and continue driving until further notice

E   No specific precautions after an isolated seizure

10.43   A 25-year-old female nurse is admitted to the Acute Medical Admissions Unit after a self-terminating generalised seizure. There is no evidence of any persistent neurological deficit, and an outpatient CT head scan has been requested. What advice should she be given about driving?

A   Advise to inform DVLA and avoid driving for 1 year

B   Advise to inform DVLA and avoid driving for 6 weeks

C   Advise to inform DVLA and avoid driving lifelong

D   Advise to inform DVLA and continue driving until further notice

E   No specific precautions after an isolated seizure

10.44   A 28-year-old man is admitted to the Acute Medical Admissions Unit after a short-lived generalised seizure that terminated spontaneously on arrival at hospital. There are no signs of neurological deficit, and an outpatient CT head scan has been arranged. What advice is most important to be given before discharge from hospital?

A   Inform DVLA and continue driving until further notice

B   Avoid cycling for 6 months

C   Avoid taking a bath for 1 year

D   Advise to avoid swimming or boating for 1 week

E   No specific precautions after an isolated seizure

10.42   Answer: C

No PSV or HGV licence permitted if any seizure has occurred after 5 years of age, unless seizure-free for 10 years off anti-epileptic medications and there is no structural epileptogenic focus.

10.43   Answer: A

Normally, if no further seizures have occurred during the 1 year period, a full licence will be restored.

10.44   Answer: B

Advise to inform DVLA and avoid driving for 1 year; licence can be restored if seizure-free. Should be advised to take only shallow baths, and to be accompanied if undertaking swimming or boating activities. If the patient insists on cycling, then they should be accompanied if possible, heavy traffic avoided and a helmet must be worn.

Neurology answers

10.45 A 33-year-old woman has had recurrent generalised seizures and has been diagnosed with epilepsy. What treatment would be most appropriate?

   ☐ **A** Carbamazepine

   ☐ **B** Clonazepam

   ☐ **C** Ethosuximide

   ☐ **D** Gabapentin

   ☐ **E** Phenytoin

10.46 A 32-year-old man has suffered from three separate generalised seizures over the past 4 months, and is commenced on sodium valproate. Which of the following is the most likely clinical course?

   ☐ **A** 50% mortality at 20 years after diagnosis

   ☐ **B** 50% seizure-free off medications at 20 years after diagnosis

   ☐ **C** 80% prevalence of alcoholism at 20 years after diagnosis

   ☐ **D** 90% seizure-free on medications at 20 years after diagnosis

   ☐ **E** 95% seizure-free off medications at 20 years after diagnosis

10.47 A 55-year-old man complains of weakness affecting his right arm. On examination, there is marked weakness of elbow and wrist extension and brisk biceps and triceps reflexes on the right side. Which of the following is the most likely cause?

   ☐ **A** Cerebral metastases

   ☐ **B** Guillain–Barré syndrome

   ☐ **C** Myasthenia gravis

   ☐ **D** Parkinson's disease

   ☐ **E** Thoracic spine compression

10.48 For 6 weeks, a 57-year-old woman has noticed progressive weakness of her arms, particularly affecting elbow, wrist and finger extension. On examination, there is marked muscle wasting and fasciculation in the upper limbs, associated with diminished reflexes. Which of the following is the most likely cause?

   ☐ **A** Cerebral metastases

   ☐ **B** Myasthenia gravis

   ☐ **C** Parkinson's disease

   ☐ **D** Recent stroke

   ☐ **E** Thoracic spine compression

10.45   Answer: A

Or sodium valproate. Phenytoin also effective, but greater adverse effects (acne, facial coarseness, osteomalacia and gingival hyperplasia). Ethosuximide used for absence seizures, gabapentin for partial seizures and clonazepam is an adjunctive treatment.

10.46   Answer: B

At 20 years after diagnosis, around one-third will have persisting seizures despite on-going anti-epileptic treatment.

10.47   Answer: A

Signs indicate weakness in a pyramidal distribution; hyperreflexia suggests an upper motor neurone lesion. Thoracic spine compression may cause upper motor neurone signs in the lower limbs.

10.48   Answer: B

Signs indicate weakness in a pyramidal distribution; hyporeflexia and muscle wasting and fasciculation suggest a lower motor neurone or neuromuscular junction lesion.

10.49 A 65-year-old man complains of weakness and incoordination affecting his left arm. On examination, there is minimal muscle wasting in both upper limbs, coarse resting tremor affecting his left hand and increased tone in his upper limbs, particularly noticeable on the left side. What is the most likely cause?

- [ ] A Cerebral metastases
- [ ] B Guillain–Barré syndrome
- [ ] C Myasthenia gravis
- [ ] D Parkinson's disease
- [ ] E Thoracic spine compression

10.50 A 64-year-old woman presents with increasing gait instability. When walking on flat surfaces, her legs are noted to be hyper-extended, her toes scuff along the ground and there is circumduction at the hips. What is the most likely underlying diagnosis?

- [ ] A Cerebral metastases
- [ ] B Guillain–Barré syndrome
- [ ] C Myasthenia gravis
- [ ] D Parkinson's disease
- [ ] E Thoracic spine compression

10.51 A 57-year-old man is noted to have a tremor at rest, affecting only his right forearm and hand. It diminishes with focussed movements of the right arm, such as picking up a cup. What is the most likely cause?

- [ ] A Alcoholic myopathy
- [ ] B Cerebellar ataxia
- [ ] C Motor neurone disease
- [ ] D Parkinsonism
- [ ] E Wernicke's encephalopathy

10.49   Answer: D

Increased tone and tremor (combined give cog-wheel rigidity),
typically affecting upper more than lower limbs, are characteristic of
Parkinsonism. Muscle wasting is usually mild, reflexes may be slightly
increased or decreased and there is bradykinesia.

10.50   Answer: E

These features are strongly suggestive of upper motor neurone
lesions affecting both lower limbs ('pyramidal' gait), ie spastic
paraparesis. Cerebral metastases may be accompanied by upper
motor neurone lesions affecting the upper and lower limbs (often
asymmetric), seizures and features of raised ICP.

10.51   Answer: D

Rest tremor is pathognomonic of parkinsonism, lessened by
concentration, and worsened by augmentation/distraction
techniques.

10.52 A 48-year-old woman is noted to have a fine, rapid tremor affecting both upper limbs that is most pronounced when the fingers and arms are outstretched. Which of the following is the most likely explanation?

- ☐ **A** Alcohol toxicity
- ☐ **B** Atenolol therapy
- ☐ **C** Cerebellar ataxia
- ☐ **D** Parkinsonism
- ☐ **E** Theophylline treatment

10.53 A 61-year-old female complains of sensory loss affecting her left leg. On examination, there is impaired pain and temperature discrimination distal to the left knee, but preservation of joint position and vibration senses. What is the most likely site of involvement?

- ☐ **A** Left-sided corticospinal tract lesion at thoracic level
- ☐ **B** Left-sided spinothalamic tract lesion at thoracic level
- ☐ **C** Left-sided dorsal column lesion at thoracic level
- ☐ **D** Right-sided dorsal column lesion at thoracic level
- ☐ **E** Right-sided spinothalamic tract lesion at thoracic level

10.54 A 59-year-old man complains of sudden onset of sensory loss affecting his right arm and leg, and the left side of his face. Involvement of which anatomical site is most likely to cause these findings?

- ☐ **A** Left side of the medulla
- ☐ **B** Left side of the mid-brain
- ☐ **C** Left side of the thoracic spine
- ☐ **D** Right side of the mid-brain
- ☐ **E** Right side of the medulla

10.52   Answer: E

Action tremor can be physiological, and exaggerated by anxiety, thyrotoxicosis, drugs (eg salbutamol, theophylline, caffeine), fatigue and alcohol withdrawal.

10.53   Answer: D

Spinothalamic pain and temperature sensory fibres synapse with 2nd order neurones, which cross in the spinal cord and ascend in the contralateral spinothalamic tract. Vibration and proprioceptive signals ascend in the ipsilateral dorsal column, and synapse with 2nd order neurones in the brainstem before crossing the midline.

10.54   Answer: B

Spinothalamic and dorsal column fibres have crossed the midline at this site, so as to cause hemisensory loss of all modalities in the arm and leg.

10.55 A 41-year-old man is rushed to the Emergency Department after a motor vehicle accident. His consciousness level is reduced. On examination, he opens his eyes in response to pain, demonstrates abnormal flexor responses to pain, and is making incomprehensible sounds. What is his Glasgow Coma Scale (GCS)?

- A 2
- B 4
- C 6
- D 8
- E 10

10.56 A 66-year-old left-handed man is admitted with sudden onset of expressive dysphasia and mild right arm weakness. What is the most likely anatomical site giving rise to these findings?

- A Left side of the mid-brain
- B Left temporoparietal lobe
- C Right temporal lobe lesion
- D Right medullary lesion
- E Right-sided mid-brain lesion

10.57 A 71-year-old man has had progressive memory impairment over the past 9 months, and is thought to have mild to moderate dementia. Which of the following investigations would be most important?

- A Brain biopsy
- B CT head scan
- C Electroencephalography
- D HIV serology
- E Lumbar puncture

10.55   Answer: C

GCS allows serial comparison of consciousness, and is a useful prognostic indicator in trauma patients. Other scoring systems may be more appropriate in different patient groups, eg poisoning severity score (PSS) after drug overdose.

10.56   Answer: B

Dysphasia indicates a dominant temporal (receptive) or parietal (expressive) lobe lesion. This is the left cerebral cortex in virtually all right-handed people and around two-thirds of left-handed people. Simultaneous right arm weakness confirms involvement of the left anterior circulation.

10.57   Answer: B

Routine investigations to identify treatable causes also include vitamin B_{12}, thyroid function tests, VDRL, chest X-ray and antinuclear antibody tests. Detailed investigations are reserved for selected patients, eg those aged < 50 years at onset, or rapidly progressive history.

10.58 A 63-year-old man has had progressively worsening memory problems over the past 8 months. A diagnosis of Alzheimer's disease is suspected. Which of the following would most strongly suggest an alternative explanation for his symptoms?

- [ ] **A** Apathy and poor food intake
- [ ] **B** Ataxia and urinary incontinence
- [ ] **C** Inability to recall home address
- [ ] **D** Preservation of long-term memory
- [ ] **E** Social isolation

10.59 A 51-year-old man is admitted with sudden onset of dysarthria associated with head tremor and truncal ataxia. What is the most likely cause of his speech defect?

- [ ] **A** Basal ganglia infarction
- [ ] **B** Bulbar palsy
- [ ] **C** Cerebellar infarct
- [ ] **D** Pseudobulbar palsy
- [ ] **E** Pyramidal tract lesion at mid-brain level

10.60 A 57-year-old woman is admitted for investigation of progressive dysphagia and dysarthria. On examination, the tongue appears wasted and there is fasciculation. What is the most likely diagnosis?

- [ ] **A** Basal ganglia infarction
- [ ] **B** Bulbar palsy
- [ ] **C** Cerebellar infarct
- [ ] **D** Pseudobulbar palsy
- [ ] **E** Pyramidal tract lesion at mid-brain level

10.61 A 56-year-old woman complains of impairment of her vision. Confrontational visual field assessment shows that there is a bitemporal hemianopia. What is the most likely cause for this disturbance?

- [ ] **A** Bilateral optic neuritis
- [ ] **B** Dominant occipital lobe tumour
- [ ] **C** External compression of the optic chiasm
- [ ] **D** Parietal lobe infarction
- [ ] **E** Wernicke's encephalopathy

10.58 Answer: B

Suggest the possibility of 'normal-pressure hydrocephalus'. Apathy, poor self-caring and social isolation are common features, but may also suggest the possibility of depression.

10.59 Answer: C

Also associated with limb ataxia, nystagmus and incoordination.

10.60 Answer: B

Bilateral involvement of cranial nerves 9–12 can cause dysphagia and dysarthria. Bulbar palsy arises from lower motor neurone lesion. Pseudobulbar palsy (upper motor neurone lesion) causes brisk jaw jerk and small, contracted tongue.

10.61 Answer: C

Often caused by pituitary lobe tumours.

10.62 A 46-year-old man complains of visual disturbance. He is found to have a partial ptosis of his left eye, with lateral and inferior deviation of left eye gaze. Pupil sizes and reactions appear normal. What is the most likely diagnosis?

   A Complete left 3rd nerve palsy

   B Complete right 3rd nerve palsy

   C Grave's ophthalmopathy

   D Partial left 3rd nerve palsy

   E Retro-orbital tumour

10.63 A 63-year-old woman is admitted due to acute confusional state. She is noted to have a small, irregular pupil on the left, which accommodates normally but fails to constrict on direct illumination. What is the most likely diagnosis?

   A Argyll–Robertson pupil

   B Glaucoma

   C Holmes–Adie syndrome

   D Partial left 3rd nerve palsy

   E Previous trauma to the left eye

10.64 A 48-year-old man is complaining of excess sweating and occasional palpitations. On examination, he is found to have swelling of the optic disc. Which of the following is the most likely explanation for this sign?

   A Amyloidosis

   B Cerebral abscess

   C Severe hypertension

   D Non-Hodgkin's lymphoma

   E Sarcoidosis

10.62 Answer: D

Sparing of pupil responses indicates partial, rather than complete ipsilateral 3rd nerve palsy (autonomic pupillary innervation remains intact).

10.63 Answer: A

Lesion is at the dorsal mid-brain region, and usually due to tertiary syphilis. Holmes–Adie syndrome gives a dilated pupil that fails to accommodate but usually reacts to light.

10.64 Answer: C

The others are recognised causes, albeit uncommon. Optic disc swelling is often a sign of raised intracranial hypertension. Alcohol excess is a very common cause of unexplained sweating, and often contributes to hypertension.

10.65 A 41-year-old woman with established multiple sclerosis is complaining of a burning pain sensation across both legs and lower back. On examination, light touch is exquisitely tender. Which of the following is most likely to be effective in controlling her symptoms?

- [ ] **A** Baclofen
- [ ] **B** Carbamazepine
- [ ] **C** Clonazepam
- [ ] **D** Methylprednisolone
- [ ] **E** Physiotherapy

10.66 A 45-year-old woman with established multiple sclerosis has been suffering from progressively declining mobility over the past 6 weeks due to increasing lower limb spasticity. Which of the following is most likely to be effective in reducing her spasticity?

- [ ] **A** Amitriptyline
- [ ] **B** Carbamazepine
- [ ] **C** Intrathecal baclofen
- [ ] **D** Methylprednisolone
- [ ] **E** Phenytoin

10.67 A 46-year-old woman has been diagnosed with multiple sclerosis for 8 years. Over the past 2 days, she has had rapidly progressive leg weakness that is affecting her ability to live independently. Which one of the following statements is correct in relation to the use of corticosteroid treatment?

- [ ] **A** Acute dysphoria is a recognised adverse effect
- [ ] **B** Chronic administration reduces relapse rate
- [ ] **C** High-dose treatment reduces relapse severity but not duration
- [ ] **D** Short-term treatment reduces long-term morbidity
- [ ] **E** Treatment should normally be given for 1–2 weeks

10.65 Answer: B

Dysaesthesia may also respond to phenytoin, amitriptyline or gabapentin.

10.66 Answer: C

Although oral treatment is almost as effective, with fewer complications; physiotherapy, benzodiazepine and dantrolene may also be effective.

10.67 Answer: A

A short course of high-dose corticosteroids (eg methyprednisolone 1 g daily for 3 days) can lessen the duration of relapses, thereby minimising functional impairment. Multiple courses should be avoided due to the long-term adverse effects, eg osteoporosis, obesity, type 2 diabetes and increased susceptibility to infection.

10.68 A 45-year-old man has been diagnosed with multiple sclerosis, with a relapsing–remitting pattern over the past 6 years. Which one of the following statements is true regarding long-term treatment of this condition?

- A Azathioprine increases 5-year survival by around 30%
- B Beta-interferon substantially reduces long-term disability
- C Ciclosporin reduces relapse rate by around 50%
- D Hyperbaric oxygen reduces relapse rate by around 25%
- E Linoleic acid diet supplements have no effect on relapse rate

10.69 A 47-year-old man presents with rigidity of his upper limbs, associated with bradykinesia and a coarse resting tremor. Which of the following is the most important investigation for a possible underlying cause?

- A 24-h urinary copper estimation
- B CT head scan
- C Early morning urinary lead concentration
- D MRI head scan
- E Serum iron concentration

10.70 A 68-year-old man complains of progressive limb weakness and difficulty swallowing. He has been treated for pneumonia on two recent occasions. On examination, he has increased muscle tone and brisk reflexes in all four limbs, and both plantar responses are extensor. Which of the following is the most likely diagnosis?

- A Amyotrophic lateral sclerosis
- B Multiple sclerosis
- C Polymyositis
- D Progressive bulbar palsy
- E Progressive muscular atrophy

10.68 Answer: E

Immune modulation can reduce relapse rate, eg up to 30% reduction with β-interferon, but has a minimal effect on long-term outcome/disability. A number of other treatments and special diets offer no proven benefits.

10.69 Answer: A

In a young patient (< 50 years), differential diagnoses of Parkinson's disease should be investigated, including Wilson's disease (high serum caeruloplasmin and 24-h urinary copper excretion).

10.70 Answer: A

Form of motor neurone disease in which upper motor neurone pyramidal tract signs predominate. In progressive bulbar palsy, dysarthria and dysphagia are early features, whilst in progressive muscular atrophy there is predominant spinal neurone involvement with prominent wasting and fasciculation.

10.71 Over the past 6 months, a 35-year-old woman has noticed intermittent drooping of both eyelids, and progressive facial weakness on speaking and upper limb weakness whilst typing. A diagnosis of myasthenia gravis is suspected. Which of these investigations would most strongly establish the diagnosis?

- ☐ **A** Abnormal spike activity on resting EMG
- ☐ **B** Anti-acetylcholine receptor antibodies
- ☐ **C** Anti-skeletal muscle antibodies
- ☐ **D** Inducible fatigue on repetitive upper limb exercise
- ☐ **E** Rapid improvement in muscle power after edrophonium chloride

10.72 A 45-year-old man has been treated for HIV infection for 8 years, and was treated for *Pneumocystis carinii* infection 8 months ago. He now presents with progressive memory impairment, weakness of his right arm and leg and marked dysphasia. MRI head scan shows diffuse white matter abnormalities. What is the most likely diagnosis?

- ☐ **A** Cryptococcal meningitis
- ☐ **B** HIV encephalitis
- ☐ **C** Herpes simplex encephalitis
- ☐ **D** *Pneumocystis carinii* cerebral abscess
- ☐ **E** Progressive multifocal leukoencephalopathy

10.73 For the past 6 weeks, a 54-year-old woman has received co-amoxiclav treatment for chronic sinusitis. She is admitted via the Emergency Department complaining of severe pain over the right maxilla, and is observed to have a short-lived self-limiting generalised seizure shortly after arrival. What is the most likely explanation for the seizure?

- ☐ **A** Adverse drug reaction
- ☐ **B** Febrile convulsion
- ☐ **C** Herpes simplex encephalitis
- ☐ **D** Sub-dural empyema
- ☐ **E** Tricyclic antidepressant overdose

10.71   Answer: E

Anti-ACh antibodies present in 85% of cases; anti-skeletal muscle antibodies often positive, especially if thymoma present. Resting EMG typically normal, but characteristic decremental response with repetitive stimulation. Edrophonium is a short-acting cholinesterase inhibitor that potentiates neuromuscular ACh concentrations.

10.72   Answer: E

Due to oligodendrocyte infection by JC human polyomavirus, a complication of AIDS, carcinomatosis, leukaemia and lymphoma. Often rapidly progressive with high mortality.

10.73   Answer: D

Often arises as a complication of chronic sinusitis, osteomyelitis, middle ear disease or trauma. Focal signs suggest abscess formation; requires contrast CT head for detection.

10.74 A 41-year-old man with established AIDS presents with progressive headache, drowsiness, nausea and vomiting. On examination, temperature is 37.8°C, pulse rate is 48 per min and blood pressure 188/90 mmHg. Which of the following is most likely to account for his symptoms?

- [ ] **A** Acute pancreatitis
- [ ] **B** Bacterial meningitis
- [ ] **C** Fungal meningitis
- [ ] **D** Migraine
- [ ] **E** Raised intracranial pressure

10.75 Which of the following is the most characteristic feature of type 2 neurofibromatosis?

- [ ] **A** Axillary freckling
- [ ] **B** Bilateral acoustic neuromata
- [ ] **C** Multiple cutaneous café au lait spots
- [ ] **D** Prominent cutaneous neurofibromata
- [ ] **E** Scoliosis

10.76 A 59-year-old woman has previously received treatment for small cell lung carcinoma. Over the past 6 weeks, she has developed progressive ataxia and vertigo, and is found to have vertical nystagmus. Which antibody test most strongly suggests paraneoplastic cerebellar degeneration?

- [ ] **A** Anti-double-stranded DNA antibody
- [ ] **B** Anti-Hu antibody
- [ ] **C** Anti-Jo 1 antibody
- [ ] **D** Antinuclear antibody
- [ ] **E** Anti-Yo antibody

10.74   Answer: E

Characteristic features include headache, impaired consciousness, papilloedema, vomiting, bradycardia and hypertension. This could be due to obstruction of CSF flow by fungal meningitis, or a mass lesion, eg lymphoma or cerebral abscess.

10.75   Answer: B

Type 1 accounts for around 75% of cases, and involves predominantly peripheral features, whereas type 2 is characterised by acoustic neuroma, optic nerve glioma, meningioma and spinal neuromata, with few or no cutaneous features.

10.76   Answer: E

Anti-Yo and anti-Hu antibodies are strongly suggestive; anti-Hu antibody is also detectable in a number of other paraneoplastic syndromes, eg subacute motor neuropathy, myelitis and sensory neuropathy. Anti-Jo 1 is associated with dermatomyositis and polymyositis, which may be associated with underlying lung, breast and ovarian cancer.

11. OPHTHALMOLOGY

11.1   Which of the following extraocular muscles is most likely to be affected by a lesion involving the fourth cranial nerve?

☐ **A**   Inferior oblique

☐ **B**   Lateral rectus

☐ **C**   Medial rectus

☐ **D**   Superior oblique

☐ **E**   Superior rectus

11.2   A 49-year-old woman presents to the Emergency Department with sudden deterioration of the vision in her right eye. Fundoscopy shows changes characteristic of retinal vein occlusion. Which of the following is most likely to predispose to this condition?

☐ **A**   Asthma

☐ **B**   Breast cancer

☐ **C**   Diabetes

☐ **D**   Hypertension

☐ **E**   Varicose veins

11.3   You are asked to see a 65-year-old man in the Emergency Department, who has presented with sudden visual disturbance affecting his left eye only. During fundoscopy, you think the appearances are those of a branch retinal vein occlusion. What feature most strongly supports this diagnosis?

☐ **A**   Arterio–venous nipping

☐ **B**   Dense cataracts bilaterally

☐ **C**   Multiple retinal haemorrhages

☐ **D**   Preservation of afferent pupillary responses

☐ **E**   Pupil is small and irregular

11.1   Answer: D

The others listed are supplied by the third cranial nerve (IO, IR, MR, SR) and sixth cranial nerve (LR).

11.2   Answer: D

Diabetes is also recognised, albeit less commonly. Other causes are hyperviscosity states (myeloma, Waldenström's macroglobulinaemia) and vasculitides.

11.3   Answer: C

Characteristic feature due to superficial haemorrhage in the nerve fibre layer, also associated with cotton wool spots, retinal vein dilatation and neovascularisation.

11.4 A 63-year-old man attends the Emergency Department with a history of dizziness, headache and blurred vision. On examination, he is found to have loss of his superior–temporal visual field in his right eye. What is the most likely cause?

☐ **A** Acute conjunctivitis

☐ **B** Acute stroke

☐ **C** Branch retinal artery occlusion

☐ **D** Episcleritis

☐ **E** Glaucoma

11.5 A 54-year-old woman is referred to the Hypertension Clinic, having been found by her employer to have readings of 182/86 and 184/82 mmHg. On examination, dipstick urinalysis is positive for glucose and protein, and fundoscopy shows multiple tiny haemorrhages and a small number of cotton wool spots. What is the most likely diagnosis?

☐ **A** Accelerated hypertension

☐ **B** Aortic valve incompetence

☐ **C** Diabetic retinopathy

☐ **D** Grade II hypertensive retinopathy

☐ **E** Grade III hypertensive retinopathy

11.6 Which of the following factors is most likely to be associated with branch retinal artery occlusion?

☐ **A** Asthma

☐ **B** Atrial fibrillation

☐ **C** Diabetes mellitus

☐ **D** Family history of glaucoma

☐ **E** Hypertension

11.4   Answer: C

Often painless, this can cause variable visual field defects depending on the extent of retinal involvement. Unlike stroke, the visual field loss is uniocular, rather than bitemporal.

11.5   Answer: E

Grade I is characterised by arteriolar narrowing, grade II is associated with AV nipping, whereas grade IV (accelerated hypertension) is associated with papilloedema.

11.6   Answer: B

Due to increased risk of occlusive embolic disease. Can also be associated with underlying arteritis or raised intracranial pressure. Note that hypertension and diabetes are associated with an increased risk of branch retinal vein occlusion.

11.7 A 56-year-old man attends an annual follow-up appointment in the Diabetes Outpatient Clinic. On fundoscopy, you find haemorrhages and exudates in a pattern suggestive of diabetic retinopathy. Which of the following statements is correct regarding this condition?

- A   It is a macrovascular complication of poorly controlled diabetes
- B   Platelet adhesiveness is generally diminished
- C   Rare cause of blindness in adults
- D   Risk of retinopathy is related to the duration of diabetes
- E   Smoking cessation does not delay progression

11.8 A 57-year-old woman attends the Medical Outpatient Department for follow-up assessment of her diabetes. The presence of which feature is most strongly indicative of background retinopathy?

- A   Absence of exudates
- B   Flame-shaped haemorrhages
- C   Impaired central visual acuity
- D   Multiple exudates involving and around the macula
- E   Neovascularisation around the optic disc

11.9 A 62-year-old woman with retinitis pigmentosa attends for her annual ophthalmology review in clinic. Which one of these statements best describes the visual defect associated with this condition?

- A   Features are normally due to impaired retinal cone function
- B   Loss of central vision is predominant feature
- C   Night-blindness is a prominent feature
- D   Pigmentation of the optic disc
- E   Red–green colour blindness predisposes to the condition

11.10 A 62-year-old man is referred to the Ophthalmology Outpatient Department for assessment of cataracts, which have caused impaired vision over the past year. Which one of the following would most strongly indicate the need for corrective surgery?

- A   Bilateral cataracts
- B   Family history of cataract disease
- C   Fundus cannot be seen to assess progression of diabetic retinopathy
- D   History of corticosteroid treatment
- E   White reflex

11.7   Answer: D

Commonest cause of blindness in young adults. Present in 80% of patients who have had type 2 diabetes for 20 years. Treatment involves smoking cessation advice and good control of blood pressure and diabetes.

11.8   Answer: B

Non-proliferative (background) retinopathy is usually associated with normal vision and is therefore only detected by fundoscopy screening. Characteristic features include microaneurysms and exudates. Diabetic maculopathy involves extensive exudates around the macula.

11.9   Answer: C

Inherited in autosomal or X-linked patterns. Features arise predominantly from retinal rod dysfunction (cones affected in late stages) to cause night-blindness and loss of peripheral vision.

11.10   Answer: C

An additional indication is severe functional impairment, eg recurrent falls.

11.11 A 21-year-old man is referred to the Ophthalmology Clinic because his GP thought he had 'unusual looking eyes' during a routine check-up for asthma. Slit-lamp examination shows downward dislocation of both lenses. What is the most likely diagnosis?

    A Corticosteroid treatment

    B Diabetes mellitus

    C Homocysteinuria

    D Marfan's syndrome

    E Trauma

11.12 A 37-year-old woman is referred to the General Medical Outpatient Department for assessment of blurred vision and generalised weakness. The GP did not find any physical abnormality, and has requested a second opinion. On examination, there is reduced visual acuity affecting the left eye associated with a central field defect. Pupil sizes are equal, but there is a relative afferent pupillary defect on the left. What is the most likely diagnosis?

    A Acute glaucoma

    B Acute stroke

    C Graves' ophthalmology

    D Optic neuritis

    E Retinal artery occlusion

11.13 A 58-year-old businessman with longstanding hypertension is found to have pale optic discs during routine fundoscopy. What is the most likely cause for this appearance?

    A Diabetes mellitus

    B Diltiazem

    C Hyperlipidaemia

    D Previous papilloedema

    E Smoking

11.11   Answer: C

Also seen in Ehlers–Danlos syndrome, with uveal tumours and after trauma (less likely cause in absence of history). Marfan's syndrome is typically associated with upward, outward dislocation of the lens.

11.12   Answer: D

The other possible causes listed are retinal artery occlusion (less likely in young adult with no predisposing factors) or acute glaucoma (less likely in absence of other signs.

11.13   Answer: D

This may have been in the setting of papilloedema due to accelerated hypertension. Other causes of optic atrophy include post-traumatic, neoplastic and metastatic infiltration.

11.14 A 24-year-old woman is referred for investigation of long-standing headaches. Seated blood pressure is 128/72 mmHg and pulse 74 per minute. Fundoscopy shows bilateral papilloedema. What is the most likely cause of this appearance?

- [ ] **A** Benign intracranial hypertension
- [ ] **B** Carbon dioxide retention
- [ ] **C** Diabetes mellitus
- [ ] **D** Multiple sclerosis
- [ ] **E** Posterior fossa tumour

11.15 A 47-year-old man self-presents to the Ophthalmology Emergency Department with an acutely painful left eye. On examination, the left eye looks red and inflamed with excess lacrimation. What is the most likely diagnosis?

- [ ] **A** Acute bacterial conjunctivitis
- [ ] **B** Acute viral conjunctivitis
- [ ] **C** Anterior uveitis
- [ ] **D** Graves' ophthalmopathy
- [ ] **E** Optic neuritis

11.16 A 56-year-old man is referred as an urgent case to the Ophthalmology Clinic by his GP because of deteriorating vision in his left eye. He is otherwise asymptomatic. On examination, pupils appear normal sized but there is a relative afferent pupillary defect affecting the left eye. What is the most likely underlying diagnosis?

- [ ] **A** Acute glaucoma
- [ ] **B** Acute scleritis
- [ ] **C** Branch retinal artery occlusion
- [ ] **D** Keratoconjunctivitis
- [ ] **E** Posterior uveitis

11.14   Answer: A

Most commonly found in young females, especially if co-existent obesity. Carbon dioxide retention can cause papilloedema in severe cases, eg sleep apnoea, but conscious level would be expected to be reduced. Posterior fossa tumour can increase ICP, but less likely in absence of other clinical features.

11.15   Answer: C

Conjunctivitis is rarely uniocular, even if asymmetric, and such a diagnosis should raise suspicion. Anterior uveitis can be a feature of ankylosing spondylitis, sarcoidosis, inflammatory bowel disease and Reiter's disease.

11.16   Answer: C

All of the above conditions can cause acute deterioration in visual acuity, but A, B, D and E are generally painful.

11.17 A 46-year-old woman with longstanding Graves' disease is referred to the Ophthalmology Outpatient Department because of deterioration in vision affecting her left eye. Examination findings include a relative afferent pupillary defect affecting the left eye, and pallor of the left optic disc. What is the cause of these findings?

- [ ] A Branch retinal artery occlusion
- [ ] B Keratoconjunctivitis
- [ ] C Optic nerve compression
- [ ] D Proptosis
- [ ] E Superior sagittal sinus thrombosis

11.18 A 27-year-old man with long-standing respiratory symptoms has recently been diagnosed with sarcoidosis. He is referred to the Ophthalmology Department for review. What is the most likely ocular manifestation in this disease?

- [ ] A Cataract formation
- [ ] B Granulomatous infiltration of lacrimal glands
- [ ] C Mononeuritis multiplex causing palsy of cranial nerves III, IV or VI
- [ ] D Optic nerve atrophy
- [ ] E Retinal artery branch occlusion

11.19 A 52-year-old woman self-presents to the Emergency Department with an acutely painful and inflamed right eye. The Emergency Department Senior House Officer considers a diagnosis of acute glaucoma, and contacts the Ophthalmology Department for advice. What feature most strongly supports the diagnosis of glaucoma?

- [ ] A Established bilateral cataracts
- [ ] B History of short-sightedness
- [ ] C Homonomous visual field defect
- [ ] D Intraocular pressure is 18 mmHg
- [ ] E Severe eye pain and vomiting

11.20 Which one of the following medications is most likely to increase the risk of developing cataracts in later life?

- [ ] A Chlorpromazine
- [ ] B Ethambutol
- [ ] C Isoniazid
- [ ] D Quinine
- [ ] E Thyroxine

11.17   Answer: C

This can be a complication of Graves' ophthalmopathy due to retrobulbar soft tissue inflammation and swelling, or may be due to lymphoma (increased incidence in Graves' disease).

11.18   Answer: B

Therefore associated with sicca syndrome, and patients should be treated with 'artificial tears' lubrication to preserve corneal integrity. Cataract is more prevalent, and may be a late complication of sarcoidosis.

11.19   Answer: E

This is more often encountered in acute glaucoma than other causes of a painful red eye. Patients with long-sightedness are at greater risk, and intraocular pressure is usually significantly higher than normal (> 22 mmHg).

11.20   Answer: B

Also corticosteroid treatment, particularly if prolonged courses at high dose. Quinine is a recognised cause of retinal toxicity, isoniazid can cause optic neuritis, and ethambutol can cause retrobulbar neuritis.

12. PSYCHIATRY

12.1 A 48-year-old woman with a past history of mania attends the outpatient department for review. Which of the following statements is most accurate with regard to this condition?

- ☐ A Delusions and hallucinations are recognised features
- ☐ B Increased somnolescence is a characteristic feature
- ☐ C It is the commonest mood disorder in Westernised societies
- ☐ D Mood is typically low during acute episodes
- ☐ E Patients often experience only a single episode

12.2 You are asked to review a 52-year-old man on a General Medical Ward, who presented with weight loss, reduced appetite and fatigue. Gastrointestinal investigations have been unhelpful, and you consider the possibility of depression. Which of the following would be most helpful in establishing this diagnosis?

- ☐ A Family history of depression
- ☐ B History of nocturnal insomnia
- ☐ C Hospital Anxiety and Depression Scale
- ☐ D Night sweats
- ☐ E Recurrent palpitations

12.3 One of the patients attending your Diabetic Outpatient Department has symptoms suggestive of unipolar depression. You are contemplating initiation of anti-depressant treatment. Which of the following would most strongly indicate that referral to a specialist psychiatric service is indicated?

- ☐ A Auditory hallucinations
- ☐ B Depressive symptoms have persisted more than 9 months
- ☐ C Family history of suicide
- ☐ D Sleep disturbance
- ☐ E Symptoms and signs suggestive of co-existent anxiety

12.1   Answer: A

Mania and hypomania (milder variant) are characterised by abnormally elevated mood, overactivity and reduced need for sleep. Most patients have recurrent episodes, and often develop depressive episodes. Unipolar depression is the commonest mood disorder.

12.2   Answer: C

Anxiety or depression scores of > 10 indicate a probable mood disorder, and provide a useful screening tool. Night sweats suggest a number of aetiologies, including alcohol excess.

12.3   Answer: A

Referral to a psychiatrist is recommended when the patient is at risk of suicide, psychotic symptoms are present or if they have bipolar depression.

12.4   You are asked to review a 24-year-old man in the Emergency
Department, who presented with evidence of deliberate self-harm.
On examination, he is found to have superficial cuts across both
wrists. In determining his suicide risk, which of the following factors
is *least* likely to be of importance?

- ☐ A History of alcohol abuse
- ☐ B History of personality disorder
- ☐ C Low socio-economic class
- ☐ D Recent loss of a job
- ☐ E Recent split from his girlfriend

12.5   You are asked by one of your psychiatry colleagues to medically
assess a 46-year-old man with major depressive disorder before he
undergoes electroconvulsive therapy (ECT). Which of the following
statements is correct regarding ECT?

- ☐ A Administration of ECT should separated by at least 1 week
- ☐ B Antidepressant medications should be stopped for 1 week before
ECT
- ☐ C It is an alternative to antidepressant medication in elderly patients
- ☐ D It is associated with early remission in around 70–75% of patients
- ☐ E Psychotic symptoms are a contraindication

12.6   You are asked for advice by a 24-year-old woman who is concerned
about her risk of developing schizophrenia because of a strong
family history. Which of the following is correct regarding
schizophrenia?

- ☐ A Genetic screening is characteristically helpful in determining risk
- ☐ B It is more common in those with high socio-economic status
- ☐ C It is not a genetic condition and she should be reassured
- ☐ D Perinatal and antenatal complications do not influence future risk
- ☐ E Recreational drug use increases risk

12.4   Answer: C

Recent fall in socio-economic class or employment status, established psychiatric illness, family history of suicide, previous suicide attempts, and drug abuse are other important factors.

12.5   Answer: D

ECT generally reserved for severe depression, not responsive to medication, and usually repeated administration required (eg bicranial 3 times in 1 week). Heart failure, raised ICP, severe COPD, recent stroke and severe ischaemic heart disease are associated with greater adverse effects of ECT.

12.6   Answer: E

Heritability is as high as 80%, and a number of distinct genetic mutations (eg coding for COMT) have been identified in a small number of patients. Prematurity, prolonged labour and fetal hypoxia appear to increase risk. It is more prevalent in those of low socio-economic status.

12.7 You are asked to review a 46-year-old man by the Emergency Department SHO, who thought that the patient's longstanding symptoms and signs suggested a diagnosis of schizophrenia. Which one of the following symptoms is most unlikely to be a feature of schizophrenia, and might suggest an alternative diagnosis?

- ☐ A Delusions of grandeur
- ☐ B Disorganised thinking
- ☐ C Impairment of attention
- ☐ D Social withdrawal
- ☐ E Visual hallucinations

12.8 Which of the following features is a 'negative' symptom characteristic of schizophrenia?

- ☐ A Auditory hallucinations
- ☐ B Disordered speech
- ☐ C Inability to focus on tasks
- ☐ D Loss of interest in academic pursuits
- ☐ E Persecutory delusions

12.9 Which of the following statements regarding antipsychotic medications is correct?

- ☐ A Adverse effects are less troublesome with 'atypical' antipsychotics
- ☐ B All antipsychotics modify central dopaminergic neurotransmission
- ☐ C Atypical antipsychotics carry a greater risk of tardive dyskinesia
- ☐ D Therapeutic effects appear due to nigrostriatal D_2 receptor blockade
- ☐ E 'Typical' antipsychotics are more effective in treating type 2 symptoms

12.7   Answer: E

Delusions and auditory hallucinations are characteristic features ('positive' symptoms). Visual hallucinations can occur in organic brain disease, eg alcohol withdrawal, encephalopathy. Other features include cognitive and affective symptoms. Grandiose delusions might also suggest mania.

12.8   Answer: D

'Positive' (type 1) symptoms are abnormal by their presence (eg delusions, hallucinations), 'negative' (type 2) symptoms are the absence of normal behaviours (eg social withdrawal, flat affect). Impaired attention is a recognised sign of cognitive impairment.

12.9   Answer: B

Therapeutic effects appear due to D_2 blockade of mesolimbic neurones, whereas nigrostriatal D_2 blockade causes extrapyramidal symptoms (EPS). Atypical antipsychotics seem more effective in treating type 2 symptoms, have lower risk of tardive dyskinesia and EPS, but cause increased weight gain, eg clozapine carries risk of agranulocytosis (1%) and seizures (2–5%).

12.10 A 32-year-old man has suffered from periodic auditory hallucinations and depressive episodes over the past 9 months, and has become increasingly socially isolated. He is diagnosed with schizophrenia, and commenced on treatment. Which of the following statements is correct, regarding this condition?

- ☐ **A** A combination of typical and atypical antipsychotics is the optimal initial treatment
- ☐ **B** Around 10% of patients commit suicide
- ☐ **C** Clinical course is typically one of progressive deterioration
- ☐ **D** Substance misuse is present in around 5% of patients
- ☐ **E** There is no need for the patient to inform the DVLA

12.11 You review a 39-year-old woman with suspected anxiety disorder. Which of the following features would most strongly suggest an alternative underlying physical diagnosis?

- ☐ **A** Breathlessness
- ☐ **B** Chest pain
- ☐ **C** Heat intolerance
- ☐ **D** Insomnia
- ☐ **E** Palpitations

12.12 A 46-year-old man attends the Outpatient Department for assessment of suspected panic attacks. For the past 6 months, he has suffered intermittent episodes of anxiety associated with throbbing headaches, palpitations and excessive sweating. Resting pulse is 94 bpm, and blood pressure is 164/108 mmHg seated and 146/92 mmHg standing. Which of the following investigations would be most helpful?

- ☐ **A** 24-h urinary catecholamines
- ☐ **B** Cranial CT scan with contrast medium
- ☐ **C** Dexamethasone suppression test
- ☐ **D** Exhaled CO_2 measurement
- ☐ **E** Thyroid function tests

12.10   Answer: B

Suicide is common, particularly during the active phase of the illness. Cardiovascular and accidental deaths are also more common. Substance misuse is present in around 30%, and most patients have a relapsing–remitting course. The DVLA must be informed in all cases.

12.11   Answer: C

Heat intolerance suggests hyperthyroidism. Other symptoms of anxiety disorder include tremor, sweating, headache, dizziness, diarrhoea and poor concentration.

12.12   Answer: A

The history is strongly suggestive of phaeochromocytoma, typically associated with excess norepinephrine, vasoconstriction, hypertension and postural BP instability. Hyperthyroidism, hypoglycaemia, paroxysmal arrhythmia and alcohol withdrawal can also mimic anxiety disorder.

12.13 You are asked to review a 43-year-old woman in the Emergency Department, who is complaining that she is unable to move her left arm. Reflexes are normal and symmetrical in her upper limbs, and other examination findings are entirely normal. Her behaviour seems somewhat odd, and she is comparatively unconcerned about this disability. Which one of the following diagnoses might most fully account for her symptoms?

   A Brachial plexus compression

   B Dissociative disorder

   C Partial anterior circulation stroke

   D Phobic anxiety disorder

   E Somatisation disorder

12.14 A 19-year-old girl is referred to the Medical Outpatient Department for investigation of amenorrhoea. She appears emaciated, and her weight is 48 kg, and BMI 14.8 kg/m². You suspect a diagnosis of anorexia nervosa. Which of the following features would most strongly support this diagnosis?

   A Hirsutism

   B Patient expresses concerns about looking too thin

   C Preoccupation with food

   D Prominent fatigue symptoms

   E Steatorrhoea

12.15 A 19-year-old man is admitted for assessment after taking a deliberate drug overdose. Which of the following factors most strongly indicates risk of future suicide?

   A Alcohol ingestion at time of overdose

   B Antisocial personality disorder

   C Background depressive illness

   D Family history of drug dependence

   E Recent bereavement

12.13 Answer: B

Dissociative (conversion) disorder commonly presents with gait disturbance, loss of limb function, aphonia, pseudoseizures or blindness. Characteristically, there is apparent unconcern, despite significant physical disability.

12.14 Answer: C

Often physically overactive, may abuse laxatives and diuretics. Patients perceive themselves to be overweight, and deny problems. Features can include bradycardia, hypotension and lanugo hair on trunk. Steatorrhoea suggestive of pancreatic insufficiency.

12.15 Answer: C

Background psychiatric illness is a major risk factor. Other risk factors include recent unemployment, bereavement, social withdrawal, previous self-harm, drug or alcohol dependence, chronic physical illness, age > 45 years and violent means.

12.16 A 68-year-old man is brought to the Emergency Department by the police, having been found confused and disorientated in the streets late at night. Which of the following features would most strongly suggest underlying dementia, rather than an acute confusional state?

- ☐ A   Decreased attention span
- ☐ B   Delusional thoughts
- ☐ C   Flat affect
- ☐ D   Fluctuating conscious level
- ☐ E   Visual hallucinations

12.17 A 42-year-old woman presents to her GP with a history suggestive of generalised anxiety disorder. Which one of the following features would be most strongly supportive of this diagnosis?

- ☐ A   Breathlessness and palpitations
- ☐ B   Early morning wakening
- ☐ C   Fatigue and lack of interest
- ☐ D   Loss of libido
- ☐ E   Excessive sweating

12.18 You admit a 46-year-old man to the General Medical Ward for investigation of vomiting and abdominal pain. Which of the following features would most strongly suggest alcohol withdrawal syndrome?

- ☐ A   Altered taste sensation
- ☐ B   Fine symmetrical resting tremor
- ☐ C   Gait instability
- ☐ D   Nausea
- ☐ E   Visual hallucinations

12.16   Answer: C

Dementia is often associated with blunted affect and depressive features. Fluctuating conscious level strongly suggests an acute confusional state.

12.17   Answer: A

Excessive sweating is a recognised feature, but less specific (eg thyrotoxicosis, alcohol excess). The other stems are more characteristically associated with depressive illness.

12.18   Answer: E

Other features include coarse tremor, sweating, anxiety and, in severe cases, seizures.

12.19 A 52-year-old woman regularly drinks 8–12 units of alcohol daily. She is admitted to hospital for elective laparoscopic sterilization procedure, and you consider the possibility of alcohol withdrawal. Which one of the following is most accurate with regard to alcohol withdrawal-related seizures?

- [ ] **A** Epilepsy does not confer increased risk
- [ ] **B** Risk is greater in females than males
- [ ] **C** Risk is greatest at 12–24 h after withdrawal
- [ ] **D** Risk is increased by hyperkalaemia
- [ ] **E** They occur in 5–15% of alcohol-dependent people

12.20 A 26-year-old man is admitted to hospital with a fever of 38.7°C, tachycardia, altered consciousness, and muscle rigidity. He had recently started treatment with olanzapine. Biochemical tests show creatinine kinase of 1800 IU/l, and you diagnose neuroleptic malignant syndrome (NMS). Which of the following statements best describes this condition?

- [ ] **A** Common feature of antipsychotic overdose
- [ ] **B** Dialysis is useful for patients not responding to other treatment
- [ ] **C** High blood pressure is strongly indicative of the diagnosis
- [ ] **D** Mortality rates are between 25 and 30%
- [ ] **E** Renal failure indicates a 50% mortality risk

12.21 A 65-year-old lady has reported a number of varied symptoms for which no physical basis has been identified. On further questioning it becomes evident that she is suffering from early morning waking, increased irritability, loss of appetite, and poor concentration. She has lost interest in gardening, which she had previously enjoyed, and has had a non-specific feeling of guilt. What is the most likely underlying diagnosis?

- [ ] **A** Anaemia
- [ ] **B** Anxiety disorder
- [ ] **C** Chronic major depression
- [ ] **D** Hypothyroidism
- [ ] **E** Moderate depression

12.19   Answer: E

Risk of seizures after alcohol withdrawal is greatest at around 48 h post-withdrawal, and is increased in the setting of hypoglycaemia, hypomagnesaemia, hypokalaemia, subdural haematoma and pre-existing epilepsy.

12.20   Answer: E

Overall mortality has fallen in recent years to around 10%. Risk of NMS is not related to duration of exposure, or to toxic overdose. Common features include fever, rigidity, elevated CK and altered conscious level.

12.21   Answer: E

Criteria for a moderate depressive episode are: depressed mood most of day, for most days (at least 2 weeks), diminished interest or pleasure and loss of energy or fatigue. Other features include reduced concentration and attention, reduced confidence and self-esteem, self-reproach or guilt, recurrent thoughts of death or suicide, pessimistic views of the future, and insomnia.

12.22 A single man, aged 24, complains of feeling irritable and dissatisfied with his life. He was made redundant 4 weeks ago, and he broke up with his girlfriend because of debts he had accrued. He now lives with a friend, and binges on alcohol up to 20 units per night. He uses cannabis occasionally. What is the most likely underlying cause of his low mood?

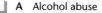

    A Alcohol abuse

    B Drug intoxication

    C Early dementia

    D Korsakoff's psychosis

    E Vitamin B_{12} deficiency

12.23 A 35-year-old woman is admitted to hospital during an acute episode of mania. She has been treated for the past 2 years with lithium and olanzapine for bipolar affective disorder with psychotic symptoms. Which of the following statements is most correct regarding bipolar affective disorder?

    A Almost 40% commit suicide

    B Antidepressant therapy should be stopped during acute mania

    C Auditory hallucinations suggest an alternative diagnosis of schizophrenia

    D Lamotrigine is effective during acute manic episodes

    E Rapid cycling bipolar disorder occurs in 20% of patients

12.24 A 25-year-old woman has recently given birth to her first child, and has been increasingly tearful, not eating or sleeping well, and the midwife has reported that she has failed to bond with her new baby. Which of the following factors most strongly supports the diagnosis of post-natal depression?

    A History of physical abuse

    B Low family income

    C Low level of social support

    D Lower occupational status

    E Obstetric complications

12.22 Answer: A

Depressive symptoms and alcohol abuse are often found together. Treatment includes advice and support regarding alcohol abstinence.

12.23 Answer: E

10–20% commit suicide, mainly during depressive or mixed episodes, and auditory and visual hallucinations are recognised features. Antidepressant cessation during a manic episode should be gradual to avoid side effects. Rapid cycling disorder occurs in up to 20% of patients: characterised by four or more acute episodes per year.

12.24 Answer: C

Strongest risk factors are past psychiatric illness or psychological disturbance, recent life events, low social support, and poor marital relationship. Other associations are obstetric complications, low family income, history of abuse, and lower occupational status.

12.25 A 35-year-old woman was involved in a road traffic accident 6 weeks ago in which she suffered minor whiplash injuries. Her car was badly damaged. She is referred to the Psychiatry Outpatient Clinic because she has been feeling very anxious, and finds that at times her thoughts are interrupted by vivid and distressing recollection of the accident. During these episodes, she feels that her heart is 'jumping out of her chest' and finds it difficult to breathe calmly. What is the most likely diagnosis?

- [ ] **A** Acute stress disorder
- [ ] **B** Adjustment disorder
- [ ] **C** Mild depressive episode
- [ ] **D** Normal reaction
- [ ] **E** Post-traumatic stress disorder (PTSD)

12.26 A 20-year-old man is brought to the Emergency Department by police. He was picked up off the street in a very agitated state and is uncooperative. He is not forthcoming with information, and is becoming increasingly withdrawn and suspicious. A relative explains that he has recently been diagnosed with schizophrenia. Which of the following features is most likely to be associated with a favourable outcome?

- [ ] **A** Auditory hallucinations
- [ ] **B** Family history of depression
- [ ] **C** Insidious onset of symptoms
- [ ] **D** Predominantly negative symptoms
- [ ] **E** Previous episode of depression requiring hospitalisation

12.27 A 48-year-old man is brought to hospital in a confused state. He appears agitated and is not forthcoming with any history. He requires treatment with haloperidol and lorazepam to control agitation. There is no obvious tremor; plantar responses show bilateral dorsiflexion, and reflexes are brisk and symmetrical. CT head is normal and CSF shows raised protein concentration, normal glucose concentration and a small number of lymphocytes. What is the most likely diagnosis?

- [ ] **A** Acute alcohol intoxication
- [ ] **B** Acute relapse of schizophrenia
- [ ] **C** Catatonic stupor
- [ ] **D** HSV encephalitis
- [ ] **E** Neurosyphilis

12.25   Answer: E

PTSD is characterised by intensely intrusive imagery, and recurring distressing dreams; other features include persistent anxiety, irritability, insomnia and poor concentration, avoidance of reminders of the events, detachment, numbness, and diminished interest in activities.

12.26   Answer: B

Factors predicting a poor outcome in schizophrenia include insidious onset, prolonged duration of first episode, previous psychiatric history, negative symptoms, younger age at onset.

12.27   Answer: D

Agitation and seizures are recognised features, along with hyperreflexia, low-grade fever and cranial nerve abnormalities. HSV is the most commonly identified cause of encephalitis in the UK and should be treated with intravenous aciclovir whilst awaiting lab confirmation (CSF PCR).

12.28 Which of the following features would be best described as a 'first-rank symptom' in schizophrenia?

◻ A Aggressive behaviour

◻ B Low mood

◻ C Social withdrawal

◻ D Thought broadcasting

◻ E Visual hallucinations

12.29 You are asked to provide an urgent psychiatric assessment of a 31-year-old man in the Emergency Department, who is very agitated and becoming increasingly verbally abusive. Which of the following symptoms is most strongly suggestive of schizophrenia rather than acute confusional state?

◻ A Third person auditory hallucinations

◻ B Delusions of grandeur

◻ C Flat affect

◻ D Nystagmus

◻ E Visual hallucinations

12.30 A 24-year-old man is brought to the Emergency Department in a confused state. There is no reported history of alcohol or illicit drug use. Which one of the following symptoms would most strongly suggest a diagnosis of mania?

◻ A Feelings of worthlessness

◻ B Increased attention span

◻ C Low mood

◻ D Over-expansive responses to questions

◻ E Reduced libido

12.28   Answer: D

(i) auditory hallucinations (echo, third person or commentary), (ii) delusions of thought control, (iii) delusions of passivity (eg thought insertion, thought withdrawal, thought broadcast), and (iv) delusional perception.

12.29   Answer: A

Delusions of grandeur might suggest mania, whilst nystagmus suggests underlying organic disease (eg Wernicke's encephalopathy). Visual hallucinations often indicate an underlying physical cause.

12.30   Answer: D

Features include elevated mood (occasionally depressed mood), pressure of speech, poor attention span, irritability, easily distracted, insomnia, overactivity, risk-taking behaviour and increased libido. Delusions are a recognised feature and are congruent with mood (grandiose or persecutory).

12.31 You review a 68-year-old woman in the Medical Outpatient Department, who you suspect might have early dementia. Which of the following features most strongly supports this diagnosis?

- A Able to give coherent and detailed history
- B Impairment of recent memory more than past events
- C Patient complains of poor memory
- D Poor cooperation and effort with psychomotor tests
- E Rapid progression over the past 2 months

12.32 A 57-year-old woman is taken to the Emergency Department because of apparent weakness affecting her left arm. During initial assessment, she is uncooperative but appears to have normal neurological function in all four limbs. The nursing staff report that she was verbally abusive earlier, but she is now refusing to speak to medical staff. Which of the underlying disorders is most likely?

- A Alcohol withdrawal
- B Alzheimer's disease
- C Depression
- D Generalised anxiety disorder
- E Schizophrenia

12.33 You see a 48-year-old woman in the General Medical Outpatient Clinic who complains of recurrent episodes of extreme anxiety. These have happened on at least six occasions over the past 2 months whilst she has been shopping and have been associated with nausea, palpitations, sweating and numbness around the fingers. Which of the following disorders would best explain these features?

- A Generalised anxiety disorder
- B Hyperthyroidism
- C Hyperventilation syndrome
- D Panic attacks
- E Phaeochromocytoma

12.31 Answer: B

The other features are more strongly suggestive of underlying depression.

12.32 Answer: C

Although highly atypical, depression in elderly patients can present in a number of bizarre ways. Hypochondriacal delusions and worries, histrionic behaviour, and pseudodementia are more common features than in younger patients.

12.33 Answer: D

Short-lived episodes of intense fear associated with at least four of the following: palpitation, sweating, fear of loss of control, trembling, choking sensation, fear of dying, abdominal discomfort, chest pain, dizziness, derealisation, numbness around lips and fingers, chills and hot flushes.

12.34 A 17-year-old woman is referred to the Medical Outpatient Department for assessment of abdominal bloating symptoms. On examination she appears very thin, and you consider an underlying eating disorder. Which of the following features would most strongly support a diagnosis of anorexia nervosa?

☐ A BMI 19.4 kg/m²

☐ B Extreme avoidance of high-fat foods

☐ C Guilt about overeating

☐ D Puberty aged 14 years

☐ E Regular scanty periods

12.35 A 55-year-old man has been attending the General Medical Outpatient Department for investigation of weight loss, apathy and fatigue over the past 6 months. He is taking lisinopril for hypertension, and has no known drug allergies. Thyroid function tests and upper and lower GI endoscopy tests are normal, and a coeliac screen is negative. You consider that his symptoms are due to depression. Which would be the most appropriate initial treatment to consider?

☐ A Fluoxetine

☐ B Olanzapine

☐ C Phenelzine

☐ D St John's wort

☐ E Venlafaxine

12.36 You are asked to review a 29-year-old man in the Emergency Department who had presented overnight with a short episode of central chest pain. He smells strongly of stale alcohol, cardiovascular examination is normal, and his ECG and chest X-ray are normal. Which of the following features would most strongly suggest a diagnosis of alcohol dependence syndrome?

☐ A Family history of heavy alcohol use

☐ B Palpable liver edge

☐ C Patient wishes to leave the Emergency Department to go to the pub

☐ D Sleep disturbance

☐ E Spider naevae on the anterior chest wall

12.34   Answer: B

Criteria are (i) loss of > 15% of normal body weight (usually BMI < 17.5 kg/m²), self-induced by vomiting, purging and exercising, (ii) overvalued ideas and preoccupation about food, morbid fear of fatness, and (iii) amenorrhoea > 3 months or loss of potency in male.

12.35   Answer: A

Phenelzine (selective monamine oxidase inhibitor: MAOI) is normally reserved for patients who have not responded to SSRI treatment. Venlafaxine is contraindicated in patients with hypertension, angina or ECG abnormalities because of its tendency for cardiotoxicity; it is also more likely to cause seizures and death in overdose.

12.36   Answer: C

Features are sense of compulsion to drink, drink-seeking behaviour, stereotyped drinking pattern and reinstatement after abstinence, increased alcohol tolerance, withdrawal symptoms and drinking to avoid withdrawal symptoms.

12.37 A 41-year-old woman is admitted to hospital after being found collapsed in the street and drowsy. You are called to review her overnight because she has become increasingly agitated and appears confused. On examination, she is sweaty and tachycardic with a coarse tremor in both upper limbs, and she is experiencing vivid visual hallucinations. Which of the following is the most likely cause of her agitation?

- A Acute schizophrenia
- B Alcohol withdrawal
- C Delirium tremens
- D Pneumonia
- E Thyroid storm

12.38 A 55-year-old man is referred to the Outpatient Department for assessment of suspected dementia. Which of the following risk factors would most strongly suggest a diagnosis of Alzheimer's disease?

- A Hypercholesterolaemia
- B Hypertension
- C Normal conscious level
- D Regular smoking
- E Right arm and leg weakness

12.37   Answer: C

In addition to alcohol withdrawal (tremor, nausea, sweating, anxiety, agitation, tinnitus), there are features of delirium tremens (visual hallucination, delusion, tremor, agitation, pyrexia, altered conscious level).

12.38   Answer: C

Disturbance of multiple cortical functions, but conscious level is not diminished. The other stems listed (A, B, D, E) are risk factors for cerebrovascular disease and multi-infarct dementia (smoking appears protective against Alzheimer's disease and Parkinson's disease).

13. RESPIRATORY

13.1 A 32-year-old postman presents with progressive shortness of breath. He is taking diclofenac for back pain, but no other medications. CXR shows bilateral upper lobe fibrosis. What is the most likely diagnosis?

- [ ] **A** Ankylosing spondylitis
- [ ] **B** Asthma
- [ ] **C** Bronchiectasis
- [ ] **D** Diclofenac-induced pulmonary fibrosis
- [ ] **E** Extrinsic allergic alveolitis

13.2 A 13-year-old male refugee presents with a history of pyrexia. Further questioning reveals a history of chronic productive sputum and weight loss with diarrhoea. Examination reveals a very thin male, clubbed with scattered coarse crepitations in the chest. There is tenderness over the maxillary and frontal sinuses. What is the most likely organism responsible?

- [ ] **A** *Legionella pneumophila*
- [ ] **B** *Moraxella catarrhalis*
- [ ] **C** *Mycobacterium tuberculosis*
- [ ] **D** *Pseudomonas aeruginosa*
- [ ] **E** *Streptococcus pneumoniae*

13.3 Which of the following is most likely to be associated with *Mycoplasma pneumoniae* infection?

- [ ] **A** Bullous myringitis
- [ ] **B** Cryoglobulinaemia
- [ ] **C** Eaton–Lambert syndrome
- [ ] **D** Erythema nodosum
- [ ] **E** Warm autoimmune haemolytic anaemia

13.1   Answer: A

The combination of a young male with back pain and upper lobe fibrosis points to a diagnosis of ankylosing spondylitis. Other causes of upper lobe fibrosis include pneumoconiosis, allergic bronchopulmonary aspergillosis, post-radiotherapy, TB, extrinsic allergic alveolitis and sarcoidosis.

13.2   Answer: D

A young boy with a history of chronic purulent sputum and chronic diarrhoea (pancreatitis) points to a diagnosis of cystic fibrosis, supported by involvement of the upper airways. Treatment of *Pseudomonas* is with tobramycin and ceftazidime to prevent emergence of resistance. Many patients need continuous anti-staphylococcal treatment.

13.3   Answer: A

Other recognised associations are Guillain–Barré syndrome, autoimmune haemolytic anaemia, aseptic meningitis, hepatitis, pancreatitis, erythema multiforme. Cryoglobulinaemia can be a feature of infection with hepatitis C.

13.4 Which of these best describes the normal anatomical location of the azygous lobe?

- A Left lower lobe
- B Left upper lobe
- C Right middle lobe
- D Right lower lobe
- E Right upper lobe

13.5 A 45-year-old male smoker is diagnosed with α-1 antitrypsin deficiency. Which of the following statements is most correct regarding this condition?

- A Administration of α-1 antitrypsin is an effective treatment
- B Genetic counselling is not required
- C Pulmonary function tests show an obstructive defect and reduced KCO
- D Pulmonary function tests show a restrictive defect and reduced KCO
- E Smoking cessation will not alter the prognosis

13.6 You notice a cavity on the chest X-ray of a patient admitted with clinical features of acute pneumonia. What organism is most likely to be responsible?

- A *Haemophilus influenzae*
- B *Klebsiella pneumoniae*
- C *Mycoplasma leprae*
- D *Pneumococcus pneumoniae*
- E *Streptococcus pneumoniae*

13.7 A 75-year-old male smoker presents with fever, and has signs of pulmonary consolidation overlying the right lower chest. Which of the following tests is most useful in assessing the severity of his pneumonia?

- A Arterial blood gas
- B Electrocardiogram
- C Plain chest X-ray
- D Sputum microcopy
- E Urea and electrolytes

13.4   Answer: E

The azygous lobe is a normal variant, seen as the 'inverted comma sign' on the chest X-ray near the right hilum. It is not a true lobe, as it does not have its own bronchus, it is produced by an invagination of the azygous vein.

13.5   Answer: C

Alpha-1 antitrypsin deficiency is a hereditary condition accounting for 2% of all cases of emphysema, and genetic counselling should be offered. Neutrophil elastase (protease) activity is increased, resulting in destruction of alveolar cell walls.

13.6   Answer: B

Other recognised causes of cavitating lung lesions are: *Staphylococcus aureus*, anaerobic infections, *Pseudomonas aeruginosa*, *Legionella*, *Mycobacterium*.

13.7   Answer: A

British Thoracic Society criteria for severe pneumonia are: confusion (MMS < 8), urea > 7.0 mmol/l, respiratory rate > 30/min, blood pressure < 90/60 mmHg and > 65 years age.

13.8 A 36-year-old factory worker is a life-long non-smoker, and presents with shortness of breath and wheeze. Symptoms generally worsen throughout the week and improve over the weekends. Which test would be most appropriate for establishing the underlying diagnosis?

A Bronchial provocation testing

B Full pulmonary function tests (with reversibility)

C PEFR monitoring both at work and at home

D Total IgE levels

E Tryptase levels

13.9 A patient presents to you with an exacerbation of COPD. At discharge you are asked about possibility of oxygen at home for this candidate, which of the following most strongly indicates a need for long-term oxygen therapy?

A FEV1 < 3.0

B PaO_2 < 8.0 kPa on air

C PaO_2< 10 kPa on 28% oxygen

D PaO_2 7.3–8.0 kPa with evidence of nocturnal hypoxaemia

E Raised $PaCO_2$ on air

13.10 A 70-year-old male smoker, with a history of intermittent claudication presents with chest pain radiating down the left arm. On examination there is enophthalmos and miosis of the left eye. Further examination reveals wasting of the small muscles of the left hand. What is the likely diagnosis?

A Eaton–Lambert syndrome

B Pancoast tumour

C Peripheral vascular disease

D Subclavian artery aneurysm

E TIA

13.8 Answer: C

Over 200 materials have been identified to cause occupational asthma (eg isocyanates, flour, wood dust, pharmaceuticals, stainless steel etc). It is often justification for industrial compensation. PEFR monitoring will confirm an association, the offending agent can then be identified using *specific* IgE levels or bronchial provocation testing.

13.9 Answer: D

The patient *must* have stopped smoking. They must have PaO_2 of 7.3–8.0 kPa and evidence of either pulmonary hypertension/ peripheral oedema or nocturnal hypoxaemia, or $PaO_2 < 7.3$ kPa on air, with either a normal or elevated $PaCO_2$ and an FEV1 < 1.5 l.

13.10 Answer: B

Tumour at the thoracic inlet, presenting with pain along the medial aspect of the foream (compression of C8/T1 nerve roots), there may be an associated Horner's syndrome. Chest X-ray will reveal an apical shadow.

13.11 A 42-year-old iv drug abuser presents with shortness of breath. On examination he is thin and pyrexial with temperature 39.3°C. Blood tests show Hb 100 g/l, WCC 3.5 × 10⁹/l, neutrophils 2.0 × 10⁹/l, platelets 165 × 10⁹/l, CD4 count 50/mm³ (normal: 600–1200/mm³). What is the most likely cause?

- ☐ **A** CMV pneumonitis
- ☐ **B** *Pneumocystis carinii* pneumonia
- ☐ **C** Pneumothorax
- ☐ **D** Pulmonary embolus
- ☐ **E** Staphylococcal pneumonia

13.12 A 57-year-old woman presents to the Asthma Clinic complaining of foot drop. She has a past history of allergic rhinitis, asthma and depression. Investigations show Hb 146 g/l, WCC 6.2 × 10⁹/l (eosinophils 2.1 × 10⁹/l), urea 7.0 mmol/l, creatinine 136 μmol/l, glucose 9.3 mmol/l, ESR 49 mm/h and CRP < 5. What is the most likely diagnosis?

- ☐ **A** Allergic bronchopulmonary aspergillosis
- ☐ **B** Churg–Strauss syndrome
- ☐ **C** Sarcoidosis
- ☐ **D** Steroid-induced neuropathy
- ☐ **E** Wegener's granulomatosis

13.13 A 67-year-old lady presents with persistent cough. On examination she appears cushingoid with evidence of generalised hyperpigmentation. She has been a heavy smoker for many years and consumes a moderate amount of alcohol. Which of the following is likely to be the underlying diagnosis?

- ☐ **A** Addison's disease
- ☐ **B** Adenocarcinoma of the lung
- ☐ **C** Squamous cell bronchial carcinoma
- ☐ **D** Small cell lung cancer
- ☐ **E** Tuberculosis

13.11   Answer: B

The low CD4 count indicates susceptibility to opportunistic infections. Desaturation on minimal exertion and pyrexia suggest the diagnosis; this is an AIDS-defining illness. CXR is normal in 25%. Cytomegalovirus more commonly presents with ocular or gastrointestinal infection.

13.12   Answer: B

Triad of rhinitis, asthma and vasculitis, with an associated eosinophilia. p-ANCA (antineutrophil cytoplasmic antibody) is often positive, and usually responds well to corticosteroid treatment.

13.13   Answer: D

A heavy smoker presenting with a persistent cough suggests lung carcinoma. Cushingoid appearance with hyperpigmentation suggests ectopic ACTH secretion, which is a recognised feature of small cell lung cancer.

13.14 A 40-year-old man with a BMI of 36 kg/m² presents with daytime somnolence and poor concentration. He has been trying to lose weight over the past 12 months with little success. His wife has complained to him about excessive snoring at night. A sleep study indicates significant periods of oxygen desaturation. Which is the next best management step?

- A Advise weight loss diet
- B Continuous positive airways pressure
- C ENT referral
- D Polysomnography
- E Uveopalatopharyngoplasty

13.15 A patient known to have COPD is rushed to the Emergency Department with an exacerbation of breathlessness. She has a GCS of 15 and oxygen saturations of 85% on pulse oximetry. Arterial blood gases whilst breathing 28% FiO$_2$ show pH 7.13, PaO$_2$ 6.9 kPa, PaCO$_2$ 10.8 kPa, HCO$_3^-$ 32 mmol/l. What is the most appropriate treatment?

- A BiPAP
- B CPAP
- C Doxapram infusion
- D Endotracheal intubation
- E High flow oxygen

13.16 A patient presents with shortness of breath, and plain chest X-ray shows patchy pulmonary infiltrates. He has been taking medications for long-term treatment of atrial fibrillation, hypertension, and ischaemic heart disease. Which of the following drugs might be most likely to contribute to his current presentation?

- A Amiodarone
- B Atenolol
- C Digoxin
- D Glyceryl trinitrate
- E Simvastatin

13.14 Answer: B

Obstructive sleep apnoea is more common in obese males. Weight loss is the first step in management. Continuous positive airways pressure (CPAP) improves quality of life. ENT referral is appropriate if mandibular positioning or tonsillectomy is required. Uveopalatopharyngoplasty is of little benefit.

13.15 Answer: A

Bi-level positive airways pressure (BiPAP). The raised bicarbonate is a chronic component; however, the low pH is a feature of acute decompensation. Doxapram is a short term measure with limited benefit. BiPAP or non-invasive positive pressure ventilation (NIPPV) may prevent the need for intubation and would be the next best intervention. CPAP is less effective in allowing restoration of normal acid-base status.

13.16 Answer: A

Amiodarone is a recognised cause of reversible and irreversible lung fibrosis, and pneumonitis. Both dose-dependent and idiosyncratic pulmonary complications are recognised.

13.17 A male 46-year-old lifelong smoker is found to have an abnormal chest X-ray during a routine health screen. Subsequent investigations confirmed the presence of lung cancer. Which of the following findings would most strongly contraindicate surgical resection?

☐ A Abnormal liver biochemistry

☐ B Background history of asthma

☐ C FEV1 < 1.0 l

☐ D Haemoptysis

☐ E Pleural effusion

13.18 A 37-year-old lady who is taking the oral contraceptive pill has just returned from New Zealand by flight. She presents to you with tachypnoea and tachycardia, and is complaining of right-sided pleuritic chest pain. What is the definitive investigation of choice to confirm pulmonary embolus?

☐ A Arterial blood gas

☐ B CT pulmonary angiogram

☐ C Echocardiogram

☐ D Lung perfusion scan

☐ E Plain chest X-ray

13.19 Which of the following organisms would be *least* likely to cause extrinsic allergic alveolitis?

☐ A *Aspergillus clavatus*

☐ B *Aspergillus fumigatus*

☐ C *Chlamydia psittaci*

☐ D *Micropolyspora faeni*

☐ E Thermophilic *Actinomycetes*

13.20 Which of the following drugs would be most likely to cause pulmonary fibrosis?

☐ A Bendroflumethiazide

☐ B Ciclosporin

☐ C Enalapril

☐ D Hydrocortisone

☐ E Methotrexate

A

13.17   Answer: C

Other contraindications to surgical resection include: stage III B and above, malignant pleural effusion (rather than other causes of effusion, eg pneumonia), phrenic/recurrent laryngeal nerve involvement, SVC obstruction, involvement of mediastinum or contralateral hilar or mediastinal nodes, and distant metastases.

13.18   Answer: B

Pulmonary angiography is the gold standard in the investigation for pulmonary embolus, which has been superseded by CTPA. Echocardiogram may be used as an immediate bedside tool in severe cases where the patient shows signs of haemodynamic compromise.

13.19   Answer: B

Extrinsic allergic alveolitis is a hypersensitivity pneumonitis, usually IgG mediated. The offending agent is usually some form of organic dust, examples include: farmer's lung (*M. faeni* and *Thermoactinomyces vulgaris*), pigeon-fancier's lung (*C. psittaci*), malt-worker's lung (*A. clavatus*) and bagasossis (*T. sacchari*).

13.20   Answer: E

Other recognised causes are amiodarone, methotrexate, nitrofurantoin, sulfasalazine, busulphan, bleomycin, cyclophosphamide and gold.

13.21 A 38-year-old school teacher presents with recurrent haemoptysis over the past 2 weeks, and intermittent symptoms of wheeze, headache and flushing. She is a non-smoker and denies weight loss. Chest X-ray shows right lower lobe collapse. Which of the following investigations would be most appropriate?

- [ ] **A** Bronchoscopy
- [ ] **B** CT-guided lung biopsy
- [ ] **C** CT thorax
- [ ] **D** Pulmonary function tests (with reversibility)
- [ ] **E** V/Q scan

13.22 A 41-year-old man of Afro-Caribbean descent presents with erythema nodosum overlying both shins. Investigations show hypercalcaemia and normal renal function. What chest X-ray findings most strongly support a diagnosis of sarcoidosis?

- [ ] **A** Bilateral hilar lymphadenopathy
- [ ] **B** Cavity in the upper lobe
- [ ] **C** Pleural calcification
- [ ] **D** Pleural effusion
- [ ] **E** Widened mediastinum

13.23 Which antibiotic would be expected to be most useful in the treatment of post-influenza pneumonia?

- [ ] **A** Amoxicillin
- [ ] **B** Cefuroxime
- [ ] **C** Erythromycin
- [ ] **D** Flucloxacillin
- [ ] **E** Metronidazole

13.24 A 58-year-old ex-smoker presents to you in the Chest Clinic. He has recently been started on inhaled tiotropium and enquires about its mechanism of action. Which of the following best describes this?

- [ ] **A** Antimuscarinic
- [ ] **B** Combination of corticosteroid and anticholinergic
- [ ] **C** Inhaled corticosteroid
- [ ] **D** Long-acting β_2 agonist
- [ ] **E** Short-acting β_2 agonist

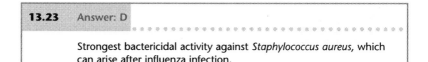

13.21   Answer: A

The scenario points to a diagnosis of bronchial carcinoid.
Bronchoscopy would best identify a centrally-placed lesion in a main
bronchus proximal to the lung collapse.

13.22   Answer: A

Staging of pulmonary sarcoidosis, based on chest X-ray appearances:

0 normal chest X-ray
1 bilateral hilar lymphadenopathy (BHL)
2 BHL + interstitial infiltrates
3 interstitial infiltrates only
4 diffuse fibrosis

13.23   Answer: D

Strongest bactericidal activity against *Staphylococcus aureus*, which
can arise after influenza infection.

13.24   Answer: A

Tiotropium is used in maintenance of COPD remission. It is long-
acting, allowing once daily administration.

13.25 The analysis of pleural fluid shows: pH 7.67, neutrophils < 1/mm³, lymphocytes 34/mm³, total protein 63 g/l, glucose 2.3 mmol/l, LDH 665 IU/l, triglycerides < 0.1 mmol/l, amylase not detected. What is the most likely explanation?

- A Liver cirrhosis
- B Lung carcinoma
- C Pneumonia
- D Rheumatoid arthritis
- E SLE

13.26 An 84-year-old man presents with an episode of collapse; on examination he is hypoxic with chest signs. You request a chest X-ray which shows evidence of calcification. Which of the following is this patient most likely to have had in the past?

- A Aspergillosis
- B Berylliosis
- C Coxsackievirus
- D Shingles
- E Tuberculosis

13.27 A 29-year-old man is referred for further investigation of wheeze, eosinophilia and abnormal chest X-ray. Which of the following diagnoses best explains these features?

- A Aspergillosis
- B Asbestosis
- C Extrinsic allergic alveolitis
- D Sarcoidosis
- E Tuberculosis

13.28 A 72-year-old ex-joiner is diagnosed with asbestos-related lung disease. Which of the following is *least* likely to be a pulmonary complication of asbestos exposure?

- A Benign pleural effusion
- B Benign pleural plaques
- C Mesothelioma
- D Progressive massive fibrosis
- E Progressive pulmonary fibrosis

13.25 Answer: B

The findings indicate an exudate; absence of neutrophils makes infection less likely. Low glucose can be seen in effusions associated with infection, malignancy, rheumatoid.

13.26 Answer: E

Other causes of pulmonary calcification on plain chest X-ray include sarcoidosis, asbestos, previous varicella pneumonia, silicosis, previous empyaema or haemothorax, and carcinoid tumours.

13.27 Answer: A

Other causes of eosinophilia with an abnormal chest X-ray include: eosinophilic pneumonia, Churg–Strauss syndrome, tropical pulmonary eosinophilia and eosinophilic leukaemia.

13.28 Answer: D

Progressive massive fibrosis is normally a complication of coal worker's pneumoconiosis. The other listed items are all recognised complications of asbestos exposure.

13.29 A patient presents with sudden exacerbation in shortness of breath. Examination reveals stony dullness and decreased air entry at the left base. Transthoracic aspiration of fluid shows a haemorrhagic effusion. Which of the following conditions is most likely to be associated with aspiration of clear fluid with protein concentration of 12 g/l?

- [ ] A Heart failure
- [ ] B Lung carcinoma
- [ ] C Parapneumonic effusion
- [ ] D Pulmonary infarction
- [ ] E Tuberculosis

13.30 A middle-aged woman presents to the Emergency Department with breathlessness. Blood gases on air are as follows: pH 7.52, $PaCO_2$ 3.0 kPa, PaO_2 12.6 kPa, HCO_3^- 22 mmol/l. What is the most likely explanation for these results?

- [ ] A Acute asthma
- [ ] B Hyperventilation syndrome
- [ ] C Lactic acidosis
- [ ] D Pulmonary embolus
- [ ] E Pulmonary oedema

13.31 A 31-year-old man with asthma presents with an acute exacerbation of his symptoms. Despite nebulisers, oxygen and intravenous steroids he remains tachypnoeic with respiratory rate 40/min, and he is unable to speak in sentences. Which would be the most appropriate additional therapy?

- [ ] A Aminophylline
- [ ] B CPAP
- [ ] C Magnesium sulphate
- [ ] D Doxapram
- [ ] E Salbutamol

13.29   Answer: A

The other listed conditions more typically cause exudative effusions; malignancy and pulmonary infarction are more commonly associated with a haemorrhagic pleural effusion.

13.30   Answer: B

There is respiratory alkalosis but no hypoxia, suggesting hyperventilation. An alternative explanation might be early salicylate toxicity, which produces respiratory alkalosis before metabolic acidosis.

13.31   Answer: C

British Thoracic Society guidelines advocate use of magnesium in asthma. Aminophylline is becoming a less popular choice with little evidence for benefit and unacceptable adverse effect profile.

13.32 A 56-year-old man presents with a large left-sided pleural effusion. You insert a chest drain, and send fluid for analysis. Laboratory results indicate an abnormally high LDH concentration. What is the most likely explanation?

☐ A   Malnutrition

☐ B   Myxoedema

☐ C   Nephrotic syndrome

☐ D   Sarcoidosis

☐ E   Sjögren's syndrome

13.33 A patient with major burns is admitted to Intensive Care with suspected diagnosis of adult respiratory distress syndrome. Which of the following most strongly support this diagnosis?

☐ A   Bilateral fluffy infiltrates on chest film

☐ B   Ejection fraction < 50% on echocardiogram

☐ C PaO_2 of < 7.5 kPa on FiO_2 of 0.5

☐ D   Pulmonary artery capillary wedge pressure 34 mmHg

☐ E   Reduced lung compliance during mechanical ventilation

13.34 A 35-year-old woman with long-standing SLE complains of reduced exercise capacity and breathlessness. Which of the following pulmonary complications is most likely to be responsible?

☐ A   Bronchiectasis

☐ B   Caplan's syndrome

☐ C   Obliterative bronchiolitis

☐ D   Rheumatoid nodules

☐ E   Shrinking lung syndrome

13.35 A patient with known bronchiectasis presents with exacerbation of breathlessness associated with high-grade fever. Arterial blood gas results confirm type II respiratory failure. Which of the following would be the most appropriate initial management?

☐ A   Antibiotics

☐ B   High flow humidified oxygen via non-re-breathable mask

☐ C   Intravenous dobutamine

☐ D   Nebulised salbutamol

☐ E   Urgent physiotherapy

13.32   Answer: E

High LDH concentration (> 250 IU/l) is suggestive of an exudate, often accompanied by a high protein concentration (typically > 30 g/l). The other listed conditions typically cause transudate pleural effusion.

13.33   Answer: E

ARDS involves non-cardiogenic pulmonary oedema, and LV systolic function is preserved. Reduced ejection fraction and increased pulmonary capillary wedge pressure suggest cardiogenic shock. Recognised causes of ARDS are trauma, sepsis, DIC, pancreatitis, drugs, inhalation injury and near-drowning.

13.34   Answer: E

Shrinking lung syndrome is a feature of SLE that arises through abnormally poor movement of the diaphragm. The other items are more characteristic complications of rheumatoid arthritis.

13.35   Answer: E

Bronchiectasis patients produce copious tenacious sputum and are highly prone to mucus plug formation and distal lung collapse. Whereas humidified oxygen, bronchodilators and antibiotics are all useful, the most important intervention is to restore airway patency; bronchoscopy may also be indicated for the same reason.

13.36 A 72-year-old male smoker presents with gradually declining exercise tolerance limited by shortness of breath. A chest X-ray shows diaphragmatic calcification. Which of the following is the most likely diagnosis?

- A   Asbestos-related lung disease
- B   Miliary tuberculosis
- C   Pneumoconiosis
- D   Sarcoidosis
- E   Silicosis

13.37 Which of the following anti-tuberculous treatments is most likely to cause irreversible visual impairment?

- A   Ethambutol
- B   Isoniazide
- C   Pyrazinamide
- D   Rifampicin
- E   Streptomycin

13.38 A 23-year-old lady presents to you after having visited Pakistan on vacation. She is worried that she may have contracted TB after being in close proximity with her grandmother, who has recently been diagnosed with sputum smear positive tuberculosis. She undergoes a Heaf test which shows a grade 3 response. A BCG scar is seen on her left upper arm. Which of the following should you do?

- A   Perform a chest X-ray
- B   Repeat Heaf test in 6 weeks time
- C   Start chemoprophylaxis with isoniazid alone for 3 months
- D   Start chemoprophylaxis with isoniazid alone for 6 months
- E   Start full chemotherapy for 6 months

13.36 Answer: A

This is the only one likely to cause diaphragmatic calcification. All of the above conditions are associated with an increased risk of pulmonary fibrosis.

13.37 Answer: A

Ethambutol can cause a dose-related retrobulbar neuritis, and visual acuity should be documented before treatment starts. Isoniazid is known to cause a peripheral neuropathy which may be prevented by co-administration of pyridoxine (vitamin B_6). Pyrazinamide, rifampicin and isoniazid can cause hepatotoxicity and liver function tests should be monitored. Streptomycin can potentially cause vestibular nerve damage, irreversibly.

13.38 Answer: A

BTS guidelines indicate that if no prior BCG vaccination, and known contact with a sputum smear positive individual, then start chemoprophylaxis irrespective. In patients with previous BCG vaccination, and Heaf test positive, then chemoprophylaxis if chest X-ray normal, or full chemotherapy if chest X-ray abnormal. Chemoprophylaxis consists of either isoniazid alone for 6 months, or combination of isoniazid and rifampicin for 3 months. Chemotherapy consists of rifampcin/isoniazid/pyrazinamide/ethambutol or suitable alternatives.

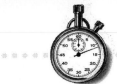

13.39 Regarding atypical mycobacteria, which of the following is true?

    A Contact tracing is not normally required in confirmed cases

    B Extra-pulmonary disease is not a recognised feature

    C *M. avium* complex is most common in HIV-infected patients, causing 50% of mycobacterial infections

    D *M. kansasii* is the most common atypical infection in immunocompromised patients in the UK

    E Treatment is as for typical mycobacterial tuberculosis

13.40 In which one of the following conditions is chest drain insertion normally avoided?

    A Empyema

    B Malignant pleural effusion

    C Rheumatoid pleural effusion

    D Secondary pneumothorax

    E Traumatic haemopneumothorax

13.41 A 69-year-old regular smoker presents with weight loss, shortness of breath and haemoptysis. A chest X-ray reveals a spiculated opacification, and blood tests show anaemia and hypercalcaemia. A bone scan is normal. What is the most likely underlying diagnosis?

    A Adenocarcinoma

    B Bronchogenic carcinoma with bony metastases

    C Sarcoidosis

    D Small cell lung cancer

    E Squamous cell lung cancer

13.42 A 56-year-old lifelong smoker presents with an ataxic gait, down-beat nystagmus, tremor and disdiadochokinesis. On further questioning he has also suffered with episodes of haemoptysis and has a persistent cough. He denies significant alcohol intake. Which of the following investigations would most help to diagnose these features?

    A ANCA

    B Anti-Purkinje antibodies

    C Vitamin B_{12} and folate levels

    D MRI brain

    E Thiamine levels

13.39 Answer: A

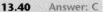

Atypical person-to-person transmission is not a recognised feature, even in sputum smear-positive individuals. *M. kansasii* is the most common atypical affecting the immunocompetent in the UK. *M. avium* complex is common in HIV patients causing over 90% of opportunistic mycobacterial infections.

13.40 Answer: C

Rheumatoid-associated effusions are normally small, and tend not to reaccumulate if disease-modifying treatment is administered. Malignant pleural effusions reaccumulate quickly so chest drain insertion reduces risk of infection associated with repeated aspiration.

13.41 Answer: E

Absence of bone metastases suggests paraneoplastic hyperealcaemia. Squamous cell carcinoma is associated with production of parathyroid hormone related protein (PTHrP). Neuroendocrine associations with small cell lung cancer include SIADH and Cushing's syndrome due to ACTH.

13.42 Answer: B

Paraneoplastic cerebellar degeneration is one of the presentations of lung cancer. Anti-Purkinje antibodies would establish the diagnosis (anti-Hu is more common in lung cancer). Other paraneoplastic syndromes associated with lung cancer include Lambert–Eaton myasthenic syndrome, dermatomyositis and nephrotic syndrome.

13.43 A 78-year-old lifelong smoker presents with shortness of breath. On examination he is clubbed. A chest X-ray reveals a cavitating mass, and you suspect cancer. Which of the following is the most likely type?

☐ **A** Adenocarcinoma

☐ **B** Alveolar cell carcinoma

☐ **C** Large cell carcinoma

☐ **D** Small cell lung carcinoma

☐ **E** Squamous cell carcinoma

13.44 Which of the following gastrointestinal disorder is most likely to be associated with fibrosing alveolitis?

☐ **A** Coeliac disease

☐ **B** Crohn's disease

☐ **C** Hepatitis B

☐ **D** Portal hypertension

☐ **E** Ulcerative colitis

13.45 A young adult presents with acute epiglottitis. Which organism is most likely to be isolated from blood cultures?

☐ **A** Adenovirus

☐ **B** *Haemophilus influenzae* type A

☐ **C** *Haemophilus influenzae* type B

☐ **D** Respiratory syncytial virus

☐ **E** Rhinovirus

13.46 A 26-year-old bakery assistant is diagnosed with Lofgren's syndrome. What feature would you be most likely to identify on a plain chest X-ray?

☐ **A** Apical fibrosis

☐ **B** Bilateral hilar lymphadenopathy

☐ **C** Cardiomegaly

☐ **D** Pleural calcification

☐ **E** Pleural effusion

13.43 Answer: E

This is the most common type of lung cancer, and shows the greatest tendency to cavitate. Clubbing is a recognised paraneoplastic feature.

13.44 Answer: E

Crohn's disease is known to produce large airway stenosis and bronchiectasis, whilst ulcerative colitis is known to do the same with added fibrosing alveolitis.

13.45 Answer: C

Epiglottitis is a potentially life-threatening illness. Intravenous cefuroxime would provide appropriate antibiotic cover.

13.46 Answer: B

Features include erythema nodosum, bilateral hilar lymphadenopathy on chest X-ray and arthralgia. It is a self-limiting form of sarcoidosis. Prognosis is excellent.

13.47 Which of the following tests is most helpful in establishing a diagnosis of asthma?

- A Peak flow monitoring for 2 weeks at work and away from work
- B Spirometry testing after methacholine challenge test
- C Spirometry testing before and after bronchodilators
- D Spirometry testing before and after exercise
- E Spirometry testing during exercise

13.48 Which of the following is the most likely explanation for a posterior mediastinal mass identified on a CT thorax investigation?

- A Dermoid cyst
- B Oesophageal carcinoma
- C Retrosternal goitre
- D Teratoma
- E Thymoma

13.49 Which of the following disorders is most likely to be associated with a raised transfer factor?

- A Anaemia
- B Asthma
- C Carbon monoxide poisoning
- D Emphysema
- E Pulmonary embolism

13.50 A 24-year-old man complains of blood-stained nasal discharge, and is found to have Hb 99 g/l, WCC 7.8 × 10^9/l, platelets 255 × 10^9/l, urea 20.2 mmol/l, creatinine 458 µmol/l and a renal ultrasound scan shows hyperechoic lesions throughout the renal cortices but no evidence of obstructive uropathy. Which of the following tests would be most helpful in confirming the underlying diagnosis?

- A ANA
- B Anti-basement membrane antibody
- C Anti-Jo antibodies
- D c-ANCA
- E p-ANCA

13.47 Answer: C

Asthma is a reversible airways disease; patients normally show improvement of 15% or more in the FEV$_1$ post-bronchodilator therapy. Spirometry testing before and after exercise may be useful in exercise-induced asthma, and regular peak flow monitoring can useful in diagnosing occupation-related asthma.

13.48 Answer: B

The other listed stems would be expected to be found in the anterior mediastinum. Middle mediastinum: aortic aneurysm, pericardial cyst, hilar lymphadenopathy. Posterior mediastinum: oesophageal cyst, neural lesions.

13.49 Answer: B

Other recognised causes are: pulmonary haemorrhage (eg Goodpasture's syndrome) and polycythaemia.

13.50 Answer: D

The combination of upper airways and renal involvement and likely glomerulonephritis are highly suggestive of Wegener's granulomatosis. Treatment is with a combination of corticosteroids and cyclophosphamide.

13.51 Which of the following would be the best initial management in treatment of acute phase Goodpasture's syndrome?

- [ ] A Cyclophosphamide
- [ ] B Interferon
- [ ] C Plasma exchange
- [ ] D Prednisolone
- [ ] E Treat underlying infection

13.52 A 22-year-old female presents with sore throat, cervical lymphadenopathy and rash. She has received a week's course of amoxicillin with no improvement. Blood count reveals thrombocytopenia. Which of the following investigations would be most helpful?

- [ ] A ASO titres
- [ ] B HIV testing
- [ ] C Monospot test
- [ ] D *Mycoplasma pneumoniae* titres
- [ ] E Streptococcal challenge test

13.53 Which of the following viruses is most likely to cause coryzal features associated with the common cold?

- [ ] A Adenovirus
- [ ] B Coronavirus
- [ ] C Influenza virus
- [ ] D Respiratory synctial virus
- [ ] E Rhinovirus

13.54 A 54-year-old woman is being investigated for fever associated with a dry cough. Which of the following organisms is responsible for development of Q fever?

- [ ] A *Bordetella pertussis*
- [ ] B *Chlamydia pneumoniae*
- [ ] C *Coxiella burnetii*
- [ ] D *Coxsackievirus*
- [ ] E *Nocardia mycetoma*

13.51   Answer: C

Goodpasture's syndrome is an autoimmune condition, p-ANCA positive in 30%, due to deposition of anti-glomerular basement membrane antibodies in the lungs and kidneys. Treatment is with immunosuppression. Goodpasture's may be precipitated by infection, but treatment of the infection will not affect outcome.

13.52   Answer: C

History suggestive of glandular fever; rash typically worsens following broad-spectrum antibiotics. Other features include petechiae, thrombocytopenia and atypical lymphocytes on blood film.

13.53   Answer: E

Rhinovirus accounts for up to one-third of cases.

13.54   Answer: C

Q fever is a zoonosis caused by *Coxiella burnetii*. Farmers, abbatoir workers and vets are predominantly affected. The illness starts with fever, myalgia, pneumonia can develop in up to 30%, hepatosplenomegaly in up to 50%. Chronic Q fever should be suspected in all culture negative cases of endocarditis. Tetracycline is the drug of choice.

13.55 Which of the following is the most characteristic feature of Pontiac fever?

- [ ] **A** It is a common cause for pulmonary fibrosis
- [ ] **B** It is caused by *Legionella pneumophilia*
- [ ] **C** It is caused by *Mycoplasma pneumoniae*
- [ ] **D** It presents with massive haemoptysis
- [ ] **E** Treatment is with benzyl penicillin

13.56 Which of the following groups of viruses is the most commonly recognised cause of severe acute respiratory distress syndrome (SARS)?

- [ ] **A** Arbovirus
- [ ] **B** Avian influenza
- [ ] **C** *Bartonella henselae*
- [ ] **D** Coronavirus
- [ ] **E** Ebola virus

13.57 A patient presents to you with a diagnosis of primary ciliary dyskinesia. Which of the following is most commonly associated with this condition?

- [ ] **A** Cilia in the retina may be affected
- [ ] **B** Dextrocardia
- [ ] **C** Hypogammaglobulinaemia
- [ ] **D** Inheritance is sporadic
- [ ] **E** Patient fertility is unaffected

13.58 Which of the following investigations would be most helpful in establishing the underlying cause of secondary bronchiectasis?

- [ ] **A** Bronchoscopy
- [ ] **B** CT thorax
- [ ] **C** Lung function tests
- [ ] **D** Skin prick testing
- [ ] **E** Sputum cytology

13.55 Answer: B

Pontiac fever is caused by a hypersensitivity reaction to
L. pneumophila. It presents with severe influenza-like symptoms with
limited chest signs but extensive involvement on chest X-ray. Extra-
pulmonary features are diarrhoea, abdominal pain, renal failure and
haematuria are recognised, and rarely pulmonary fibrosis.
Clarithromycin is the antibiotic of choice.

13.56 Answer: D

An acute viral respiratory tract infection, first identified in 2003.
Transmission is mainly via the respiratory route, though faeco–oral is
also possible. Features include high fever, myalgia and dry cough.
Diagnosis can be established by PCR testing. At present there is no
effective antiviral treatment.

13.57 Answer: B

Found in up to 50% of cases. Other recognised features are situs
inversus, male and female infertility, and autosomal recessive
inheritance. Kartagener's syndrome is ciliary dyskinesia with situs
inversus.

13.58 Answer: A

Bronchoscopy is more helpful in establishing a primary obstructive
cause of bronchiectasis. Other useful tests in establishing the
diagnosis of bronchiectasis may include *Aspergillus* precipitins,
immunoglobulin screen, sweat sodium and ciliary function test.

13.59 Which of the following is most likely to cause a leftward shift of the oxygen dissociation curve?

- A Acidosis
- B Carbon dioxide concentration
- C 2,3-diphosphoglycerate
- D High haemoglobin concentration
- E Temperature increase

13.60 Which of the following features is most closely associated with a diagnosis of Goodpasture's syndrome?

- A Cavitation on chest X-ray
- B Gas transfer is reduced
- C Haematemesis as a presenting symptom
- D Renal biopsy demonstrating crescentic glomerulonephritis
- E Women are more often affected than men

13.61 You receive a call about a patient in the wards who has become more breathless than normal. He has a background COPD, and his current oxygen saturation is only 77% on 24% inhaled oxygen by Ventura mask. Which one of the following arterial blood gas descriptions most strongly suggests a severe exacerbation of existing COPD?

- A Low $PaCO_2$, low PaO_2, normal bicarbonate, normal pH
- B Normal $PaCO_2$, low PaO_2, low bicarbonate, alkalosis
- C Raised $PaCO_2$, low PaO_2, high bicarbonate, acidosis
- D Raised $PaCO_2$, low PaO_2, high bicarbonate, picture of alkalosis
- E Raised $PaCO_2$, low PaO_2, low bicarbonate, picture of acidosis

13.62 A 61-year-old previously healthy man presents with a large pleural effusion. You insert a chest drain and aspirate milky effusion. Biochemistry confirms high lipid concentration in the effusion fluid. What is the most likely diagnosis?

- A Autoimmune disease
- B Bronchial carcinoma
- C Hepatocellular carcinoma
- D Lymphoma
- E Myeloma

13.59   Answer: D

The oxyhaemoglobin dissociation curve describes the relationship between the saturation of haemoglobin and the partial pressure of oxygen in the blood. The other factors cause a rightward shift, and therefore bind oxygen less tightly so as to liberate more oxygen to the tissues.

13.60   Answer: D

Goodpasture's syndrome typically affects young adult males, and is usually preceded by an upper respiratory tract infection. It is associated with pulmonary haemorrhage (causing haemoptysis and raised KCO[SB9]) and renal failure.

13.61   Answer: C

COPD results in a type II respiratory failure with respiratory acidosis.

Bicarbonate is raised due to renal retention, and is a chronic feature.

13.62   Answer: D

Lipaemic fluid indicates a chylothorax, suggesting thoracic duct infiltration. Commonest causes are lymphoma and tuberculosis, but may be seen with other infiltrative lung disease.

13.63 Arterial blood gas analysis shows: pH 7.47, PaO_2 8.0 kPa, $PaCO_2$ 3.42 kPa, HCO_3^- 23 mmol/l and base excess –3.5 mmol/l. What is the most likely explanation for these findings?

    ☐ **A** Anxiety state

    ☐ **B** Exacerbation of COPD

    ☐ **C** Pneumonia

    ☐ **D** Pulmonary embolus

    ☐ **E** Renal failure

13.64 Which of the following ECG findings is most commonly associated with a diagnosis of acute pulmonary embolus?

    ☐ **A** Frequent ventricular ectopic beats

    ☐ **B** Prolonged PR interval

    ☐ **C** Prolonged QT interval

    ☐ **D** Right bundle branch block

    ☐ **E** Sinus tachycardia

13.65 Which of the following statements most closely describes the features of cryptogenic fibrosing alveolitis?

    ☐ **A** CT scan with contrast is the investigation of choice

    ☐ **B** Immunosuppression shows improvement in 90% patients

    ☐ **C** Oxygen therapy improves prognosis

    ☐ **D** Peak flows should be maintained regularly

    ☐ **E** Pulmonary function tests show decreased lung and residual volumes

13.66 A patient presents with sudden onset of pleuritic chest pain and breathlessness. A chest X-ray reveals a pneumothorax with a 2 cm gap between the pleural edge and costal margin. There is no significant past medical history. What is the management of choice?

    ☐ **A** Aspiration

    ☐ **B** Discharge home with advice

    ☐ **C** In-patient observation with serial chest X-rays

    ☐ **D** Intercostal drain insertion

    ☐ **E** Outpatient follow-up with repeat chest X-ray in 6 weeks

13.63   Answer: D

The patient is hyperventilating (raised pH, low $PaCO_2$) in response to hypoxaemia. This is characteristic of a type 1 respiratory failure pattern.

13.64   Answer: E

Other features include small QRS complexes in anterior leads, T-wave inversion in the anterior leads, and the ECG can be normal in around 30%.

13.65   Answer: E

High-resolution CT scan is the investigation of choice. Peak flows are more indicative of airflow obstruction, whereas fibrosis is a restrictive defect. Oxygen offers symptomatic relief only, and up to 50% of patients will respond to steroids.

13.66   Answer: A

In a patient with a simple pneumothorax (first time presentation, with no known chronic lung disease), BTS guidelines suggest serial chest X-ray follow up as outpatient if patient is symptom free and rim less than 2 cm. If symptomatic and rim less than 2 cm, pleural aspiration, chest X-ray and discharge home with advice. If > 2 cm, for aspiration initially and consideration of intercostal chest drain.

13.67 A patient with known cystic fibrosis presents to you unwell with wheeze, eosinophilia, fever and increased plasma IgE. Chest X-ray shows diffuse opacification. Which of the following would you consider the most likely diagnosis in this scenario?

A Allergic bronchopulmonary aspergillosis

B Asthma

C Bronchiectasis

D Exacerbation of cystic fibrosis

E Pneumococcal pneumonia

13.68 Regarding treatment of malignant mesothelioma, which of the following is most appropriate?

A Chemotherapy alone

B Chemotherapy and radiotherapy combined

C Lung resection alone

D Radiotherapy alone

E Radiotherapy followed by lung resection.

13.69 A normally independent 87-year-old lady presents to you with breathlessness due to florid pulmonary oedema. You have treated her with furosemide and high flow oxygen. She is currently on a nitrate infusion, but her condition is deteriorating. Which of the following forms of ventillatory support would be most appropriate?

A BiPAP

B Bronchodilators

C CPAP

D Endotracheal intubation

E Intravenous furosemide infusion

13.67   Answer: A

Allergic bronchopulmonary aspergillosis is encountered in approximately 20% of patients with cystic fibrosis. Treatment is with high dose corticosteroids.

13.68   Answer: D

Commonly associated with asbestos. Poor prognosis (with estimated maximum 12-month survival).

13.69   Answer: C

Continuous positive airways pressure works by recruiting alveoli and so improving oxygenation, useful in pictures of type I respiratory failure. Trials have shown that patients with pulmonary oedema in the acute setting respond well to CPAP.

13.70 A 67-year-old business man has recently flown back to the UK from Thailand. He presents with sudden onset of shortness of breath and right leg swelling. Which of the following statements best describes investigation of thromboembolic disease?

    A DVT is demonstrable in 50% patients with pulmonary embolism

    B Low probability perfusion scan would exclude pulmonary embolism

    C Spiral CT can detect segmental artery clot

    D Ultrasound of leg should be conducted before a V/Q scan

    E V/Q scan is gold standard in patients with pre-existing lung disease

13.71 Which statement is most accurate regarding asbestos exposure?

    A Around 90% of people exposed to asbestos develop pleural plaques

    B Benign pleural plaques require annual chest X-ray follow up

    C Chest X-ray is the most sensitive way of detecting pleural plaques

    D Compensation is available in the form of a disability benefit

    E Pleural biopsy is required to make a definitive diagnosis

13.72 A 47-year-old Afro-Caribbean lady presents with polydipsia and a nodular rash on the lower limbs. Which of the following would be the best test to confirm an underlying diagnosis?

    A Chest X-ray

    B Plasma and urine osmolalities

    C Serum calcium

    D Serum glucose

    E Thick and thin blood films

13.73 A 35-year-old male presents with weight loss, night sweats and fever. On examination there is a widened mediastinum. Which investigation would be most helpful to confirm the diagnosis?

    A CT thorax with contrast

    B Gallium uptake scan

    C Mediastinoscopy

    D Positron emission tomography (PET)

    E Single photon emission computed tomography (SPECT)

13.70   Answer: C

Spiral CT can detect clot from pulmonary trunk to the segmental arteries. V/Q is an alternative that can be used if there is no underlying lung defect. DVT is demonstrable in about 10% cases of pulmonary embolism.

13.71   Answer: D

Those with pleural plaques secondary to asbestos exposure are entitled to financial compensation: industrial injuries disability benefit in the UK. Around 50% develop plaques after exposure; high-resolution CT scan is more sensitive than plain chest X-ray, and benign plaques require no follow-up.

13.72   Answer: A

The clinical scenario suggests sarcoidosis complicated by erythema nodosum and thirst due to hypercalcaemia or diabetes insipidus.

13.73   Answer: C

This is the only investigation which will allow histopathological confirmation of diagnosis, although CT scanning would normally be undertaken in the first instance.

13.74 A 56-year-old man attends the Respiratory Clinic for review of his chronic obstructive airways disease. Recently, he has suffered fever symptoms, watery diarrhoea and intermittent abdominal cramps. He is a heavy smoker but has no further medical history. Which of the following is most likely to account for his symptoms?

- [ ] **A** Bowel obstruction
- [ ] **B** Coeliac disease
- [ ] **C** Crohn's disease
- [ ] **D** Cystic fibrosis
- [ ] **E** Ulcerative colitis

13.75 An 86-year-old lady presents with respiratory distress 4 days after surgical repair of her fractured neck of femur. Respiratory rate is 45/min, temperature is 38°C, Glasgow Coma Scale is 9, and there is a petechial rash over her lower limbs. Which of the following would best explain the above findings?

- [ ] **A** Acute respiratory distress syndrome
- [ ] **B** Disseminated intravascular coagulation
- [ ] **C** Fat emboli
- [ ] **D** Meningococcal meningitis
- [ ] **E** Pulmonary embolus

13.76 Your colleague calls you for advice about a patient with very advanced rheumatoid arthritis who has developed breathlessness. Which of the following patterns of lung function test abnormalities would be most consistent with a diagnosis of bronchiolitis obliterans?

- [ ] **A** Raised FEV_1
- [ ] **B** Reduced FEV_1
- [ ] **C** Reduced residual volume
- [ ] **D** Reduced total lung volume
- [ ] **E** Reduced vital capacity

13.74 Answer: E

Ulcerative colitis is more common in smokers, whereas in Crohn's disease smoking appears to be protective.

13.75 Answer: C

ARDS and DIC can be the result of a fat embolus but do not offer the most precise underlying explanation. Fat embolus most commonly occurs 3–10 days post-fracture.

13.76 Answer: B

Bronchiolitis obliterans is a picture of progressive small distal airways inflammation, resulting in an obstructive picture (reduced FEV_1) with raised residual volume.

14. RHEUMATOLOGY

14.1   Which of the following statements most correctly describes the clinical features of osteoarthritis?

- [ ] **A**   Characteristic distribution is asymmetric
- [ ] **B**   It is more common in Afro-Caribbean populations
- [ ] **C**   Radiological features are present in most people > 60 years age
- [ ] **D**   The prevalence is gradually declining
- [ ] **E**   There are no effective interventions to delay disease progression

14.2   Which of the following is most likely to predispose to the development of generalised osteoarthritis?

- [ ] **A**   Atrophy and loss of peri-articular bone
- [ ] **B**   Decreased local production of interleukin-1
- [ ] **C**   Inhibition of matrix metalloproteinases
- [ ] **D**   Irregular cartilage surface due to disordered osteoblast function
- [ ] **E**   Repetitive jogging in youth

14.3   A 56-year-old woman is referred to the General Medical Outpatient Department for review of joint deformity affecting both hands. On examination, there are painless bony swellings affecting the distal and proximal interphalangeal joints of both hands. Which of the following is the most likely explanation?

- [ ] **A**   Acute osteoarthritis
- [ ] **B**   Nodal osteoarthritis
- [ ] **C**   Psoriatic arthropathy
- [ ] **D**   Rheumatoid arthritis
- [ ] **E**   Systemic lupus erythematosus

14.4   You see a 52-year-old woman in the Medical Outpatient Department who has nodal osteoarthritis affecting both hands. Which of the following is a recognised feature of this condition?

- [ ] **A**   Family members are not affected
- [ ] **B**   More common in men
- [ ] **C**   Poor prognosis for functional outcome
- [ ] **D**   Typically develops between 20 and 30 years of age
- [ ] **E**   Usually associated with osteoarthritis of knee, hip and spine

14.1   Answer: C

Clinical features are less prevalent, most common in Caucasian and Western populations. Weight loss can delay disease progression in certain patients.

14.2   Answer: E

Repetitive joint use, trauma (particularly involving articular discontinuity), obesity and joint hypermobility predispose to osteoarthritis. Increased metalloproteinase activity contributes to cartilage destruction. Chondrocyte activity is often disordered.

14.3   Answer: B

This is associated with Bouchard's nodes (PIP joints) and Heberden's nodes (DIP joints). Often associated with carpometacarpal and metacarpophalangeal osteoarthritis of the thumb.

14.4   Answer: E

Develops in late middle age, more common in women, and a strong familial component. Polyarticular hand involvement with good functional prognosis.

14.5 Which of the following factors is most likely to be associated with significant pain in patients with osteoarthritis affecting the knee?

- [ ] **A** Depression
- [ ] **B** Cartilage abnormalities shown on MRI scan
- [ ] **C** Family history of joint disease
- [ ] **D** Fissures and surface erosion seen on arthroscopy
- [ ] **E** Loss of joint space on plain X-ray

14.6 You are asked to review a 64-year-old man in the General Medical Outpatient Clinic. He has longstanding osteoarthritis and is complaining of significant pain in his right knee. Which of the following factors would most strongly indicate the need for surgical joint replacement?

- [ ] **A** Joint space < 1 mm on plain X-ray
- [ ] **B** History of peptic ulcer disease
- [ ] **C** Patient's willingness to pay for private treatment
- [ ] **D** Previous successful left knee joint replacement
- [ ] **E** Symptoms uncontrolled despite maximal medical therapy

14.7 A 54-year-old man presents to the local Emergency Department with spontaneous onset of acute pain and swelling of his left knee. On examination, there is local erythema and limitation of movement. Plain X-ray appearances are normal. Which of the following diagnoses is most likely?

- [ ] **A** Acute osteoarthritis
- [ ] **B** Haemarthrosis
- [ ] **C** Reactive arthritis
- [ ] **D** Rheumatoid arthritis
- [ ] **E** Septic arthritis

14.8 Which of the following statements is correct in relation to rheumatoid arthritis?

- [ ] **A** Affects around 10% of adults
- [ ] **B** HLA-DR4 phenotype is found in 98% of patients
- [ ] **C** Incidence in post-menopausal women is similar to age-matched men
- [ ] **D** Most cases present at 50–60 years of age
- [ ] **E** Oral contraceptive pill use provokes earlier disease onset

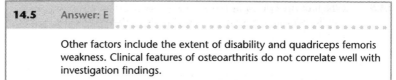

14.5   Answer: E

Other factors include the extent of disability and quadriceps femoris weakness. Clinical features of osteoarthritis do not correlate well with investigation findings.

14.6   Answer: E

The key considerations are the severity of symptoms and the extent of disability.

14.7   Answer: E

Haemarthrosis is less likely in the absence of trauma; acute psoriatic arthritis should also be considered. The other disorders listed typically present as an inflammatory polyarthritis.

14.8   Answer: C

Affects 1–2% of the population, and the commonest age of onset is 30–50 years. OCP use appears to delay disease onset, and incidence is 2- to 3-fold higher in premenopausal women than age-matched men. HLA-DR4 is found in 60–70% of patients.

14.9 Which of the following factors is most relevant to the development and progression of joint abnormalities in patients with rheumatoid arthritis?

   ☐ **A** Development of anti-TNFα antibodies

   ☐ **B** Impaired secretion of IL-1 and IL-8

   ☐ **C** Production of autoantibodies directed at the Fab portion of IgG

   ☐ **D** Synovial atrophy and thinning

   ☐ **E** TNFα-mediated bony erosion

14.10 A 38-year-old woman attends the Rheumatology Outpatient Department for assessment of symmetrical joint pains and stiffness affecting both wrist and hands, for around 8 weeks. Which of the following most strongly indicates a diagnosis of rheumatoid arthritis?

   ☐ **A** Characteristic radiographic changes

   ☐ **B** Morning stiffness

   ☐ **C** Raised erythrocyte sedimentation rate (ESR)

   ☐ **D** Rheumatoid factor positive

   ☐ **E** Subcutaneous nodules

14.11 A 45-year-old woman attends the General Medical Outpatient Clinic. She has previously been diagnosed with rheumatoid arthritis, which has been quiescent for the past 8 years. Which of the following features most strongly suggests active rheumatoid disease?

   ☐ **A** Anaemia

   ☐ **B** Presence of rheumatoid nodules

   ☐ **C** Rheumatoid factor strongly positive

   ☐ **D** Soft tissue swelling and bony erosion on plain X-ray

   ☐ **E** Tenderness on palpation overlying interphalangeal joints

14.9   Answer: E

Rheumatoid factor is present in around 70% of patients, which is an autoantibody directed at the Fc portion of IgG, and stimulates cytokine release by macrophages.

14.10   Answer: A

American College of Rheumatology criteria are 4 or more of:

Morning stiffness > 1 h (> 6 weeks)
Arthritis affecting more than 2 joints (> 6 weeks)
Arthritis of hand and wrists (> 6 weeks)
Symmetrical arthritis (> 6 weeks)
Positive rheumatoid factor
Subcutaneous nodules
Typical radiological changes

14.11   Answer: E

Other features include heat overlying affected joints, and raised ESR and C-reactive protein. Anaemia can be a feature of acute rheumatoid arthritis but is a non-specific marker of disease activity.

14.12 A 56-year-old woman with longstanding rheumatoid arthritis presents with progressive breathlessness. Which of the following disorders is most likely to be an extra-articular manifestation of rheumatoid arthritis?

◻ A Emphysema

◻ B Fibrosing alveolitis

◻ C Pleural effusion

◻ D Streptococcal pneumonia

◻ E Tuberculosis

14.13 A 42-year-old man with longstanding rheumatoid arthritis is referred to the Medical Outpatient Department for assessment of progressive peripheral sensory loss affecting both upper and lower limbs. Which of the following should be considered the most likely diagnosis?

◻ A Addisonian crisis

◻ B Atlanto–axial subluxation

◻ C Mononeuritis multiplex

◻ D Sulfasalazine toxicity

◻ E Vasculitis affecting the *vasa nervorum*

14.14 A 34-year-old man has been investigated for chronic pain affecting his wrists, hands and shoulders and has been diagnosed with rheumatoid arthritis. His symptoms are inadequately controlled with regular paracetamol and ibuprofen. Which of the following would be the most appropriate next step in his management?

◻ A Intramuscular gold injections

◻ B Oral ciclosporin

◻ C Oral prednisolone

◻ D Oral sulfasalazine

◻ E Refer for physiotherapy

14.12   Answer: B

Other manifestations include pleural nodules and obstructive bronchiolitis. Effusion is less specific but it can be a complication of rheumatoid-mediated pleural serositis.

14.13   Answer: E

Mononeuritis multiplex and compression neuropathies (eg carpal tunnel syndrome) are also recognised.

14.14   Answer: D

Early use of disease-modifying anti-rheumatic drugs is recommended. Sulfasalazine is better tolerated than gold in most patients, but typically causes nausea and reversible azoospermia. Around 50% of patients respond within 3–6 months.

14.15 A 51-year-old woman has been suffering from rheumatoid arthritis for the past 3 years. Recently, she has been experiencing increasing pain and stiffness of her left shoulder despite persisting with regular analgesia. Which of the following statements regarding local intra-articular corticosteroid administration is correct?

A Avoids systemic adverse effects of corticosteroids

B Injections should be repeated at regular intervals

C Semi-crystalline preparations are commonly used

D Symptom relief is usually sustained for 4–6 months

E They are generally less effective than high dose oral corticosteroids

14.16 A 43-year-old man is referred to the Outpatient Department for assessment of pain and stiffness affecting the sacro-iliac joints and lower back. On examination, there is severe limitation of lumbar spine movement. The GP letter states that 'rheumatoid factor is negative'. Which of the following disorders is the most likely to account for his symptoms?

A L4–L5 disc prolapse

B Osteoarthritis

C Polymyositis

D Psoriatic arthropathy

E Rheumatoid arthritis

14.17 A 28-year-old man has recently been diagnosed with ankylosing spondylitis. His GP has referred him to be seen urgently in the Ophthalmology Department with severe pain, photophobia and blurred vision. Which of the following is the most likely explanation for his symptoms?

A Acute conjunctivitis

B Acute glaucoma

C Anterior uveitis

D Cerebral vasculitis

E Hypertensive encephalopathy

14.15   Answer: C

These provide effective symptom relief, but it is often short-lived. They may be associated with fewer systemic complications but do not avoid them completely. They should only be used where other treatments are ineffective.

14.16   Answer: D

Features suggest a seronegative spondyloarthropathy. Other causes include ankylosing spondylitis, reactive arthritis and enteropathic arthritis seen in inflammatory bowel disease.

14.17   Answer: C

Strongly associated with ankylosing spondylitis and the HLA-B27 genotype. Patients with AS should be asked to report immediately if they develop a painful red eye.

14.18 A 37-year-old man has a past history of psoriasis, which has been quiescent for several years. He presents to the Rheumatology Outpatient Department with a symmetrical polyarthropathy affecting both hands and wrists. Which of the following statements is correct regarding treatment of this condition?

- [ ] A   Ciclosporin is the initial treatment of choice
- [ ] B   Intra-articular corticosteroids are ineffective
- [ ] C   Methotrexate controls skin lesions but not joint involvement
- [ ] D   Non-steroidal anti-inflammatory drugs prevent future relapses
- [ ] E   Sulfasalazine delays progression of joint disease

14.19 A 22-year-old man attends the Rheumatology Outpatient Department with back pain and stiffness and a diagnosis of reactive arthritis is considered. Which of the following factors would most strongly suggest an alternative diagnosis?

- [ ] A   Conjunctivitis
- [ ] B   Exfoliative rash on soles
- [ ] C   Involvement of MTP joints
- [ ] D   Nail dystrophy
- [ ] E   Syndesmophytes on lumbar spine X-ray

14.20 A 56-year-old man attends the Emergency Department with a sudden onset of pain and swelling of the first metacarpophalangeal joint of his left foot. Which of the following would most strongly suggest a diagnosis of acute gout?

- [ ] A   Demonstration of urate crystals in joint fluid
- [ ] B   Normal appearance of plain X-ray
- [ ] C   Previous acute gout 1 year before
- [ ] D   Raised circulating neutrophil count
- [ ] E   Serum uric acid 520 µmol/l

14.18 Answer: E

NSAIDs and analgesics are effective for symptomatic relief. Methotrexate and ciclosporin delay progression of both skin and joint involvement in psoriasis.

14.19 Answer: E

This is strongly suggestive of ankylosing spondylitis. Other features of reactive arthritis include circinate balanitis, large joint effusion and heel pain.

14.20 Answer: A

Serum urate concentrations are poor indicators: majority of patients with acute gout have 'normal' serum values at presentation. Fewer than 10% of patients with chronic hyperuricaemia ever develop an episode of acute gout.

14.21 A 61-year-old man presents with an acutely painful, swollen right knee. Aspiration of joint fluid reveals neutrophils 1500/mm³, and needle-shaped crystals that are negatively birefringent. Which of the following is the most likely diagnosis?

◻ **A** Acute gout

◻ **B** Chondrocalcinosis

◻ **C** Chronic tophaceous gout

◻ **D** Pseudogout

◻ **E** Septic arthritis

14.22 A 56-year-old woman presents to the Emergency Department with a hot, swollen and painful left knee. Joint aspiration reveals a watery yellow fluid, which is cloudy but no crystals are seen on microscopy, and neutrophil count is 5200/mm³. Which of the following is the most likely diagnosis?

◻ **A** Acute gout

◻ **B** Chondrocalcinosis

◻ **C** Pseudogout

◻ **D** Rheumatoid arthritis

◻ **E** Septic arthritis

14.23 A 52-year-old man is referred to the Rheumatology Outpatient Department with sudden onset of pain in his left knee. On examination, the joint is swollen and red, with limited movement due to pain. Aspiration of joint fluid reveals a turbid, blood-stained yellow fluid, and microscopy shows neutrophil count of 85,000/mm³. Which of the following is the most likely diagnosis?

◻ **A** Acute gout

◻ **B** Chondrocalcinosis

◻ **C** Pseudogout

◻ **D** Rheumatoid arthritis

◻ **E** Septic arthritis

14.21 Answer: A

This is the characteristic microscopic appearance of urate crystals.

14.22 Answer: D

Presents acutely in around 15% of cases. Typically, white cell count is increased to 2000–40,000/mm³ and rheumatoid factor may be positive.

14.23 Answer: E

Such a high white cell count is highly suggestive of infection. Diagnosis might be confirmed by Gram stain and culture of aspirated fluid, and there may raised systemic white blood count and positive blood cultures.

14.24 A 59-year-old woman presents to the Emergency Department with an acutely swollen and tender right knee. Microscopy of aspirated joint fluid shows a neutrophil count of 3280/mm³ and the presence of rhomboid crystals that are weakly positively birefringent. Which of the following is the most likely diagnosis?

- [ ] **A** Acute gout
- [ ] **B** Chondrocalcinosis
- [ ] **C** Pseudogout
- [ ] **D** Rheumatoid arthritis
- [ ] **E** Septic arthritis

14.25 A 70-year-old woman is referred to the Rheumatology Outpatient Department with progressive pain in her left knee, which has begun to limit the distance she can walk. Plain X-rays of both knee joints show narrowing of the joint space, predominantly affecting the left side. In addition, there is patchy linear calcification within the joint-space cartilage. Which of the following is the most likely diagnosis?

- [ ] **A** Acute gout
- [ ] **B** Chondrocalcinosis
- [ ] **C** Pseudogout
- [ ] **D** Rheumatoid arthritis
- [ ] **E** Septic arthritis

14.26 An 18-year-old man presents to the Emergency Department with sudden onset of pain in his right elbow. On examination, there is redness and swelling, and passive movement is exquisitely painful. Which of the following tests is most likely to clearly establish the diagnosis?

- [ ] **A** Blood cultures
- [ ] **B** Chest X-ray
- [ ] **C** Microscopy of joint aspiration fluid
- [ ] **D** Peripheral blood count
- [ ] **E** X-ray of the affected joint

14.24 Answer: C

Microscopy appearance suggests calcium pyrophosphate crystals. These are distinct from the needle-shaped, negatively birefringent urate crystals seen in acute gout.

14.25 Answer: B

Condition characterised by calcium pyrophosphate deposition in the cartilage; can manifest as pseudogout, osteoarthritis-like features or a rapidly destructive arthritis.

14.26 Answer: C

The most likely diagnosis is septic arthritis, which is usually associated with normal X-ray appearances. There may be increased peripheral white cell count and positive blood cultures. Diagnosis is best established by positive identification of organisms in the joint aspiration fluid.

14.27 A previously well 17-year-old woman presents with sudden onset of a painful and swollen right knee. The joint appears diffusely swollen and red, and a diagnosis of septic arthritis is suspected. Which of the following is the most appropriate initial step in her management?

- [ ] **A** Blood cultures
- [ ] **B** Intravenous antibiotics before undertaking other investigations
- [ ] **C** Joint aspiration and urgent microscopy
- [ ] **D** Peripheral blood count
- [ ] **E** X-ray of the right knee

14.28 A 68-year-old man presents to the Emergency Department complaining of severe left hip pain. He admits to regular excess alcohol intake, but denies any recent falls or trauma. On examination, temperature is 37.8°C, he is thin, and movement of his left hip appears very tender. Plain X-ray is normal, and septic arthritis is suspected. Which of the following is the most likely causative organism?

- [ ] **A** *Haemophilus influenzae*
- [ ] **B** *Mycobacterium tuberculosis*
- [ ] **C** *Neisseria meningitides*
- [ ] **D** *Staphylococcus aureus*
- [ ] **E** *Treponema pallidum*

14.29 A 42-year-old man presents to the local Emergency Department with severe pain affecting his left knee joint. The joint appears red and swollen, and a suspected diagnosis of septic arthritis is made. Which of the following would be the most appropriate Initial treatments?

- [ ] **A** Intravenous high-dose flucloxacillin
- [ ] **B** Intravenous high-dose benzylpenicillin
- [ ] **C** Intravenous ciprofloxacin
- [ ] **D** Oral co-amoxiclav
- [ ] **E** Oral erythromycin

14.27 Answer: B

This should be given immediately on diagnosis, even before other investigations have been performed.

14.28 Answer: B

1% of TB patients have bone/joint disease. Risk factors include alcohol abuse, debility and immunocompromise, and patients suffer sweats, fever and weight loss.

14.29 Answer: A

The most common organism is *Staphylococcus aureus*; an alternative to flucloxacillin is high dose intravenous erythromycin or clarithromycin. Oral fucidic acid is often co-administered. Gonococcal arthritis is a common cause in young patients.

14.30 A 45-year-old farmer is referred to you because of recent symptoms suggesting arthritis of his knees and wrists. He had been treated several months earlier for a febrile illness associated with headache and unusual rash. You suspect a diagnosis of Lyme disease. Which of the following tests would be most appropriate for confirming this?

☐ **A** Detection of *Borrelia burgdorferi* in blood culture

☐ **B** Detection of *Borrelia burgdorferi* in joint aspirate

☐ **C** IgE antibodies to *Borrelia burgdorferi*

☐ **D** IgM antibodies to *Borrelia burgdorferi*

☐ **E** Peripheral eosinophilia

14.31 Which of the following confers the greatest likelihood of developing SLE?

☐ **A** Affected first-degree relative

☐ **B** Age > 50 years

☐ **C** Male gender

☐ **D** HLA-B27 genotype

☐ **E** Suppressed B-lymphocyte function

14.32 A 54-year-old woman is referred to the Rheumatology Outpatient Department for investigation of a symmetrical arthropathy affecting both hands. On examination, the joints of both hands are tender, and the patient has facial erythema overlying her cheeks and nasal bridge. The GP letter reports that anti-double-stranded DNA antibody is undetectable. Which of the following is the most likely diagnosis?

☐ **A** Drug-induced lupus

☐ **B** Psoriatic arthropathy

☐ **C** Reactive arthritis

☐ **D** Rheumatoid arthritis

☐ **E** Systemic lupus erythematosus

14.30   Answer: D

25% of cases develop oligoarthritis; 20% of these progress to a chronic arthritis. Treatment with antibiotics is effective for early disease, and prolonged therapy may be effective in chronic arthritis.

14.31   Answer: A

Around 3% risk; 25% concordance in monozygotic twins. Risk greater in females, those aged 20–40 years and the HLA-B8 and DR3 genotypes.

14.32   Answer: A

SLE typically affects younger patients, and anti-DS DNA antibody is normally positive. In drug-induced lupus, raised titres of anti-DNA histone antibody are often detectable.

14.33 A 56-year-old man is treated with hydralazine and nitrate therapy for heart failure. Three months after commencing treatment, he complains of aches and pains across many joints. Examination shows an erythematous scaly rash and lymphadenopathy, and a plain chest X-ray shows diffuse pulmonary infiltration. Which one of the following statements regarding hydralazine-induced lupus is correct?

   ☐ **A** Corticosteroid treatment is contraindicated

   ☐ **B** People with HLA-B27 antigen are at significantly greater risk

   ☐ **C** Rapid acetylators are at greatest risk

   ☐ **D** Remission usually occurs after drug withdrawal

   ☐ **E** Renal involvement is a characteristically prominent feature

14.34 A 28-year-old woman is referred to the Rheumatology Outpatient Department for assessment of chronic inflammatory symptoms affecting the joints of both hands, wrists and shoulders. Which of the following features would be most strongly suggestive of SLE as the underlying diagnosis?

   ☐ **A** Alopecia with scarring

   ☐ **B** Nail bed infarcts

   ☐ **C** Negative rheumatoid factor test

   ☐ **D** Positive antinuclear antibody

   ☐ **E** Scaly, erythematous skin rash overlying both knees

14.35 You are asked to review a 37-year-old woman in the Rheumatology Outpatient Department. She has had SLE for around 8 years. Which of the following findings would be the strongest indicator of poor prognosis?

   ☐ **A** Livedo reticularis seen overlying both lower limbs

   ☐ **B** Mild depression

   ☐ **C** Nail bed infarcts

   ☐ **D** Protein + on dipstick urinalysis

   ☐ **E** Serum creatinine 186 μmol/l

14.33   Answer: D

HLA-DR4 and slow acetylator phenotype are risk factors. Unlike SLE, renal and CNS involvement is uncommon. Treatment with corticosteroids may be helpful.

14.34   Answer: A

Present in around 50% of cases. Positive ANA test in SLE, rheumatoid arthritis and other conditions. Nail bed infarction is non-specific, and occurs after trauma and in patients with vasculitis of any origin.

14.35   Answer: E

Kidney involvement confers a very poor prognosis, particularly where there is evidence of impaired renal function or nephrotic syndrome (typically associated with heavy proteinuria).

14.36   A 38-year-old woman attends the General Medical Outpatient Department with a suspected diagnosis of Raynaud's syndrome. She describes blanching and pain of her extremities following exposure to cold weather. Which of the following is most likely to be an effective treatment?

A   Atenolol

B   Clopidogrel

C   Misoprostol

D   Nicardipine

E   Sumatriptan

14.37   A 52-year-old woman is referred to the Rheumatology Outpatient Clinic with shiny and atrophic skin overlying her fingers, with ulceration of a number of her fingertips. She is noted to have facial telangiectasia. Which of the following diagnoses is most likely to account for these features?

A   Discoid lupus

B   Pseudogout

C   Psoriatic arthropathy

D   Scleroderma

E   SLE

14.38   A 45-year-old man has been diagnosed with systemic sclerosis for 5 years. He is referred to the General Medical Outpatient Department for investigation of progressive dyspepsia and gastro-oesophageal reflux over the past 4 weeks. Which of the following disorders is most likely to account for his symptoms?

A   Achalasia of the oesophagus

B   Adenocarcinoma of the distal oesophagus

C   Chronic pancreatitis

D   Oesophageal dysmotility

E   Peptic ulceration

14.36 Answer: D

Dihydropyridine calcium channel blockers cause smooth muscle relaxation and oppose the vasoconstriction in Raynaud's disease (eg nifedipine). Beta-blockers (eg atenolol) tend to cause peripheral vasoconstriction and reduced cardiac output, which might exacerbate the condition.

14.37 Answer: D

Typically presents between 30 and 50 years. May also be calcinosis, and erythema and dilated capillaries in the proximal nail folds.

14.38 Answer: D

The gastrointestinal tract is involved in most patients. Reflux is commonly due to loss of normal peristalsis (local sclerosis) and hiatus hernia.

14.39   A 52-year-old woman with longstanding systemic sclerosis presents with progressive breathlessness over the past 4 months. Which of the following investigations would be most helpful in establishing the cause of her breathlessness?

- [ ] A   Arterial blood gas analysis
- [ ] B   High-resolution CT thorax
- [ ] C   Measurement of anti-topoisomerase I titres
- [ ] D   Plain chest X-ray
- [ ] E   Pulmonary function tests

14.40   A 46-year-old woman is referred to the General Medical Outpatient Department for investigation of progressive limb girdle weakness over the past 2 months, associated with mild pain and stiffness affecting the wrists and hands. Rheumatoid factor is negative, antinuclear antibody is mildly elevated, and ESR is 28 mm/h. Which one of the following is most likely to account for these features?

- [ ] A   Cushing's syndrome
- [ ] B   Paraneoplastic myositis
- [ ] C   Polymyalgia rheumatica
- [ ] D   Polymyositis
- [ ] E   SLE

14.41   Which of the following statements is correct with regard to Paget's disease of the bone?

- [ ] A   Affects around 10% of patients over the age of 50 years
- [ ] B   Diagnosis is unlikely if serum calcium concentration is normal
- [ ] C   High serum phosphate is a characteristic finding
- [ ] D   It confers a 30-fold increased risk of osteosarcoma
- [ ] E   Plain X-ray investigations are usually normal

14.42   A 67-year-old man has bowing of both tibia, and a diagnosis of Paget's disease is suspected. Which of the following findings is most strongly suggestive of this diagnosis?

- [ ] A   Dense osteosclerosis detected by bone scan
- [ ] B   Discrete punched out lytic skull lesions
- [ ] C   Mixed osteolytic and osteosclerotic changes on a pelvic X-ray
- [ ] D   Multiple osteophytes on lumbar spine X-ray
- [ ] E   Raised serum alkaline phosphatase

14.39   Answer: B

Pulmonary fibrosis occurs in many patients with systemic disease. Presence of anti-topoisomerase I (anti-Scl 70) antibody is suggestive of pulmonary involvement. Recurrent infection is a recognised complication, particularly in patients with significant gastro-oesophageal reflux.

14.40   Answer: D

Onset insidious over several months associated with weight loss, fever and proximal muscle weakness in the acute phase. Can also involve respiratory muscle weakness (associated with anti-Jo1 antibodies), and oesophageal muscles resulting in dysphagia.

14.41   Answer: D

0.5–1.0% of cases. Serum calcium and phosphate are typically normal, while alkaline phosphatase is significantly raised. X-ray changes can show lytic lesions or sclerotic lesions and thickening of bony trabecula.

14.42   Answer: C

Discrete osteolytic lesions suggestive of myeloma. Bone scanning is unable to distinguish from metastatic carcinoma (eg prostate). Raised alkaline phosphatase is found in a number of skeletal and liver disorders.

14.43 A 72-year-old woman is referred to the Medical Outpatient Clinic for investigation of progressive breathlessness. She has been diagnosed with Paget's disease several years before. Which of the following diagnoses is most likely to account for her current symptoms?

A High output cardiac failure

B Hypercalcaemia

C Myocardial ischaemia

D Phrenic nerve compression

E Pulmonary fibrosis

14.44 You have been attending a 66-year-old woman who presented with headache and cranial nerve deafness. CT head scan revealed bone abnormalities consistent with severe Paget's bone disease. Which of the following drugs is most likely to be beneficial in long-term treatment of this condition?

A Alfuzosin

B Aluminium hydroxide

C Ciclosporin A

D Pamidronate

E Risedronate

14.45 A 56-year-old man is referred to the General Medical Outpatient Department with a 4-month history of progressive lower limb weakness and vague hip and knee pains. Examination shows proximal muscle weakness and tenderness, and investigations show corrected calcium 1.98 mmol/l, phosphate 0.8 mmol/l, alkaline phosphatase 230 IU/l and alanine transferase 24 IU/l. Which of these is the most likely diagnosis?

A Osteomalacia

B Osteoporosis

C Paget's disease

D Polymyalgia rheumatica

E Polymyositis

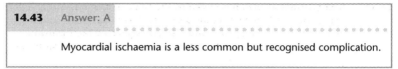

14.43   Answer: A

Myocardial ischaemia is a less common but recognised complication.

14.44   Answer: E

Bisphosphonates are the mainstay therapy in Paget's disease. Pamidronate is only available as an intravenous preparation.

14.45   Answer: A

Raised alkaline phosphatase (ALP) is the characteristic finding in this condition, secondary to raised PTH. Calcium is low to normal.

14.46 A 65-year-old woman is referred to the General Medical Outpatient Department following a recent traumatic hip X-ray. Plain X-rays showed marked osteopenia, and reports suggested osteoporosis. Which of the following is the strongest risk factor for osteoporosis?

- [ ] **A** Alcohol excess
- [ ] **B** Cigarette smoking
- [ ] **C** Diabetes mellitus
- [ ] **D** Female gender
- [ ] **E** Low dietary calcium intake

14.47 A 64-year-old woman is recovering from a recent osteoporotic hip fracture after minor trauma. She is making good progress and you are considering steps to reduce the risk of further fractures. Which of the following is likely to be most effective?

- [ ] **A** Alendronate
- [ ] **B** Hormone replacement therapy
- [ ] **C** Nasal calcitonin
- [ ] **D** Oral low-dose prednisolone
- [ ] **E** Vitamin D and calcium

14.48 A 48-year-old man is admitted to the Medical Assessment Unit with an 8-week history of fever, weight loss and generalised myalgia. On examination, blood pressure is 186/94 mmHg. Investigations show ESR 52 mm/h, WCC 13.2×10^9/l and dipstick urinalysis shows proteinuria ++ and haematuria +++. Which of these is the most likely underlying diagnosis?

- [ ] **A** Paraneoplastic myopathy
- [ ] **B** Phaeochromocytoma
- [ ] **C** Polyarteritis nodosa
- [ ] **D** Polymyalgia rheumatica
- [ ] **E** Polymyositis

14.46   Answer: D

The others are also important risk factors; others include early menopause, family history and advancing age.

14.47   Answer: A

Hormone replacement therapy (HRT) may also be effective, but is usually reserved for those patients with post-menopausal symptoms. Vitamin D and calcium supplementation is less effective but may be a suitable alternative if bisphosphonates are not tolerated. Calcitonin has been shown to reduce only vertebral fracture rate.

14.48   Answer: C

Can also involve CNS, abdominal viscera, heart and skin. Angiography demonstrates pathognomonic multiple microaneurysms.

14.49 A 56-year-old woman is undergoing in-patient investigations of weight loss, fever and rash. Skin biopsy of an affected site shows inflammation consistent with a small vessel vasculitis. Antineutrophilic cytoplasmic antibody (ANCA) test is negative. Which of the following is the most likely explanation for these findings?

- A Churg–Strauss granulomatosis
- B Henoch–Schönlein purpura
- C Kawasaki's disease
- D Microscopic polyangiitis
- E Wegener's granulomatosis

14.50 A 60-year-old man is referred to the General Medical Outpatient Clinic with a short history of severe pain and stiffness affecting both shoulder girdles, lumbar spine and hips. His symptoms are usually worst in the mornings. Which of the following is the most likely diagnosis?

- A Cushing's syndrome
- B Grave's disease
- C Osteomalacia
- D Polymyalgia rheumatica
- E Polymyositis

14.51 A 64-year-old woman is referred to the General Medical Outpatient Clinic with suspected polymyalgia rheumatica. Which of the following investigations is most useful in confirming this diagnosis?

- A Alkaline phosphatase
- B Creatinine kinase
- C ESR
- D Serum calcium
- E Temporal artery biopsy

14.49   Answer: B

Kawasaki's disease is associated with medium to large vessel vasculitis. The others are typically associated with positive c-ANCA (Wegener's) or p-ANCA (Churg–Strauss and microscopic polyangiitis).

14.50   Answer: D

Although some features overlap with the other conditions, the symptoms and diurnal variation make polymyalgia rheumatica the most likely.

14.51   Answer: C

Invariably high, and can be used to monitor response to treatment. Temporal artery biopsy shows giant cell arteritis in only 20–30% of cases.

14.52 You review a 71-year-old woman in the Medical Assessment Unit, who presents with new onset of left-sided headache associated with blurred vision. Neurological examination of her limbs is normal. ESR is 68 mmol/l. Which of the following is the best initial treatment?

- ☐ **A** Amitriptyline
- ☐ **B** Co-amoxiclav
- ☐ **C** High-dose prednisolone
- ☐ **D** Intramuscular morphine
- ☐ **E** Nimodipine

14.53 A previously well 38-year-old man presents with 12-week history of progressively worsening dry eyes and dry mouth. He is taking no regular medications. Which of the following is the most likely diagnosis?

- ☐ **A** Allergic conjunctivitis
- ☐ **B** Hypothyroidism
- ☐ **C** Rheumatoid arthritis
- ☐ **D** Sjögren's syndrome
- ☐ **E** Stevens–Johnson syndrome

14.54 A 42-year-old woman is admitted with sudden onset of left arm weakness and left homonomous hemianopia. On examination, she has a soft systolic murmur. ESR and full blood count are normal. Which of the following tests would best establish an underlying cause for stroke?

- ☐ **A** Anti-double-stranded DNA antibody
- ☐ **B** Anticardiolipin antibodies
- ☐ **C** Coagulation screen
- ☐ **D** Coomb's test
- ☐ **E** Lupus anticoagulant

14.52   Answer: C

These features suggest giant cell arteritis. Ophthalmic artery involvement is associated with the risk of permanent blindness and urgent corticosteroid treatment is required, eg prednisolone 60–100 mg daily.

14.53   Answer: D

Xerostomia and dry eyes (keratoconjunctivitis sicca), in the absence of rheumatoid arthritis or autoimmune disease. Can be associated with Raynaud's phenomenon, arthralgia, neuritis and renal tubular defects.

14.54   Answer: B

Diagnostic for antiphospholipid syndrome, which accounts for a quarter of strokes < 45 years. May be associated with lupus anticoagulant antibodies and positive Coomb's test.

14.55 A 34-year-old woman is admitted via the Emergency Department with sudden onset of left leg pain, 6 weeks after a spontaneous abortion. On examination, the leg is cold and pale with absent pulses beyond the popliteal artery. Which of the following disorders is most likely to be responsible?

A   Addison's disease

B   Antiphospholipid syndrome

C   Disseminated intravascular coagulation (DIC)

D   Polycythaemia rubra vera

E   SLE

14.56 A 43-year-old woman is referred to the Outpatient Department with pain and stiffness of her joint associated with a facial rash. The GP letter has suggested a diagnosis of SLE. Which of the following would most strongly suggest an alternative diagnosis?

A   Cranial nerve palsy

B   Finger clubbing

C   Normocytic anaemia

D   Pleural effusion

E   Raynaud's phenomenon

14.57 A 31-year-old woman attends the Medical Outpatient Department for investigation of exertional breathlessness. She has recently been diagnosed with SLE, and has a characteristic facial rash. Which of these investigations would most strongly suggest pulmonary involvement?

A   Anti-Jo1 antibody

B   ESR > 45 mm/h

C   High antinuclear antibody titres

D   Peak expiratory flow rate 85% of predicted

E   Rheumatoid factor positive

14.55   Answer: B

Arterial and venous thrombosis; 30% of woman with recurrent miscarriages have antiphospholipid antibody syndrome. May also be associated with migraine, thrombocytopenia, livedo reticularis and valvular heart disease.

14.56   Answer: B

The others are characteristic findings, along with vasculitis and skin, pulmonary and cardiac involvement.

14.57   Answer: A

Around 60% of patients have lung involvement: pleurisy, pleural effusion, pneumonitis and restrictive lung defect with reduced lung volumes.

14.58 A 49-year-old woman is referred for measurement of bone mineral density. Which of the following clinical factors most strongly suggests underlying osteoporosis?

- ☐ **A** Alcoholism
- ☐ **B** Longstanding asthma
- ☐ **C** Obesity
- ☐ **D** Prolonged corticosteroid treatment
- ☐ **E** Regular cigarette smoking

14.59 A previously well 64-year-old woman presents to the Emergency Department with sudden onset of lumbar back pain. Plain X-rays of the lumbar spine indicate wedge-type fractures affecting L3 and L4 vertebrae. Which of the following statements is correct regarding her management?

- ☐ **A** Bisphosphonate therapy will reduce her long-term fracture risk
- ☐ **B** Bone biopsy should be performed
- ☐ **C** Constipation is most likely due to hypercalcaemia
- ☐ **D** Hormone replacement therapy should be commenced
- ☐ **E** Radiotherapy of the lumbar spine should be arranged

14.60 A 34-year-old woman with longstanding asthma is referred to the General Medical Outpatient Department for investigation of pulmonary infiltrates noted on a recent chest X-ray. Full blood count shows a raised eosinophil count, and ESR is normal. Which of the following diagnoses is most likely?

- ☐ **A** Acute exacerbation of chronic obstructive airways disease
- ☐ **B** Chronic lymphocytic leukaemia
- ☐ **C** Churg–Strauss syndrome
- ☐ **D** Goodpasture's syndrome
- ☐ **E** Pneumoconiosis

14.58   Answer: D

Other risk factors include inflammatory bowel disease, lack of physical exercise, immobility, female gender and advanced age.

14.59   Answer: A

Osteoporotic crush fracture most likely cause. Underlying metastases or myeloma important but uncommon. Transient constipation is common, due to entrapment of parasympathetic nerves.

14.60   Answer: C

Characteristic features also include allergic rhinitis, cardiac involvement and often p-ANCA positive.

14.61 A 46-year-old patient is admitted to the Emergency Department with breathlessness. He has a history of asthma and allergic rhinitis, and his plain chest X-ray shows diffuse pulmonary infiltration. Which of these findings would most strongly support a diagnosis of Churg–Strauss syndrome?

   A Anti-double-stranded DNA antibody positive

   B Antinuclear antibody positive

   C c-ANCA positive

   D p-ANCA positive

   E Raised blood lymphocyte count

14.62 A 59-year-old man is referred for investigation of pain and swelling of his nose associated with significant tenderness. There is no history of trauma. Investigations show ESR 45 mm/h, and urinalysis shows protein ++ and blood ++. Which of the following diagnoses best explains these findings?

   A Dermatomyositis

   B Polymyalgia rheumatica

   C Polymyositis

   D Relapsing chondritis

   E SLE

14.63 A 54-year-old woman is referred to the General Medical Outpatient Department for investigation of proximal muscle weakness and facial rash. The GP letter suggests a diagnosis of dermatomyositis. Which of the following features would most strongly suggest an alternative diagnosis?

   A Electromyography shows delayed axonal conduction

   B Heliotropic rash over the upper eyelids

   C Periorbital oedema

   D Positive rheumatoid factor

   E Raised antinuclear antibody titres

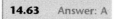

14.61   Answer: D

Also associated with high eosinophil count. c-ANCA more strongly suggestive of Wegener's granulomatosis.

14.62   Answer: D

Classically involves relapsing course with inflammation of the pinna or nasal cartilage. Can result in permanent damage, eg saddle nose deformity. Associated with anti-type II collagen antibody.

14.63   Answer: A

This suggests a peripheral neuropathy.

14.64 A 56-year-old woman has recently been diagnosed with dermatomyositis. Which of the following statements is most accurate regarding the clinical course in this condition?

- [ ] **A** A relapsing–remitting pattern is most common
- [ ] **B** Corticosteroids are an effective treatment
- [ ] **C** Joints are typically spared
- [ ] **D** The ESR is elevated in around two-thirds of patients
- [ ] **E** There is a 10-fold increased risk of underlying malignancy

14.65 A 55-year-old man has been diagnosed with asymptomatic hyperuricaemia. Which of the following factors is most likely to predispose to high serum urate concentrations?

- [ ] **A** Bendroflumethizide
- [ ] **B** Ibuprofen
- [ ] **C** Sedentary lifestyle
- [ ] **D** Triamterene
- [ ] **E** Type 1 diabetes

14.66 A 45-year-old man is referred to the General Medical Outpatient Department because of progressive pain in both knees, which is limiting mobility. On examination, his weight is 108 kg, blood pressure is 176/92 mmHg, there is mild swelling of both knee joints and there are active striae across the abdominal wall. Which of the following is most likely to account for his joint pains?

- [ ] **A** Avascular necrosis
- [ ] **B** Chondrocalcinosis
- [ ] **C** Haemarthrosis
- [ ] **D** Osteoarthritis
- [ ] **E** Psoriatic arthropathy

A

14.64   Answer: B

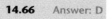

Long-term, there may be muscle contractures and a 2- to 3-fold increased risk of underlying malignancy. The ESR is high in only around 5%.

14.65   Answer: A

Type 1 diabetes typically associated with hypouricaemia, whereas type 2 diabetes, hypertension, renal impairment are associated with hyperuricaemia.

14.66   Answer: D

The clinical features suggest Cushing's syndrome and obesity; the latter is a major risk factor for premature osteoarthritis.

14.67 A 34-year-old man is referred to the Rheumatology Outpatient Department because of a symmetrical arthropathy involving the knees, ankles and wrists. You note the presence of dusky-coloured raised plaques over both shins. Which of the following is the most likely underlying diagnosis?

- A Dermatomyositis
- B Psoriatic arthropathy
- C Rheumatoid arthritis
- D Sarcoidosis
- E Tuberculous arthritis

14.68 A 48-year-old man has received immunosuppressive treatment for severe rheumatoid arthritis. Which of the following best describes the pharmacological action of these drugs?

- A Azathioprine is a pyrimidine analogue
- B Azathioprine is metabolised to 6-mercaptopurine
- C Ciclosporin A increases interleukin-1 activity
- D Cyclophosphamide acts by inhibiting folate dehydrogenase
- E Methotrexate is an alkylating agent

14.69 A 62-year-old woman presents to the General Medical Outpatient Clinic for assessment of easy bruising. She has had rheumatoid arthritis for more than 30 years, but this has been asymptomatic recently. On examination, the skin is dry and thin and there are purpura overlying the forearms and lower limbs. Which of the following is most likely to account for her symptoms and signs?

- A Autoimmune thrombocytopenia
- B Cushing's syndrome
- C Immunosuppression secondary to sulfasalazine
- D Impaired liver function
- E Lupus anticoagulant antibodies

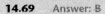

14.67 Answer: D

Also associated with bilateral hilar lymphadenopathy, and may be raised serum calcium and ACE concentrations. The rash distribution is characteristic of erythema nodosum.

14.68 Answer: B

Azathioprine is a pro-drug; both are purine analogues and are also useful in Crohn's disease. Cyclophosphamide is an alkylating agent, ciclosporin is a lymphocyte calcineurin inhibitor, and methotrexate is a folate antagonist.

14.69 Answer: B

Other features include truncal obesity, hirsutism, impotence, acne, striae, hypertension and diabetes mellitus.

14.70   A 49-year-old woman has had rheumatoid arthritis for 8 years, and is complaining of a recent exacerbation of pain and stiffness affecting her hands and wrists. Which of the following factors would most strongly suggest the need for systemic corticosteroid therapy?

- A   Effective symptom relief after previous corticosteroid administration
- B   ESR > 60 mm/h
- C   Lack of response to sulfasalazine
- D   Raised blood leukocyte count
- E   Rheumatoid factor very strongly positive

14.71   A 50-year-old woman has had diffuse muscle pain and stiffness for more than 8 months. She is found to have local tenderness overlying both biceps muscles. Serum creatinine kinase, ESR, full blood count and EMG studies are normal, and rheumatoid factor is negative. Which of these is the most likely diagnosis?

- A   Fibromyalgia
- B   Polymyalgia rheumatica
- C   Polymyositis
- D   Rhabdomyolysis
- E   Rheumatoid arthritis

14.72   A 45-year-old labourer is complaining of lumbar back pain. He had fallen from a ladder at work 2 months earlier. Which of the following features would most strongly support the diagnosis of functional low back pain?

- A   Documented history of malignant disease
- B   Loss of bladder control
- C   Night sweats
- D   Tenderness on superficial palpation over the lumbar spine
- E   Weight loss

14.70   Answer: C

Lack of pain relief with rest, NSAIDs, disease-modifying anti-rheumatic agents or local corticosteroids, or if there is life-threatening visceral disease (eg severe pericarditis) or sight-threatening ocular involvement.

14.71   Answer: A

Affects around 2% of GP attenders, 10 times more common in women. Often associated with features of anxiety and depression. Management involves exclusion of more serious pathology, reassurance and physiotherapy.

14.72   Answer: D

The other features should prompt more urgent investigation.

14.73 A 56-year-old woman is complaining of progressively worsening lumbar back pain. There is no history of trauma. Which of the following features indicate the need for urgent investigation?

- A   Limited straight leg raising
- B   Loss of bowel and bladder continence
- C   Pain aggravated by lumbar spine movements
- D   Severe pain not relieved by simple analgesia
- E   Recurrent episodes

14.74 A 52-year-old woman complains of aching and stiffness affecting both hands and wrists for the past 6 weeks. Rheumatoid factor is positive. Which of the following conditions is most likely to account for the presence of this antibody?

- A   Achalasia of the oesophagus
- B   Polyarteritis nodosum
- C   Tuberculosis
- D   Viral meningitis
- E   Wegener's granulomatosis

14.75 Which of the following statements related to bone turnover is most accurate?

- A   Bone remodelling is inhibited by thyroxine
- B   Interleukin-1 inhibits bone remodelling
- C   Osteoblasts lay down unmineralised 'osteoid' material
- D   Osteoclasts stimulate new bone formation
- E   Osteocytes are anuclear and cannot multiply by meiosis

14.76 A 30-year-old woman is suspected of having SLE. Detection of which of the following antibody tests most strongly suggests an alternative diagnosis?

- A   Anti-double-stranded DNA antibody
- B   Anti-histone antibody
- C   Antinuclear antibody
- D   Anti-ribonuclear protein antibody
- E   Anti-topoisomerase 1 antibody

14.73   Answer: A

Other signs indicating a need for urgent/emergency investigation include saddle-area sensory loss, loss of sphincter tone, bilateral leg pain and neurological deficit and finding a discrete sensory level.

14.74   Answer: C

Other non-articular causes of a 'false positive' test include Epstein–Barr virus infection, endocarditis, hepatitis and syphilis.

14.75   Answer: C

Parathyroid hormone, active vitamin D, thyroid hormone, growth hormone and IL-1 (rheumatoid arthritis) stimulate bone remodelling, whereas oestrogen, androgen and calcitonin may inhibit it. Osteoclasts are active in bone resorption.

14.76   Answer: E

This is more suggestive of systemic sclerosis. Anti-histone antibody is found in SLE (H_1, H_3, H_4) and drug-induced lupus (H_2), whilst anti-ribonuclear protein antibody is found also in mixed connective tissue disease.

INDEX

AS
Pneumonia
Lung Carcinoma
Occupational Asthma
PE
AF
Pneumothorax

COPD